Contents

Preface to Third Edition   v

Acknowledgements   vi

Introduction   vii

Chapter 1: Reception   1
Winning the client ● Client reception ● Clinic records ● Booking an appointment ● Professional ethics ● Client relaxation, conversation and preparation ● Self check

Chapter 2: Learning about the Skin   12
Deciding treatment ● Skin cleansing ● Manual skin cleansing ● Manual cleansing removal sequence ● Cleansing tools and techniques ● Brush cleansing ● Skin inspection ● Skin diagnosis ● Recognition of basic skin types ● Skin toning ● Cosmetic preparations ● Self check

Chapter 3: Facial Anatomy   33
Facial proportions ● Bones of the cranium and face ● Muscles of the face and neck ● Blood circulation of the head and neck ● Regional lymph nodes and vessels of the face and neck ● The nerves of the face and neck ● The skin ● Appendages of the skin ● Functions of the skin ● Self check

Chapter 4: Facial Massage   53
Indications for massage treatment ● Contra-indications to massage ● Manual massage movements ● Massage technique ● Hand mobility exercises ● The basic facial massage routine ● Pore treatment massage routine ● The Continental facial massage (face, neck and shoulder girdle) ● Self check

Chapter 5: Skin Diseases and Disorders   85
Dermatological terms ● Bacterial-based problems ● Fungal diseases ● Viral skin conditions ● Parasitic skin problems ● Allergic skin disorders ● Pigmentary disorders Skin gland disorders ● Skin cancer ● Self check

Chapter 6: Mask Therapy   99
Mask applications ● Setting masks ● Application and removal of clay masks ● Phytotherapy masks ● Natural product masks ● Specialised masks: peel off masks, thermal/mineral masks, paraffin wax masks, warm oil masks (using infra-red or radiant heat irradiation) ● Self check

Chapter 7: Lash and Brow Treatment   113
Minor facial treatments ● Eyebrow shaping ● Eyebrow and lash tinting ● Application of semi-permanent individual lashes ● Permanent eyeline and eyebrow colour ● Self check

Chapter 8: Makeup — 124

Makeup techniques ● Makeup products: moisturisers, foundations ● Makeup products: eye makeup ● Makeup products: lipstick ● Photographic, evening and high-fashion makeup ● Correction and emphasis of eye shapes ● Makeup for the dark and non-European skin ● Cosmetic camouflage ● Self check

Chapter 9: Electrical Treatment — 150

Indications for electrical treatment ● General contra-indications to electrical treatment ● Safety points in the application of electrical treatment ● Steaming ● Vibratory treatment ● Brush massage ● Abrasive peeling treatment ● Facial vacuum/suction treatment ● Pulsed air–vacuum massage ● Muscle toning (passive muscle contraction) ● High-frequency treatment ● Ultraviolet treatment ● Galvanic treatment (desincrustation and iontophoresis) ● Desincrustation ● Iontophoresis ● Self check

Chapter 10: Treatment Plans — 190

Purpose and choice of treatment ● Treatment plan for normal skin ● Treatment plan for combination/oily skin ● Treatment plan for the oily/acneic skin ● Treatment for the dry skin ● Treatment for the dehydrated skin ● Treatment for the mature skin ● Rejuvenation treatment ● Treatment for the sensitive skin ● Treatment for the couperose skin ● Specialised treatments ● Self check

Chapter 11: Treatment of the Arms and Legs — 217

Anatomy of the hands and forearms ● Structure and function of the nails ● Manicure ● Recognition of nail diseases and disorders ● The manicure treatment ● Hand and arm massage ● Organisation of the manicure trolley ● Paraffin wax treatment ● Nail repairs and extensions ● Anatomy of the foot, ankle and lower leg ● The pedicure treatment ● Foot and leg massage ● Self check

Chapter 12: Depilatory Treatments — 265

Consultation ● Depilatory methods available (temporary) ● Permanent hair removal methods available (destruction of the active follicle) ● Depilatory hot waxing ● Under-arm waxing (hot wax method) ● Bikini wax (hot wax method) ● Warm waxing ● Bikini wax (warm wax method) ● Abdominal waxing (warm wax method) ● Underarm waxing (warm wax method) ● Arm wax (warm wax method) ● Lip and chin waxing (warm wax method) ● Eyebrow waxing (warm wax method) ● Lip and chin waxing (hot wax method) ● Self check

Chapter 13: Health, Hygiene and Safety — 286

Image projection ● Public hygiene ● Personal hygiene ● Client hygiene ● Salon hygiene ● Methods of sterilisation ● Waste disposal ● Self check

Chapter 14: Business Organisation, Salon Procedure and Equipment Choice — 296

Methods of work ● General salon work, beauty clinic ● In-store salon ● Home visiting practice ● The health hydro ● Television makeup artist ● A career in sales ● Leisure centre ● Teaching ● Beauty therapist on board ship ● Treatment planning and promotion ● Setting up the facial cubicle ● Home visiting practice equipment ● Beauty therapy qualifications and methods of training available ● Professional bodies and awards ● Benefits of professional membership ● Useful addresses ● Self check

Conversion Tables — 321

Index — 325

Preface to Third Edition

So many changes and advances are occurring in the beauty therapy industry at this time, that I am very pleased to be able to prepare, with the help of my co-authors, a new edition which will keep therapists up-to-date with techniques and trends. Increasingly popular electrically biased treatments, such as brush cleansing and massage, galvanic treatments and warm depilatory wax methods, are more fully illustrated for easier understanding.

Cosmetic chemistry advances, especially in phytotherapy, reflect a 'back-to-nature' trend of international popularity which provides great new scope for sales. A new chapter, *Treatment Plans*, acts as a working manual, providing the latest information on ingredients and their actions, showing how to combine them in treatment and so achieve retail sales.

With so much to learn to become proficient, information has been made more accessible to the reader, using charts and quick reference lists, also useful for revision. The more techniques the therapist is comfortable with and can use with confidence, the greater will be her success in this exciting and rewarding field.

Ann Gallant
1993

Acknowledgements

I am specially indebted to Dr Parashu Singh for sharing his very considerable cosmetic chemistry knowledge with me over the last few years, as we have worked together developing product lines. I have learnt a lot about the chemistry behind the phytotherapy and aromatherapy products, and have tried to reflect this knowledge in this new edition. We will try to provide more information in new books in time.

I am grateful to my co-authors, Jackie Howard and Kathy Gillott, for their contributions and help in ensuring that the book meets the needs of the UK colleges and training schools. They themselves would like to acknowledge the support and encouragement given by their respective families and colleagues throughout the preparation of this book. They would like to thank Kim Aldridge of ITEC for the initial introduction to Stanley Thornes, Ted Cachart for his word processing skills and each other for mutual motivation and friendship that has developed from working together.

My thanks go to the therapists around the world for their support and interest, which has encouraged me to try to learn more cosmetic science and interpret it in a form therapists can understand and use to get treatment results and make product sales. Suggestions made to me have been incorporated wherever possible – see particularly Chapter 10, *Treatment Plans*.

Introduction

The growing beauty industry provides new opportunities for the skilled and ambitious operator who is able to take on its challenge and promote its services effectively. The beauty specialist's and beauty therapist's work overlap to a large extent. The jobs have an increasing emphasis on the selling of both treatment and products with the greatest earning and career rewards relating to sales ability.

An operator who concentrates on facial therapy may be termed a beauty specialist, facial therapist or beautician. In French-speaking countries the operator is considered to be qualified in the field of aesthetics, and is known as an aestheticienne. As long as the techniques learnt are sound, and a full range of professional skills is obtained, the titles mentioned above that are recognised by the public are the ones that should be used. The confusion in job title arises from the way the industry has developed over the years, growing from modest beginnings to its present size and stature. As beauty training becomes standardised as to hours of training and practical content around the world, consistent titles will become established, reflecting the growing importance and maturity of the industry.

The beauty specialist will find her work very similar wherever she is (apart from legal and health authority restrictions in force in varying parts of the world which alter what may be undertaken). The work of the beauty specialist ranges from treatment to the associated product sales relating to the face, hands and feet. *The Principles and Techniques of the Beauty Specialist* contains all the skills needed for success in this dynamic and exciting field.

As the beauty therapy industry is mainly, but by no means exclusively, a female-oriented industry we have referred throughout to the client and therapist as she, but this is only for speed and ease of reading. We realise that men are entering the profession both as clients and therapists.

CHAPTER ONE

Reception

Winning the client

A strong international interest in personal fitness has resulted in a tremendous demand for beauty therapy services. As the general public has become more informed about the services offered by the industry, they have become more discerning in their choice of clinic. Beauty services are available at health clubs, hotels, exercise centres, slimming, sun-tanning, health and beauty clinics, hairdressing salons, fashion shops and pharmacies. With so much competition beauty therapists need to think more about 'winning the client'.

Clients demand an efficient and friendly service. They expect excellent facilities (equipment and treatments) and trained staff. Value for money and immaculate standards of hygiene will also influence a client's choice of treatment. Media exposure has heightened public awareness of the AIDS epidemic, and its implications for the population and this has affected the beauty services. (Chapter 13 discusses the implications of AIDS in more detail.)

Maintaining a friendly, professional approach will go a long way to attracting and keeping clients and this, in turn, will help make a business successful. Many of the professional treatments booked will follow a consultation so the ability to welcome a client and put her at her ease is important. Good listeners, with the patience to help solve seemingly trivial problems, will lead the way to treatment and sales success. Once the client feels at home and trusts the staff she will seldom want to change to a new clinic. So, although correct clinical appearance and ability also play a part, a pleasant, caring attitude is perhaps the greatest asset of all.

The facial specialist works in a competitive atmosphere, and learns to sell her skills and knowledge. With a lively attitude and interest in her field, the skilled operator can work anywhere in the world and always attract a good clientele. As the market grows daily, there has seldom been a better time in the beauty industry to achieve personal success.

Client reception

A client's awareness of the treatment and its results may have come from the media, personal recommendation or may be a positive result of advertising.

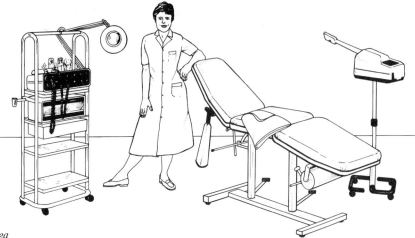

The treatment area

There are many reasons why a client will seek professional help from a beauty clinic. It may be because of a personal problem, a wish for improvement, or a desire for a new image. A consultation or a friendly discussion at reception can quickly dispel any anxieties the client may have about what the treatment involves. The time commitment, the cost and the products needed for home use to ensure the success of treatment can all be dealt with during this discussion. The client must feel that her problems have a good chance of being resolved by the treatment and that success is possible.

Initial impressions

Many factors can influence the client's decision to have treatment. These may include:

- Convenient clinic location that is easy to find with good parking or access by public transport, and with flexible business hours to suit its clients' needs.
- Attractive and spotless clinic appearance with decor suited to its location; attractive product displays and clear pricing of the treatments offered.

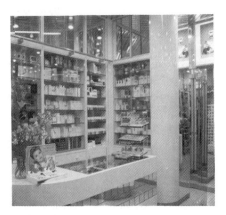

The reception area

- A professional and efficient welcome at reception to secure the appointment booking or organise a confidential initial consultation with the beauty specialist to determine the treatment required.
- Attractive and caring reception and beauty staff with immaculate, well groomed, clinical appearances, and confident, out-going, friendly manners that put clients at ease in the strange, new environment.
- An aura of calm efficiency and businesslike organisation that should be apparent to the client from her first contact with the clinic, giving her confidence in the professional skills offered.

Consultation

- The main purpose of a consultation is to confirm an appointment booking, or a course of treatment, with associated sale of cosmetic products.
- The treatment chosen can be briefly explained to the client. Details of the proposed treatment, the time involved, the cost involved and the home products required to ensure a successful result should all be discussed.
- A quiet area away from the rush of clinic services should be used for the consultation, such as an empty treatment cubicle or cabin. This ensures privacy and allows the client to overcome anxiety by letting her get to know her therapist and become familiar with the new surroundings.
- In order to complete a safe and effective treatment, certain information has to be known about the client's medical history, life style and general health. The consultation provides the opportunity to find out what the client expects from treatment. It also allows the beauty specialist time to promote clinic services and explain why the information is necessary for success. If a booking is achieved, the client's card may be filled in, ready to be added to later.
- To save time, the consultation is often incorporated into an initial treatment booking, where the condition can be discussed and viewed in confidence. Initial treatment concentrates on manual and cosmetic routines and avoids electrotherapy.
- Deciding the products required for home use to start skin improvement is a high priority of the combined consultation/initial treatment.
- If the consultation is given independent of an initial treatment and is only of a few minutes' duration, this will be a free service. If more detailed information is given and hence more time needed, then the time will be charged for as it would be for any other professional consultation.
- An atmosphere of trust should be created in a consultation. This helps the client to relax. Skilled and tactful questioning of the client can then reveal details of skin problems which can be used to help to decide the treatment plan.
- Information obtained in a consultation is recorded on the client's record card.

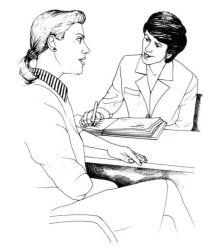

Consultation in progress

Consultations confirm bookings, sell products, and establish bonds between the client and the operator that achieve good results.

Clinic records

Keeping complete records of treatments booked, treatments applied and associated product sales achieved, has become much less time consuming with the advent of computerised record keeping. Clients' record cards are listed alphabetically and treated with strict confidentiality whether they are kept in a filing system or on a computer disc.

A full record, whether manually written or kept on computer, provides several advantages:

- It provides a detailed medical account, which could reveal reasons why a treatment should not be applied (contra-indications).
- It shows the progress achieved and problems encountered during treatment. Therefore it can point to the way to forward planning.
- A full record of the cosmetic sales made can enhance product sales turnover and reveal new areas of interest to share with the client.
- A record of cosmetics sales can also act as a reminder to check whether the client has all her home skin care needs and whether she could be needing replacements. This gives the operator an idea of what products need to be ordered.
- A computerised record can act as a stock checking device if linked to computerised lists of the actual stock held. In larger clinics purchases made at reception can then be debited directly from stock lists, providing an immediate guide to the stock position.
- Full records also act as a check against financial accounts and can be used to charge accounts, determine staff commissions and document treatments completed within a course plan.
- In times of illness or staff changes, the records provide an immediate and accurate reference on which to base continued treatment. This can often avoid the loss of a valuable customer.

Client record cards

The client's card acts as a blueprint for her physical condition, life style, and personality, and can be used to guide treatment. The record card must record:

Record cards provide fast, clear, and complete information to guide the therapist's choice of treatment.

- The client's full name and initials (to avoid errors).
- The client's address and home and work telephone numbers.
- Age and family history (number and age of any children).
- The name, telephone number and address of the client's doctor. The card should also record whether medical permission has been needed or obtained prior to treatment.
- The medical history of the client, e.g. operations, illnesses, allergies, any medication taken at present, etc.
- An assessment of the client's existing physical condition. This could reveal contra-indications that could alter treatment.
- A detailed skin assessment noting any special problems that need attention.

Health & beauty clinic prescription form

Therapy prescription for: _____

Date _____

Home address _____

Town _____ Post Code _____

Business phone no. _____

Home no. _____

Medical history _____

_____

_____

Date of birth _____

Medication taken _____

Number of children/ages _____

Personal doctor _____ Phone _____

Aesthetician/Beauty therapist _____

Skin Assessment (tick appropriate boxes)

Overall skin impression

☐ young ☐ combination ☐ oily ☐ blemished
☐ sensitive ☐ normal ☐ dry ☐ dehydrated
☐ lifeless ☐ prematurely aged ☐ mature
☐ couperose

Sensitivity

☐ general ☐ localised area ☐ temporary
☐ cause known ☐ allergies ☐ drug allergies
☐ existing couperose ☐ [_____] condition–location

Skin texture

☐ fine ☐ normal ☐ heavy ☐ open pores
☐ coarse ☐ scarred ☐ irregular

Sebaceous activity

☐ normal ☐ underactive ☐ overproductive
☐ seborrhoea ☐ confined to centre of face

Hydration levels

☐ normal ☐ superficial dehydration
☐ severe dehydration ☐ flaking
☐ skin irritated, taut skin ☐ temporary dehydration

Skincare

Skin assessment (cont.)

Skin tone

☐ firm ☐ ageing signs ☐ loss of firmness
☐ crepey skin ☐ fine lines

Skin pigmentation

☐ suntan ☐ discoloured skin ☐ vitiligo
☐ scars ☐ skin redness (erythema)
☐ sallow skin

Imperfections

☐ enlarged pores ☐ blocked pores ☐ comedones
☐ milia ☐ pustules ☐ cystic blockage
☐ superfluous hair ☐ warts ☐ moles
☐ naevi ☐ scars

Prescribed Therapy

Desired result

☐ maintain oil ☐ hydric balance ☐ increase hydration
☐ regeneration ☐ delaying ageing tendencies
☐ firming skin tone ☐ control of seborrhoea
☐ firming ☐ rehydration
☐ after acne/refining of scars ☐ control of sensitivity
☐ improve couperose ☐ increase muscle tone

Recommended Products

Chosen line _____

Day care

Cleanse _____

Tone _____

Protect _____

Night care

Cleanse _____

Tone _____

Nourish _____

Client record card

Treatment Plan

Treatment plan for _____

Chosen treatment line _____

Specific therapy _____

Date	Treatment	Products	Next appointment

Special care

Eye care _____

Ampoules _____

Mask _____

Peeling/scrub _____

Anti-ageing products _____

Repair products _____

Neck care _____

Suncare _____

Special care guidance _____
_____
_____
_____

Body care _____
_____
_____
_____

Notes and instructions _____
_____
_____
_____
_____
_____
_____
_____
_____
_____
_____
_____
_____
_____
_____
_____
_____
_____

A sample form for recording client treatments

- An assessment of the client's present life style and home skin and health routines.
- Home treatment product recommendations and sales made to the client.

The client card must provide space to record treatments, their date of completion and progress comments. It should be signed by the therapist and her client.

Booking an appointment

The normal facial of one hour duration is a good starting point and working frame for treatment and covers cleansing, toning, massage, mask and makeup. Electrically biased routines, for the younger client, may be accomplished in a half-hour period, which suits the time and finances they have available.

Appointments may be made by telephone or in person, often following a brief consultation.The way any enquiry is handled decides whether the clinic gains or retains a client. Skilled reception can build a simple treatment booking into a profitable routine by suggesting additional services such as lip waxing or perhaps eyelash tinting added to a facial.

A patient and helpful manner can help the client to make a treatment choice, or agree to come for a combined consultation and initial treatment. Attention should be given to building business through casual enquiries. These can be developed into bookings,

Beauty Clinic		Epilation
Facial cleanse and makeup		(Removal of unwanted hair)
Facial treatment		Lip and chin
Specialised facial treatments for dry, greasy or dehydrated skin conditions by consultation	For the convenience of our business clients, the Hair Salon will remain open until 7.30 p.m. on Friday evenings	15 minutes
		20 minutes
Mature skin treatment		Legs and bikini
Treatment to include muscle toning and electrical stimulation	A free consultation is advised prior to all therapy treatments to decide the most advantageous method of treating the skin or body condition. We can provide continental electrical treatments and manual massage therapy	½ hour
		1 hour
Manicure		Waxing
Pedicure		(Depilatory for hair removal)
Eyebrow shaping		Lip
Eyelash tinting		Chin
Shaping and tinting brows and lashes		Lip and chin
Lip bleach		Leg (to knee)
Course of eight or more treatments at a special price		Full leg
		Underarm
		Bikini

Salon treatment list

through conversation and use of leaflets, promotional offers and free consultations.

When a client books an appointment she should know:

- The date and time of the treatment and its duration.
- The cost of the chosen routine.
- What her cosmetic product commitment is likely to be.

The clinic needs to:

- Know the new client's name, address and telephone number in case an appointment has to be cancelled or moved for any reason.
- Ensure that no confusion exists between the clinic and the client as to the date and time of the appointment.

Professional ethics

Successful therapy relies on the beauty specialist being skilled, efficient, approachable and able to inspire confidence in and achieve results for the client. The successful beauty specialist can guide the efforts of her clients and motivate them to follow the treatment and product advice given through genuine interest in the client as an individual. Results are achieved through the client helping herself to success with the operator acting as a catalyst. This pays great dividends in terms of treatment success and clinic income.

If an operator is confident and happy with her work, this comes across in a positive way to the clients. It shows in the interaction between staff and results in a pleasant atmosphere in the clinic, making it a pleasure to visit. This can be termed a professional attitude, but is also an indication that the work is personally satisfying. Maintaining an excellent standard of service and following stringent hygiene rules then becomes a matter of personal pride rather than a chore.

Client relaxation, conversation and preparation

Client relaxation

A relaxed and pleasant atmosphere within the clinic allows the client to enjoy treatment free from tension. A salon decor which combines the clinical and luxurious aspects of therapy helps to establish the mood of intimacy, comfort and cleanliness that encourages relaxation (see Chapter 14, Business Organisation). A friendly but professional rapport develops, which builds interest and supports home efforts.

Encouraging the client to really relax and free herself from stress whilst undergoing treatment allows her to gain the full benefit of the treatment both mentally and physically. Avoid instigating topics of conversation other than those relating to treatment. If a client is determined to chat, let her, but let the conversation drift away as she relaxes.

Client conversation

Client conversation should:

- Concentrate on the client exclusively within the context of treatment. Attention should be given to her needs, interests and hopes in treatment.
- Centre on treatment, products used and progress made at home, to maximise the treatment-associated sales potential.
- Avoid controversial subjects such as politics, religion, sex, etc.
- Keep away from personal or family matters.
- Avoid the topics of other therapists and competitive clinics.

Many clients do love to talk and enjoy the human contact of visiting a caring therapist. For them, talking is itself a form of therapy, as it releases tension. Many personal facts may be revealed in the course of treatment and these must be treated with integrity. The therapist must realise that she is valuable only as a listener and with experience, little impression is retained of the client's personal problems. It is not the place of the therapist to give advice, other than in her professional capacity.

Client preparation

Good organisation is the key to ensuring that the client obtains prompt and efficient treatment and gets the best value from her visit to the clinic. A smooth client flow increases efficiency and makes best use of the space and facilities available. This allows maximum time to be spent in direct client contact. Knowledge of the day's work sequence permits preparation of record cards and the treatment area for the appointments booked.

Preparation of the working position ahead of the client's arrival minimises noise and unnecessary movement during the treatment. With everything ready, the operator is able to concentrate her energies on the client, quickly putting her at ease and robing her correctly for treatment. The gentle authority of the operator helps the client to gain the most benefit from the routine chosen. This calm professionalism soon builds an excellent personal relationship based on trust and confidence in the operator's skill.

General therapy routines

Complete therapy routines require a robing which leaves the shoulders, neck and face free for treatment. Gowning should be comfortable and modest, with no restricting underclothes which could prevent relaxation. The facial chair should be adjusted to the client's comfort and give adequate back support. A multi-position chair/lounger provides for a wide range of treatments in one cubicle or working area.

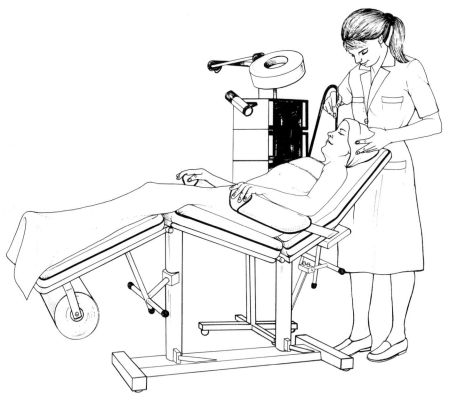

General facial treatment position

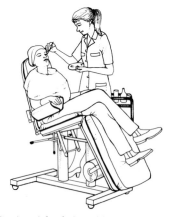

Semi-upright chair position

Cosmetic facial applications

Short duration treatments such as cosmetic facial applications, grooming routines, waxing, lash tinting and makeup can be applied in a semi-upright chair position. This is space saving and requires less preparation and client disrobing. Only simple protection of clothes is needed and this should use disposable materials where possible. The treatment should be immediately available to clients, with no delays for preparation. This enables clients to take advantage of the service whenever they have time available.

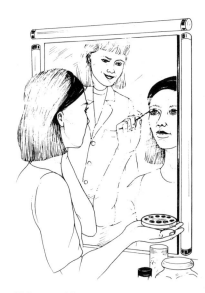

Makeup position

Makeup application

Treatments involving client participation, such as makeup instruction, require a mirror, adequate lighting and the client in a natural position. This allows a true impression of the client's facial contours and personality to be gained. In larger salons a makeup bar with lights at the sides of and above the mirror would be available. Clients can then be moved to the bar for final makeup in conjunction with a facial or hair treatment.

Self check

1 Why is it important to create a good initial impression?
2 Why do we carry out a consultation?
3 What should be included on a client's record card?
4 What are the reasons for keeping client records?

11

CHAPTER TWO

Learning about the Skin

If one knows how to read the signs, the skin can be very revealing. Such skin problems as age, the effects of physical and mental strain, over exposure to the sun, and an inclination to skin sensitivity, all register immediately. This initial assessment gives guidance as to which treatments are suitable and which are not (contra-indicated). The process starts with careful cleansing of the skin, and inspection under a magnifier. The art of the successful beauty specialist is to match the skin condition to the correct treatment and products.

Deciding treatment

The aim is to bring the skin into correct oil, hydric (water) and pH (acid/alkaline) balance. There are many ways to achieve this and a beauty specialist will need to consider the needs of the skin, the client's finances and the time available.

Of all the routines available, cleansing is the essential first step. It includes:

- The one-hour facial routine: cleansing, toning, massage, mask and makeup. This provides a good frame to work within and can include electrotherapy if needed.
- Shorter, half-hour, electrically biased routines with an emphasis on cleansing. These are very popular with the younger client.
- Skin cleansing, toning and makeup applications. These lead the client towards therapy routines and help to decide her product requirements.

The treatment plan will be based on observation, skilful questioning during consultation and initial treatment. It will, of course, consider information recorded on the client's record card and such factors as age, general health, contra-indications, home skin care routine, and the condition of the skin when first seen. The progress of the skin during the treatment will be recorded.

Skin cleansing

First, the skin is cleansed gently to reveal the skin for further inspection. A cleansing product is used which is able to remove makeup efficiently and is appropriate to the client's age and general skin type (see Cleansing products, page 31). This introduces the client to the feel and natural fragrance of the cleanser selected as suitable for home use.

If the skin is sensitive, or you suspect that it might be, use special cleansers for delicate skin until more is known about the skin. Then, as treatment progresses, changes can be made to more accurately matched products without risking skin irritation or losing the client's confidence. Skin inspection may point out a need for specialised products and equipment (such as galvanic desincrustation) to be used to cleanse the skin deeply if it is blocked. The inspection may also determine the direction treatment will take, with emphasis on corrective aspects (see Chapter 9, Electrical Treatment).

Cleansing methods

Modern therapy provides many methods of skin cleansing apart from such manual methods as using standard cosmetic cleansing milks and creams. Electrical brush cleansing and deep pore cleansing by galvanic desincrustation now form a normal part of clinic practice. The simplicity of brush cleansing makes it an ideal alternative to manual methods and will be considered here. Galvanic cleansing, which is considered in Chapter 9 covers specialised electrical work for the oily skin, though it is increasingly used to ensure very thorough and gentle cleansing for a wide range of skin conditions and to combat the effects of pollution on the younger skin.

Manual cleansing

- Manual cleansing builds an immediate rapport with the client,through the skilful massage technique, unique to the therapist.
- Direct hand contact with the skin adds further information to the assessment of the skin such as texture, firmness, existing blockage, sensitivity or dehydration.
- Manual cleansing is an ideal skin preparation for nervous, over-stressed and mature clients, as it allows them to become accustomed to the therapist's hands and personality.
- Manual cleansing is the most widely used method of cleansing and is gentle and relaxing. It uses products which suit the age and condition of the client's skin.
- A wide range of cleansing products can be employed. Oil-based creams, water-based cleansing milks, liquefied creams, etc. can all be chosen to match the skin type and the amount of makeup to be removed.
- Manual cleansing introduces the chosen cleanser to the client and allows its special properties to be discussed, building home sales.

Manual skin cleansing

Method of work

When the client is correctly prepared with hair and underclothing protected and is settled and relaxed, the cleansing stage is performed, in preparation for further facial treatment. The therapist uses the cleanser recommended for home use and introduces the client to its properties. A little quiet conversation will help to put the client at ease, and talking about the products used is an ideal tension breaker, and helps to make important product sales.

The routine of cleansing strokes deeply cleanses the surface layers of the skin. Continuous sweeping strokes distribute the cleansing medium. Rhythmical, flowing effleurage movements performed with even pressure prepare all areas that will be massaged later in treatment.

Initial stokes are superficial. The routine then repeats with careful rollpatting movements, giving special attention to areas where skin blockage could be present. The centre of the forehead, the nose and the chin all need detailed cleansing to remove old makeup and oily blockage resulting from over active sebaceous glands.

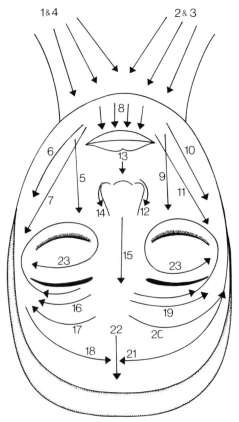

Routine of cleansing strokes

The cleansing sequence must remove any makeup quickly and effectively and leave the skin clean and gently stimulated ready for the skin inspection.

Routine of work

The entire palmar surface of the hand should be in contact with the skin wherever possible and adjustments made according to the position of the supporting bony prominences of the skull. For sensitive areas such as the upper cheeks, eyes and trachea (wind-pipe) where heavy pressure would be uncomfortable, the speed, repetition and pressure of the strokes can be altered.

The amount of the hand or fingers used for the strokes depends on the size of the therapist's hands and the area under treatment.

Rollpatting on the neck

The hands first mould around the neck, fitting its contours, lifting the platysma muscle from the base of the neck to the mandible (lower jaw bone), avoiding heavy pressure over the trachea. The movements work across the neck and chest area, from left to right, returning to the left side. The movement repeats more deeply and then the hands move on to the face from the left with contouring jawline strokes. Movements on the superficial cheek muscles follow the direction of the muscle fibres, taking care to avoid distorting the mouth or touching the nose. Movements should be more specific and controlled in the cheek area, with fewer fingers used as necessary. The position and tension present in the cheek muscles guide as to the correct pressure and repetition of the effleurage strokes.

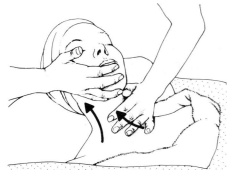

Rollpatting on the neck

Rollpatting on the cheek

Changing direction, the hands work deeply into the chin fold, and the cheek movements are repeated on the right side. Treatment of the nose follows, with detailed attention to the removal of makeup preparations in this area.

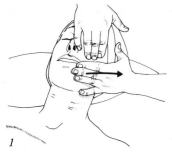
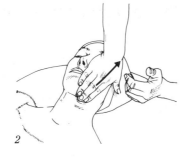
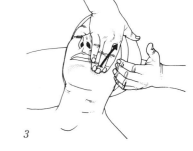

1   *2*   *3*

Rollpatting on the cheek

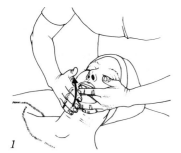
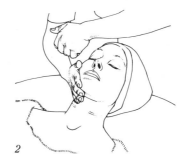
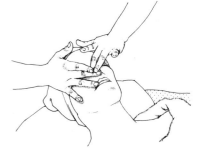

1   *2*

Crossing the chin to the other cheek   *Detailed work on the nose*

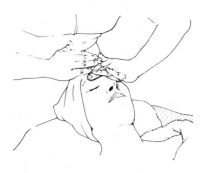

Forehead rollpatting

Forehead rollpatting

The hands progress to the forehead, the movements become lighter and the speed slows to a relaxing restful pace. Treatment on any bony area of the face should be slower, and with **considerably** less pressure than is used on the rest of the face because of the differences in distribution of adipose (fatty) tissue in the subcutaneous layers supporting the muscles of facial expression.

The routine of manual cleansing is completed by gentle circles around the eye area, releasing the tinted eye makeup and mascara, whilst endeavouring not to spread them on to the facial areas. The sequence is concluded with gentle, even, upward pressure on the temples.

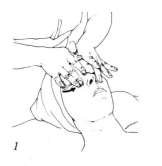
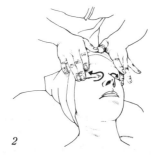
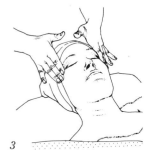

1   *2*   *3*

Slow careful strokes around the eyes

Manual cleansing removal sequence

On completion of the cleansing sequence the client should be becoming free from tension, relaxed and starting to unwind. This attitude should be maintained by avoiding harsh or sudden movements during the entire facial routine and by staying in close contact with the client.

The cleansing preparation chosen is thoroughly but gently removed to avoid over stimulation of the skin which could limit further, more active treatment planned.

Previously prepared damp cotton wool tissues are used to remove makeup. The eye and lip makeup is removed first to avoid spreading the tinted cosmetics around the face. Small, triangular cotton wool tissues are used to gently remove makeup from around the eyes to avoid irritation to the fine skin around the eye or to the eye itself. Heavy eye makeup may require the use of special eye makeup remover products or impregnated eye makeup remover pads for speedy removal avoiding irritation.

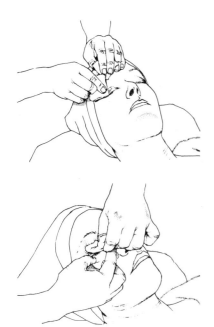

Eye makeup removal

The tissues are held, one in each hand, so that the skin is held gently but firmly, avoiding discomfort or pressure on the eye itself. One pad holds the eyebrow so that the eyelashes lift slightly, whilst the other pad sweeps gently downwards and outwards to remove the makeup with small, repeating strokes. The tissue is turned at the corner of the eye to present a clean surface and the flat area of the tissue is then lightly swept under the lashes towards the nose. Heavy mascara can be removed by repeating the under eye stroke and pausing to cleanse the lashes down on to the pad, using the second pad as a wiper. In this way the mascara is contained within the pads and does not spread on to the fine skin or get into the eye itself, causing irritation.

The removal of very heavy eye makeup or waterproof mascara will benefit from the use of special eye makeup remover products, used directly on a damp cotton wool piece, and held in place for a few seconds prior to removal. The impregnated pads are used in a similar way, pressed gently to the eye area, allowed a few seconds to act, then wiped away taking the bulk of the makeup cleanly with them. This also introduces the product to the client, for consideration for home use.

Lipstick removal

The lipstick is removed by lightly passing across the lips a just damp cotton wool tissue folded into a manageable shape. The pressure must be light and should not cause discomfort or distort the mouth. Care should be taken to avoid touching the nose. The lipstick is removed by

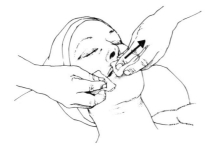
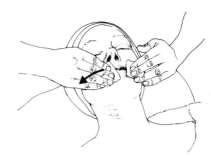

first holding one side of the mouth with a cotton wool tissue whilst the other hand passes across the mouth, removing the lipstick and cleansing preparation on to another folded shape of cotton wool. The routine is then reversed, using a fresh surface of the tissue to complete the entire cleansing sequence of the lips.

Cleansing removal sequence

The cleansing preparation may be removed either with the hands following each other, or working in unison on both sides of the face at once. The throat is completed before the routine progresses to the face, first on the left cheek, across the chin to the right cheek, then moving up the face to the nose, and on to the forehead, if the hands are following each other. With the hands working in unison, the neck is completed, followed by removal on both cheeks, then the nose and forehead. Both methods complete the sequence by circles around the eyes, finishing with gentle pressure on the temples.

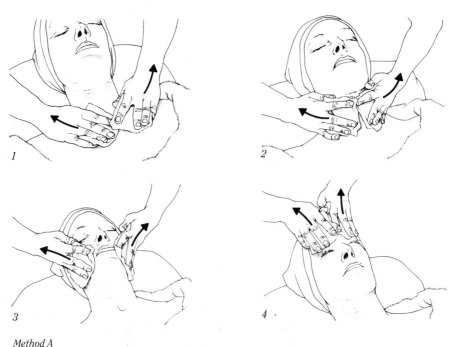

Method A

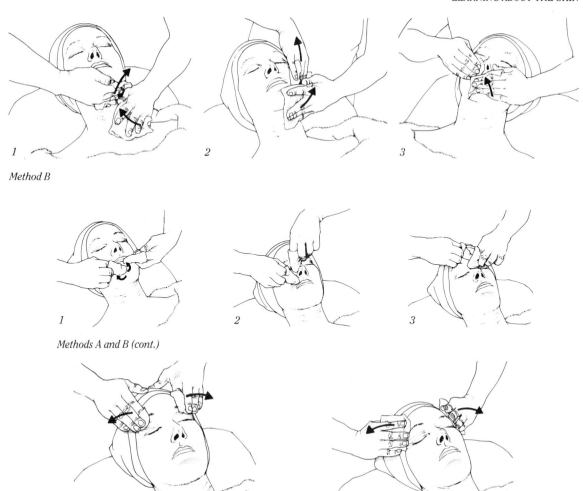

Method B

1   2   3

Methods A and B (cont.)

1   2   3

Method A (end)   *Method B (end)*

General makeup removal is completed, turning tissues and replacing them as needed to avoid spreading the tinted makeup, repeating the removal with fresh pads if necessary to ensure a thorough cleansing in the case of heavy makeup. Either method then proceeds to detailed cleansing of the centre panel, with pads firmly tucked around index fingers. Deep rolling movements are applied where blockage occurs and makeup can become trapped, even in the older skin. The strokes move up on to the forehead and become slower and more gentle. Removal should be more thorough in this area in Method B as it has not been previously cleansed. The pads are then opened out under the fingers, and eye arching completes the removal sequence for both methods.

If removal pads are still showing evidence of makeup present at the conclusion of the routine, the entire cleansing sequence and its removal may be repeated. The correct choice of cleansing preparation, selected for its ability to remove the makeup present as well as suit the skin type, should avoid this occurrence.

Cleansing tools and techniques

Certain points are of importance to achieve an efficient and thorough removal which feels comfortable to the client.

- Cotton wool pads should be controlled by the therapist during the sequence, and not allowed to flap in the client's face, or tickle, breaking the relaxation.
- The pads are normally held between the thumb and the index fingers, and the fourth finger and the little finger, spread open by the pressure of the hands against the client's skin. Alternatively the pads may be wrapped around the fingers.
- Cotton wool used for the pads should be of the very best quality, free from lumps or harsh bits that could scratch the skin; it should split into layers easily when cut into squares and moistened.
- The pads should be about 4 in. (10 cm) square. depending on the size of the therapist's hands. Any oddments can be used to make eye and lip pads.
- The pads should be wrung out firmly so that they are just damp, not wet; otherwise they will be incapable of removing the oily makeup and cleansing preparations.

Removal with sponges

In busy commercial practices, sterilised viscose sponges will often replace the cotton wool tissues as they are time saving and economic. They are used especially in combination with brush cleansing methods and electrotherapy generally. Each operator should ideally have a minimum of 30-40 soft sponges to allow for use during treatment, and the washing and sterilisation sequence. Because of the need for meticulous cleaning and sterilisation, to avoid cross infection risks, there are areas of the world where viscose sponges are not permitted by health authorities. In the training situation disposable cotton wool tissues remain the best way of avoiding problems.

Damp sponges may be used to remove the cleansing products, with the procedure repeated until the skin is thoroughly clean. Both sides of the soft viscose sponges are used, then they are put aside ready to be cleaned and sterilised. They are not rinsed and reused, as this defeats the whole purpose of the cleansing, reintroducing soiled material on to the face rather than removing it.

Brush cleansing

Electrical brush cleansing is becoming an increasingly popular alternative to manual cleansing and fits in very well with the reduced time many clients have available for completing their treatment routines. Brush cleansing is available independently or within combined facial treatment units, often in association with high frequency, galvanism, vacuum and muscle stimulation applications.

- Electrical cleansing is effective and when well applied provides a fast, professional method of deep cleansing the skin. It is popular with younger clients.
- It is normally not applied on the first treatment,to avoid over stimulation, in case the skin is very sensitive. Neither is it used on

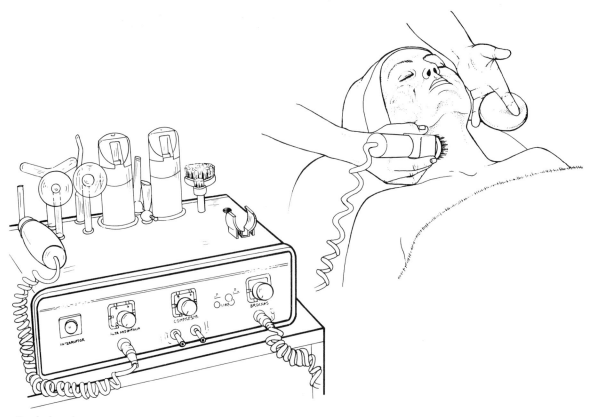

Brush cleansing

Brush cleansing can be used for both cleansing and massage applications and gives a variety in treatment to maintain client interest.

highly nervous clients for whom relaxation is the main aim of the cleansing sequence.

- It is not as personal a procedure, so does not provide so much skin information, as the hands are not in direct contact with the client's skin.
- Brush cleansing is often used within an electrically biased facial, where the time saving is valuable.
- It is applied using water-based cleansing milks for economy and easy-flowing application; removal is by viscose sponges or cotton wool tissues. (Most cleansing milks are water based.)

Application

Brush cleansing is gently stimulating and provides a thorough and fast cleansing of the skin. Cleansing milk is applied generously on the chest, cheek and forehead areas and the brush applicator is applied in a pattern over the entire area to spread the preparations and cleanse the skin (see illustrations for Removal sequence, Method A, pages 18–19 for the movements).

A range of brushes for varying skin conditions is available from soft, tapered bristles for cleansing to firm, bristle brushes in different

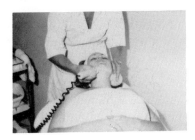

shapes for activating and abrasive massage. The brushes are powered by a variable speed motor. A flexible drive system rotates and gently vibrates the chosen applicator. A slightly damp brush applicator is attached and applied with light pressure over the area to deep cleanse the skin, remove cellular blockage and free surface adhesions (see opposite for brush cleansing sequence).

The equipment head should be contoured to the area under treatment and bony and sensitive sections treated with reduced pressure and speed and the minimum number of strokes possible to accomplish complete removal. The client should be advised to keep her eyes closed throughout the routine to prevent preparations entering them. The range of brushes and speed variations permit all but the most sensitive of skin conditions to be treated by this method.

Skin inspection

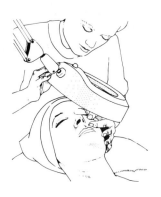

The cleansed skin is viewed through an illuminated magnifier or in natural daylight to see the different skin conditions present. If progressing to further facial treatment it is not always necessary to tone the skin at this stage as it can alter the skin pH level. However, wiping the skin gently with a diluted tonic preparation removes all traces of oiliness left from cleansing and avoids getting a false impression of the natural oil and moisture balance of the skin.

Sensitive skin which responds quickly to the stimulation of cleansing may present a false picture at this stage of inspection, appearing irritated and red but within a few minutes becoming calm and settled. This is a simple vascular response – like blushing – to the effect of the sensory nerve endings on the blood vessels.

Mature skin can sometimes look mottled, red and irritated after cleansing. This can be due to anxiety or could be associated with hormonal influences experienced by clients going through the menopause. These red flushes, especially on the neck, normally fade after a few minutes as the client relaxes. Hormonal changes occurring in the body appear to make the surface capillaries more sensitive to internal and external influences and dilation (flushing) occurs more readily. Whether of psychological (emotional) or physiological (physical) origin, evidence of this condition will require that the treatment proceeds with caution until the skin's true sensitivity is known.

Skin diagnosis

Treatment success will depend on the therapist's ability to recognise the facial conditions present and accurately match her treatment and product advice to the client on this information.

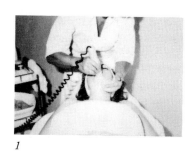

1

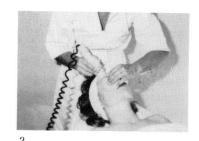

2

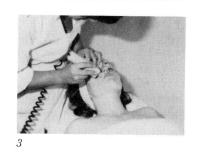

3

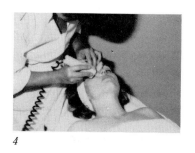

4

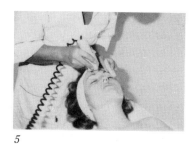

5

Brush cleansing is often completed with sponge method removal, providing a fast, thorough and popular sequence in preparation for further treatment massage, etc.

Cleansing removal with sponges

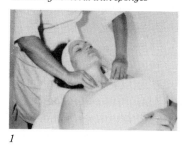

1

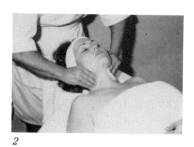

2

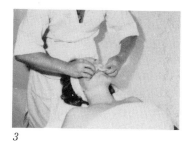

3

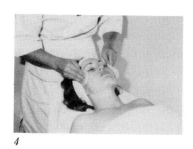

4

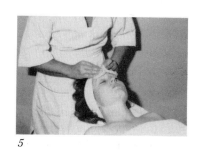

5

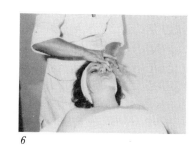

6

Although for client and sales convenience skins are referred to as different 'types', normal, oily, dry, etc., this is not accurate enough for therapy purposes. More detail is needed to avoid problems and ensure skin change and improvement.

Factors such as age, general health and well being have a major influence on skin appearance, and this holistic, or whole person, approach is widely recognised by clients. A sound knowledge of general physiology is needed so that the effects of ageing, ill health and external influences on skin tissue can be understood and explained to clients (see Chapter 3, Facial Anatomy).

Main points of diagnosis

Skin diagnosis will be built up by using verbal skills, visual observation and tactile assessment. Observing reactions to massage, cosmetic treatment, etc. will further develop this understanding of the skin.

- Age.
- Pigmentation and skin colour.
- Skin texture.
- Skin imperfections.
- Skin temperature.
- Acid/alkali balance (pH).

Age

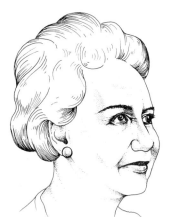

The age of the client provides the most immediate guide to treatment.

Loss of tone in the muscles of facial expression and softening of both the profile and the skin itself gives the therapist a clear indication of the client's age. As a person ages the facial bones appear more prominent and expression lines become etched. Crepey, loose skin may be seen on the neck and fine wrinkling around the eyes. Women who retain a fuller face, often due to slight overweight, look younger in the face.

The following factors affect the ageing of the skin:

- Genetic factors.
- The care received.
- Mental and physical health.
- Dietary habits.
- Life style (adequate sleep, stressful workload, career demands, etc.).
- Environmental and climatic factors (pollution, sun exposure, etc.).
- Weight loss or weight changes associated with low-fat diets, which have a detrimental effect on skin elasticity.

Correct professional treatment and home product guidance can considerably delay the effects of ageing. Medical and cosmetic research into ways of delaying ageing are receiving great attention at present. New discoveries that will become available to the industry in time must be watched for.

Pigmentation and skin colour

Skin colour and pigmentation provide valuable treatment guidance. A partial loss of colour (as in vitiligo) can indicate that skin reaction will be stronger in these areas and that cautious treatment is required.

Points that should be considered in skin diagnosis are:

- The actual colour should be recorded, i.e white, high-colour, tanned, brown, black, etc.
- Any pigmentation abnormalities of a permanent or temporary nature that could alter treatment. Amongst these are conditions such as vitiligo, lentigo, chloasma, ephelides (freckles) and pigmented moles (see Chapter 5, Skin Diseases and Disorders).
- Evenness of colour over the face and neck, which could indicate a rare 'normal' skin.
- High colour on the paler skin indicating sensitivity or existing capillary damage (couperose).
- Discolouration and its cause, whether relating to some physical condition or associated with the heavy complexion of seborrhoea (acne).
- Sallow skin colour, which is often a racial characteristic but one that can be improved through treatment to speed the skin's shedding and replacement rate.

Skin texture

Skin texture relates directly to the rate of secretion from the sebaceous glands and the hydric or moisture level in the skin. Both elements are strongly influenced by hormonal factors, stress, dietary influences and general health. A major aim of treatment is to bring these elements into correct balance.

The skin appears fine, soft and small-pored, if the oil output from the sebaceous glands and the hydric level are in balance (normal skin).

The skin appears coarse-textured and large-pored when the oil output is excessive and the moisture level low, causing the skin to be out of balance, presenting a hard, glassy appearance (seborrhoea).

Skin imperfections

Any existing imperfections must be noted as they may alter the form the treatment takes or contra-indicate certain electrical routines. To avoid further problems, medical guidance should be obtained if the beauty specialist is in any doubt as to the wisdom of applying treatment. The therapist is often the first person consulted regarding the removal of small moles, warts, etc. and has a duty to direct her clients for medical attention if required (see Chapter 5, Skin Diseases and Disorders).

The following points should be noted:

- Dilated capillaries (telangiectasia), their position and the extent of the problem, whether the blood vessels are bulbous, ruptured into the epidermal layers and presenting a thread-like appearance.
- Vascular naevi, blood spots, small birth marks.

- Skin tags, fibroma simplex and other fibrous growths need noting so that routines can be adapted around them. Some imperfections, like warts, may also contra-indicate treatment.
- Superfluous (unwanted) hair problems on the lip or chin.
- Scars, or scar tissue relating to a resolved skin problem (e.g. acne).
- Enlarged pores, blocked pores, comedones, blemishes, cystic blockage.

Skin temperature

The skin helps to control the body temperature through the dilation and constriction of surface capillaries (see Chapter 3, Facial Anatomy). This is evident by the colour and warmth of the skin's surface. The colour, texture and thickness of the skin affects how well this can be detected. In fine, pale skins the dilation can be seen clearly, whereas in darker or coarser skins temperature changes are disguised for longer. The beauty therapist must be checking constantly for changes in the temperature of the skin both visually and manually to prevent over stimulating.

Factors that can effect changes in skin temperature include:

- External stimulation.
- Internal body temperature (general health).
- Embarrassment or nervousness.
- Excitement or fear.
- Allergic reaction.

Acid/alkali balance (pH)

The pH value of the horny layer in healthy skin ranges between 5 and 5.6, showing an acid reaction compared to a neutral pH of 7. The secretions resulting from the activities of the sebaceous and sweat glands, and the process known as keratinisation of the epidermis, form the so called *acid mantle*, covering the entire skin surface. The acid mantle plays a most important role since it acts as protection against action by bacteria and micro-organisms living in the external environment, which is characterised by an alkaline pH.

The acid mantle also helps to maintain a healthy skin. In fact, a decrease in acidity in the skin tissues results in an unhealthy appearance with uneven texture.

Various factors affect the 5–5.6 pH of the skin; these include:

- Internal health of body.
- External factors.
- Environmental and climatic conditions.
- Topical applications (cosmetic products, etc.).
- Client's dietary habits (nutrition and digestion).
- Excessive perspiration.

Recognition of basic skin types

Skin diagnosis is a very important process and can directly affect the success or failure of the beauty treatment. For client and sales convenience, skin types are described under the following headings. In reality however, most skins show features of more than one type, and it is the actual assessment that must direct the treatment given.

Normal skin with correct oil and moisture balance

The normal skin has an ideal balance of oil and moisture and needs simply protection and maintenance in treatment. It is the evenness of colour that makes the normal skin easy to recognise. The texture is fine and there are no imperfections present. The skin will feel warm to the touch and have a smooth texture and firmness of tone.

Dry/dehydrated skin with reduced oil and moisture balance

The dry/dehydrated skin needs stimulation in treatment to redress the reduced oil and moisture balance. The dry/dehydrated skin condition is caused by insufficient secretion of sebum and is associated with genetic, internal and external factors that alter the hydric balance. Dry skin is more often encountered in clients of middle age or older, but areas can display dryness/dehydration at any age. Often dryness/dehydration is prematurely caused by neglect (incorrect care, suntanning, etc).

The texture of dry skin is fine with no visible pores, although flakiness may be present. Premature lines and wrinkles are evident, skin tone is soft and the skin has a thin, almost transparent appearance. The dry skin is more prone to sensitivity and broken capillaries can be a problem.

On occasions the skin may look and feel tight, possibly causing a smooth sheen which in this case indicates dehydration and is not to be confused with the shiny, oily skin.

Mature skin with ageing signs

The skin as it ages still reflects the texture and hydric balance it had in former times, and this decides the emphasis of treatment, i.e. whether stimulating, refining, calming, etc.

The mature skin which has been oily in youth starts out with its balance of oils to moisture in credit, and as it ages, the sebaceous glands produce just sufficient oily matter to produce a finely textured, firm skin in excellent health. Facial lines, where present, will tend to be etched, rather than soft and web like.

The dry/dehydrated skin obviously ages more quickly than the normal to oily skin, starting out with a disadvantage; its vulnerability to outside influences such as sun, poor care, poor diet, etc. all impact directly on the skin's texture and firmness. Fine pored, the skin lacks vitality and is often traced with superficial wrinkles. Premature ageing is in fact a big problem. The indiscriminate use of soaps and harsh products and inadequate skin protection all lead to ageing signs showing very early on.

Whatever its background, as skin ages certain things occur, and these ageing signs can be delayed through specialised skin treatment. Skin texture changes relating to menopause are evident as the desquamation rate slows and the skin becomes coarse and thickened, especially around the mouth and chin. Colour changes may also occur as the skin compacts and becomes keratinised and horny. Senile pigmentation may be evident.

The skin becomes loose and crepey, especially on the neck, and lines around the eyes, mouth and forehead are common. The elasticity and plumpness of the skin decreases as a direct result of changes occurring in the collagen fibres of the skin. The collagen fibres become cross-linked and rigid, losing their flexibility and lowering the skin's water retaining abilities. Vascular damage may be present with broken capillaries on the upper cheeks,and across the nose. Superfluous hair may also be a problem.

Oily/combination/blemished skin with overproduction of oil and low fluid balance

Oily Skin

This is a condition caused by an over secretion of the sebaceous glands. It usually occurs during adolescence due to the hormone imbalance, but areas of the face may display oiliness at any age. The skin may appear sallow or dull with a coarse, uneven texture due to the enlarged pores. Comedones, pustules and other primary lesions may be present and the skin can appear shiny and hard. Patches of dehydration may be present due to the harsh products used in an effort to combat the oiliness.

Combination skin

The classic combination skin is a modified oily skin, with a central T-zone of oiliness, with the cheeks and neck showing normal or dry characteristics. It is one of the most common skin 'types'.

Blemished/problem skin

The condition of seborrhoea can occur at any age, though is most common in youth, and can lead to acne if not correctly controlled. Sebaceous secretion is overproduced, causing dilation of the pores and a thickened, shiny skin appearance with uneven texture and variable pH levels.

Pores become blocked and blemishes can result from a build up of epidermal cells at the mouths of the follicles. This keratinisation is caused by the slowing down of the cellular growth in the basal layer of the skin.

Treatment seeks to reverse the skin blocking process through specialised cleansing routines (e.g. galvanic desincrustation).

Sebaceous glands occur in greater numbers on the face, chest, and shoulders and are most numerous on the centre part of the face, Sebum,the oily liquid produced by the sebaceous glands, contains fatty acids, lipids and cellular matter. Sebum acts to protect the skin from transient bacteria and external drying elements. Sebum is vital to the well being of the skin; only when it becomes blocked in the pores does it cause problems which result in blemishes and subsequent scars.

Sensitive skin

Sensitive skin is thin, easily stimulated and has a quick response to treatment, so caution is required. Emphasis is on calming and settling routines and products, to maintain the skin in balance. Sensitive skin can be recognised by high colour (or by warmth of skin and through discussion with darker skinned clients), evidence of dilated capillaries and dry, irritated or flaking skin areas.

Skin toning

Cleansing of the skin is always the initial practical phase; skin diagnosis commences before the cleansing, continues throughout and is completed when the skin is free from makeup and really clean. Depending on the treatment to follow, it may be desirable to tone. This will depend on the skin condition and the effect to be achieved.

If specialised cleansing is the next active stage, the skin would not be toned at this point, nor would it be within active facial routines. Toning would occur after massage, mask, etc. and at the final conclusion of the routine prior to day protection.

Within a cleanse and makeup sequence toning and moisture protection would follow immediately after cleansing. The toning has to be performed very thoroughly to allow a matt, long-lasting makeup to be applied.

Effects of skin toning

- Toning within cleanse and makeup removes final traces of cleanser.
- Within treatment plans toning removes all final traces of massage

cream, mask, etc. and prepares the skin for moisture protection and makeup.
- Refines skin texture.
- Closes the pores.
- Cools and soothes the skin.
- Within home care plans, removes all traces of cleanser and makeup and refreshes the skin.

Manual skin toning

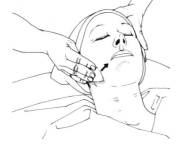

Manual skin toning

A dampened cotton wool pad folded into a spatula shape is used to manually tone the skin, using a tonic suitable for the skin type. Light, fast tapping movements are used all over the face and neck, and then the excess solution is settled into the skin using a rolling movement of the hand and an opened out tissue. Application can be adjusted to avoid sensitive areas, if present, and the alternative of a toning compress made of gauze can be used. The compress is soaked in an appropriate lotion, then applied for a few minutes to settle the skin.

An aerosol spray, containing a mineral water such as Evian water, may also be employed to refresh the skin. It is sprayed in a fine mist all over the face and neck. A paper tissue is then placed over the face and gently held against the skin to absorb excess moisture.

At conclusion the skin should feel slightly tacky to the touch, and be settled and calm in appearance.

Electrical skin toning

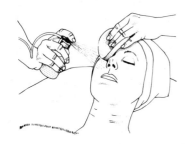

Electrical spray toning

Toning may also be accomplished electrically using a spray toner or vaporiser. A fine and evenly distributed mist of fluid produced under pressure tones the skin and is easily absorbed into it. Toning lotions appropriate for the skin type are prepared in a 10% solution with water to meet varying skin conditions. A viscose sponge or cotton wool tissue is used to protect the eyes,and catch any drips. Electrical spray toning is very professional, effective and popular with clients.

Cosmetic preparations

A sound knowledge of the cosmetic chemical function of the product used is essential if the correct result is to be achieved. Accurate matching of the skin condition against the known actions of the preparations is important, both for results and to avoid over reaction.

If sensitivity is suspected (by observation and through conversation) caution can be used in early treatment. Products for the sensitive skin can be used initially and given as samples until more is known about the skin.

Cosmetic manufacturers provide detailed information about their preparations, ingredients, actions, etc. and much can be learnt from this to enhance sales.

Cleansing products

Cleansing products have the biggest share of the cosmetic market and come in a wide range of formulations to match different skin needs. Most are water-based emulsions and include a detergent or soap constituent as these are effective cleansers. The formulation is balanced by other ingredients that prevent dehydration of the skin.

Cleansing products have to:

- Remove makeup effectively, aid desquamation and remove skin debris.
- Be easy to handle and economic to use.
- Be suitable for the client's skin, not causing irritation or over stimulation.
- Be matched to the client's taste, and financial status.
- Be appealing, having a pleasant appearance, texture, perfume and feel on the skin.
- Clean the skin effectively without stripping it of its natural protective barrier.

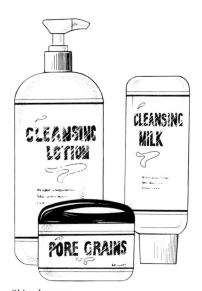

Skin cleansers

Deep cleansing by specialised products and equipment has increased the range of preparations dramatically in recent times.

Advances in cleansing products
New products available include:

- Combined cleansing and toning lotions which are popular for home use with younger clients, being swift and convenient. They are not suitable for heavy makeup removal.
- Foaming cleansers which are applied as a mousse-like cream that can then be worked up into a lather with water and rinsed off.
- Soap based desincrustation products used in combination with galvanic deep cleansing procedures which are now firmly established as part of clinic procedures.
- Cleansers based on natural ingredients which are once more back in fashion, and are helping to build new markets for 'natural' products.
- Latest research is providing cleansers based on liposomes and AHA (alpha-hydroxy acids) which have special roles to play in skin regeneration and delaying ageing signs.

Cleansers are available in many forms:

- Cleansing milk, which can be formulated for all skin types.
- Cleansing cream, which is suitable for dry and mature skins. Cream avoids skin drag and removes makeup quickly, leaving the skin supple and settled.
- Liquefying cleansing cream, normally used for removal of theatrical makeup, which requires careful toning to remove completely.

- Soapless cleanser/complexion soap, ideal as a cleanser for the younger client if makeup is not worn.
- Cleansing lotion/ combined toner, popular for repeated use in the day on the oily and combination skin.
- Cleansing pore grains, used periodically within home plans to maintain the unblocking actions achieved through clinic routines.
- Desincrustation products, based on electrically activated soap solution used in conjunction with galvanic current,within clinic routines for the oily and blemished skin (see Chapter 9, Electrical Treatment).

Skin toning products

Most skin toners are gentle in action and within home use are designed to be compatible with the cleanser, to ensure thorough removal whilst freshening the skin. In less common use are astringents and corrective lotions which in the past were alcohol based. These have fallen from popularity and the corrective or refining action required is produced using skin tonics based on natural, plant-based ingredients with corrective action. Plant extracts of camomile and calendula (soothing), ginseng and royal jelly (regenerating), rosemary, thyme and seaweed (corrective and healing), are now widely used in tonic preparations.

Skin toning products in use include:

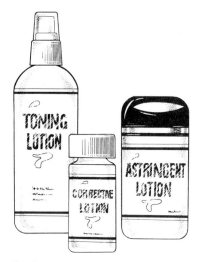

Skin toners

- Skin tonic with mild refining and freshening action, suitable for dry, dehydrated and sensitive skin and often based on flower extracts. Diluted rose water is a good example of a low cost, useful skin toner.
- Astringent products are still available but are quite changed in action from their alcohol-based predecessors. They contain herbal plant extracts and witch hazel to balance oil flow, refine and help heal the oily skin. Astringents containing any alcohol are not advised for sensitive, mature or blemished skins.
- Corrective lotions, to control seborrhoea, are based on seaweed extracts, chamomile, and other soothing plant extracts to correct the skin's oil balance and reduce or prevent the formation of blocked pores. They contain no alcohol, but rely for action on phytotherapy (plant derived ingredients).

Self check

1 List the methods of cleansing available and explain the procedure for each one.
2 Why is a skin diagnosis very important?
3 What are the main points of diagnosis?
4 Explain the significance of each point from question 3.
5 Describe how to recognise the main types of skin.
6 List the effects of skin toning.
7 State the main properties of (a) a cleanser and (b) a toner.

CHAPTER THREE Facial Anatomy

Before we proceed with further manual or electrical applications, a knowledge of underlying structures, bony supports, and the very nature of the skin itself is necessary.

Facial proportions

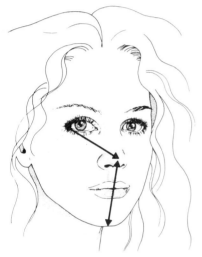

Ideal facial proportions

An ideally proportioned face is thought to be one which has equal measurements, (1) from the tip of the nose to the lowest part of the chin, and (2) from the outer corner of the eye to the tip of the nose. The facial features and expression are determined by the shape of the bony structures supporting the muscles of facial expression, and the subcutaneous fat overlying the muscles. As an individual ages, or loses weight, the true bone structure emerges and the nose, cheekbones, etc. appear more prominent.

Differences in the shape and size of the skull, due to national and inherited characteristics, determine the facial features, whilst superficial muscles provide the expression. The position and attachments of facial muscles to fascia and bones of the skull determine the massage technique and sequence of movements required.

Bones of the cranium and face

The bony framework of the head is called the skull. The skull, apart from the lower jaw (the mandible), is usually classed as the *cranium*. There are 22 bones involved in the formation of the skull, which, apart from the lower jaw, are all fixed in position. The skeleton of the face and cavity enclosing the brain are made up of 15 bones, whilst the other 7 are deeply situated and do not affect the contour.

Bones of the cranium

1 Frontal bone
Large flat bone, forms the forehead and part of the roof of the eye orbit. Contains the frontal sinuses.

Bones of the head (cranium)

1 frontal bone
2 parietal bones (right and left)
2 temporal bones
1 occipital bone
1 sphenoid bone
1 ethmoid bone

Bones of the face

2 maxillae (single maxilla)
1 mandible (lower jaw)
2 zygomatic (cheek bones)
2 nasal

Internal facial bones

2 palatine
1 vomer
2 lacrimal
2 inferior conchae

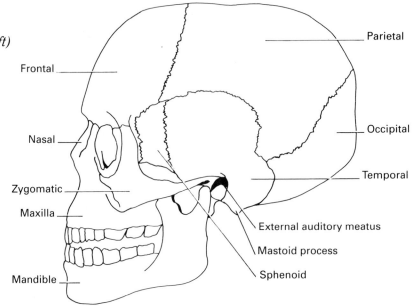

2 Parietal bones

One on either side of the head. Flat bones forming the sides and roof of the skull. Join with the frontal bone in the front and occipital in the back.

2 Temporal bones

Irregular bones which form the temples at the sides of the skull. Contain the organs of hearing. The projection at the bottom is called the *mastoid process*.

1 Occipital bone

Flat bone forming the back of the head. Heavier and stronger than other skull bones. Contains a large opening called the *foramen magnum* for the passage of the spinal cord.

1 Sphenoid bone

A bat-shaped irregular bone. Lies in the centre of the base of the cranium, contains a depression in which the pituitary gland sits.

1 Ethmoid Bone

A light, fragile bone. It forms the roof of the nose and separates the eye orbits from the nasal cavity.

Bones of the face

2 Maxillae

Two irregular bones joined in the middle to form the upper jaw. Carry the upper teeth, form part of the roof of the mouth, floor and wall of

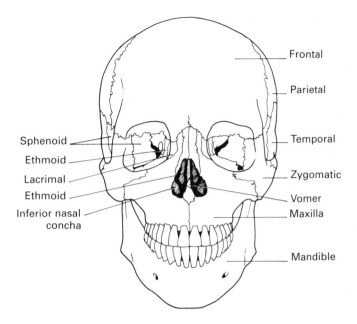

Frontal

Parietal

Temporal

Zygomatic

Vomer

Maxilla

Mandible

Sphenoid

Ethmoid

Lacrimal

Ethmoid

Inferior nasal concha

the nasal cavity and parts of the eye orbits. They are light bones containing the maxillary sinuses.

1 Mandible bone

Lower jaw bone, longest and strongest in the face. The only moveable bone in the head carries the lower set of teeth. It provides attachment for some facial muscles and contains openings for the nerves and blood vessels that supply the teeth.

2 Zygomatic bones

Two bones forming the prominence of the cheeks. They join with the zygomatic process of the temporal bone on each side.

2 Nasal bones

Small, flat bones forming the bridge of the nose. They join with the frontal bone.

Internal facial bones

2 Palatine bones

These bones aid in the formation of the floor and wall of the nasal cavity, the roof of the mouth, and the floor of the eye socket.

1 Vomer

The vomer bone forms the back and lower part of the nasal cavities.

2 Lacrimal

Two very small bones within the eye sockets.

2 Inferior conchae

These are separate bones forming part of the nose.

The bones of the adult skull, with the exception of the mandible, are joined so tightly to one another that no movement between them is possible. The serrated joints (sutures) become less evident with age, and the bones become fused. The complex nature of the facial bones is seen clearly in the orbital cavity, where six bones are involved: the *frontal, lacrimal, sphenoid, ethmoid, zygomatic* and *maxilla*.

Facial muscles

 1 *Occipitofrontalis*
 2 *Corrugator*
 3 *Procerus nasi*
 4 *Orbicularis oculi*
 5 *Nasalis*
 6 *Orbicularis oris*
 7 *Risorius*
 8 *Zygomaticus*
 9 *Buccinator*
10 *Masseter*
11 *Levators of upper lip*
12 *Depressors of lower lip*
13 *Mentalis*
14 *Triangularis*
15 *Temporalis*
16 *Platysma*
17 *Sternocleidomastoid*

Muscles of the face and neck

The muscular system of the face is concerned with the production of movement for speech, facial expression and mastication (chewing). Muscle tissue consists of cells which are capable of contraction. Although most of the muscles are attached directly to the skull, some originate from and insert into the skin, surface fascia (sheath of tissue covering muscle fibres) or other muscles.

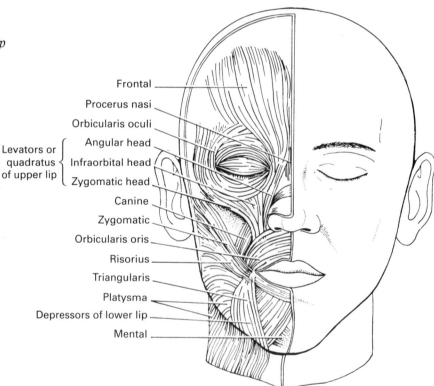

The following table shows the position, origin, insertion and action of the muscles of the face and neck. The *origin* of a muscle is the more fixed attachment, usually to a bone. The *insertion* is the more moveable attachment, often into skin, fascia or other muscle. The action of the muscle is the movement it performs.

Table 3.1

Muscle	Position	Origin	Insertion	Action
1 Occipitofrontalis (may be separated into two muscles)	Broad muscular sheet from eyebrows to the back of the head	Occipital bone and frontal bone	Aponeurosis of scalp, tissue of eyebrows	Moves the scalp and lifts the eyebrows, creates an expression of surprise or horror
2 Corrugator	A small triangular muscle between the eyebrows	Frontal bone and nasal prominence at inner end of eyebrow	Skin about halfway across eye socket	Draws eyebrows inwards and downwards causing vertical lines as in frowning
3 Procerus nasi	Covers bridge of nose between the eyebrows	Nasal bone	Skin of eyebrow and forehead	Wrinkles the nose and depresses the wider part of the eyebrows
4 Orbicularis oculi (spherical sphincter* muscle of the eyelids)	Surrounds the eye	Frontal bone and circles the eye	Frontal process of maxilla	Opens and closes the eye
5 Nasalis	Covers the tip of the nose	Maxilla	Soft tissue of the nostril	Compresses the nostril
6 Orbicularis oris (spherical sphincter* muscle of the mouth)	Circular muscle surrounding the mouth	No bony attachments – its fibres occupy the entire width of the lips		Closes and compresses the lips forward as in kissing and presses them against the teeth
7 Risorius (grinning muscle)	A triangular muscle from the angle of the mouth across the cheek	Fascia of the masseter muscle	Skin at the angle of the mouth	Pulls the corner of the mouth laterally and creates a grinning expression
8 Zygomaticus	From the cheek bone to the corner of mouth	Temporal process of the zygomatic	Skin at the corner of the mouth	Pulls the corners upwards and backwards
9 Buccinator (muscle of mastication)	Principle muscle of the cheek (deep)	Maxilla and mandible	Corner of the mouth	Keeps the cheeks stretched during opening and closing of mouth thus preventing injury during mastication
10 Masseter (muscle of mastication)	Superficial rectangular muscle of the cheek	Zygomatic arch	Mandible	
11 Levators of upper lip (labii superioris, plus anguli oris)	Surrounds the upper part of lip	Maxilla, lower margin of eye socket and zygomatic bone	Orbicularis oris and upper lip	Powerful elevator of the lower jaw, closes jaw and exerts pressure on teeth
12 Depressors of lower lip (labii inferioris, plus anguli oris)	Surrounds the lower lip	Mandible	Orbicularis oris	Draws lip outwards as in sneering
13 Mentalis (chin muscle)	Tip of chin	Mandible	Orbicularis oris (lower border)	Depresses the lower lip down one side

Table 3.1 (cont.)

Muscle	Position	Origin	Insertion	Action
14 Triangularis (muscle of mastication)	Triangular muscle of the lower lip	Mandible	Corner of mouth	Elevates the skin of the chin, turns the lower lip outwards as in pouting
15 Temporalis (muscle of mastication)	Fan-shaped muscle, extends from the eyes to the top of the ears on the sides of the head	Temporal fossa at the sides of the head	Mandible	Pulls corner of the mouth downwards and inwards
16 Platysma	Front and sides of neck	Fascia overlying pectoralis major and deltoid muscles	Mandible and subcutaneous tissue and skin	Elevates the mandible closes the mouth, aids the mastication process
17 Sternocleido-mastoid	Sides of neck	Has two heads, one from sternum and one from clavicle	Mastoid process of the temporal bone	Wrinkling of the skin of neck, depression of lower lip
18 Pectoralis major	Covers the upper half of chest wall Mammary glands lie on it	Sternum, clavicle, cartilages of first six or seven ribs	Bicipital groove of the humerus	Flexes and rotates the neck. Bows the head Adduction of the arm and medially rotates the arm
19 Trapezius	Triangular muscle which covers back and sides of neck and upper part of back	Occipital bone and spines of thoracic vertebrae	Calvicle, spine of scapula	Steadies the scapula during movements of the upper arm. Rotates, elevates the scapula
20 Deltoid	Epaulette muscle of the shoulder	Clavicle, spine of scapula	Humerus	Abduction, flexion, inward and outward rotation. Extension of the arm

*A *sphincter* has no bone attachment; it is attached to the fascia of other muscles.

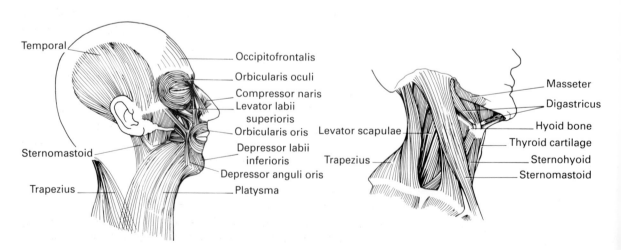

Blood circulation of the head and neck

All superficial treatments increase the blood circulation of the face and neck, causing a rise in the local skin temperature and increased colour (*erythema*). The superficial capillaries dilate to regulate the temperature, and the interchange of tissue fluids increases nutrition to the skin's surface layers.

The blood circulatory system

The blood circulatory system consists basically of the heart, arteries, veins, capillaries and the blood. The heart weighs about 250 g and is the organ that pumps blood around the body. It is divided into four chambers. The right and left sides are separated by a solid muscular structure (*septum*).

Venous blood (deoxygenated) enters the heart at the right *atrium* via the superior and inferior *venae cavae*. It passes into the right *ventricle*. It leaves this chamber via two pulmonary arteries where it travels to the lungs. At this point carbon dioxide is taken out of the blood and oxygen is taken in. The oxygenated blood then returns to the heart via the pulmonary veins to the left atrium, then it passes into the left ventricle and finally out through the *aorta* to all parts of the body.

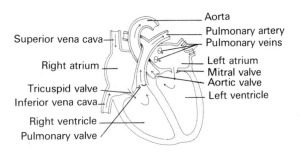

The heart

The blood

The blood is a fluid tissue contained within a closed system of vessels – the arteries, veins and capillaries – through which it is made to circulate by the pumping action of the heart.

The blood circulatory system is the chief transport system of the body, conveying nutrients and gases from one part of the body to another. It also acts as a means of communication by conveying messages in the form of hormones from the *endocrine* glands. The blood consists of a yellow liquid called *plasma,* which makes up 55% of the volume, and a large number of cells called *corpuscles,* which make up the remaining 45% of the volume.

Arteries and veins

Arteries are hollow elastic tubes which carry blood away from the heart. They become smaller as they spread through the body. As they become smaller they are known as *arterioles* and then as *capillaries*.

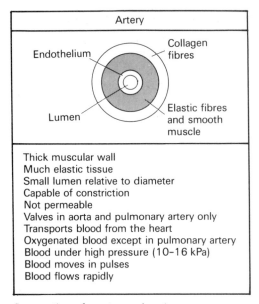

Artery	Vein
Thick muscular wall	Thin muscular wall
Much elastic tissue	Little elastic tissue
Small lumen relative to diameter	Large lumen relative to diameter
Capable of constriction	Not capable of constriction
Not permeable	Not permeable
Valves in aorta and pulmonary artery only	Valves throughout all veins
Transports blood from the heart	Transports blood to heart
Oxygenated blood except in pulmonary artery	Deoxygenated blood except in pulmonary vein
Blood under high pressure (10–16 kPa)	Blood under low pressure (1 kPa)
Blood moves in pulses	No pulses
Blood flows rapidly	Blood flows slowly

Cross sections of an artery and a vein

Veins are hollow elastic tubes which carry blood towards the heart. They are oval and their walls are thinner than arteries. They have valves to prevent back-flow of blood.

Arteries of the head and neck

Three arteries that supply the head, neck and upper limbs branch from the arch of the aorta. These are the *innominate* artery, also known as

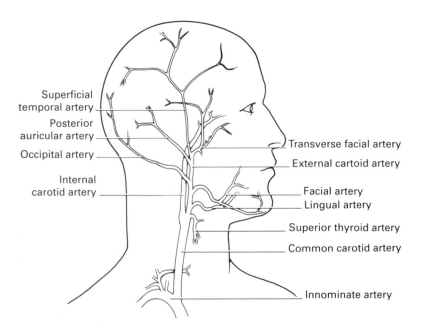

brachiocephalic artery, the left *common carotid* artery and the left *subclavian* artery.

The *external carotid* artery branches to form the:

- *Thyroid* artery.
- *Facial* artery.
- *Temporal* artery.
- *Lingual* artery.
- *Occipital* artery.
- *Maxillary* artery.

The *internal carotid* artery branches to form the:

- *Ophthalmic* artery.
- *Middle cerebral* artery.
- *Anterior* artery.
- *Posterior communicating* artery.

Venous returns from the head and neck

Superficial veins

- *Thyroid* vein
- *Facial* vein   } empty into the external jugular vein.
- *Occipital* vein

Deep sinuses

- *Superior sagittal* sinus
- *Inferior* sinus
- *Straight sagittal* sinus   } empty into the internal jugular vein.
- *Transverse sagittal* sinus

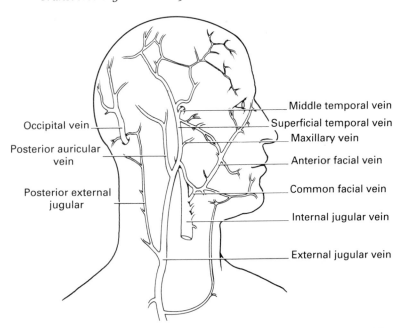

Occipital vein

Posterior auricular vein

Posterior external jugular

Middle temporal vein

Superficial temporal vein

Maxillary vein

Anterior facial vein

Common facial vein

Internal jugular vein

External jugular vein

Regional lymph nodes and vessels of the face and neck

The lymphatic system

Composition of lymph fluid

Lymphatic fluid closely resembles blood plasma in its composition, but has a much lower concentration of protein. There are also a large number of *lymphocytes* (the only living cells in the fluid) which come from the lymphatic glands.

Lymphatic capillaries and vessels

The lymphatic capillaries commence in the tissue spaces of the body as minute blind-ended tubes.

These minute capillaries join one another to form a network of very fine vessels, which drain away the fluid that has passed through the walls of the capillaries carrying blood into the tissue spaces. All lymphatic vessels open into lymphatic nodes. The lymph from the vessels drains through at least one lymphatic node before it passes eventually into one of two main lymphatic ducts, the *thoracic duct* and the right *lymphatic duct*.

Lymphatic nodes

The nodes are almond or bean-shaped structures, situated at various points in the course of the lymph vessels. The lymph nodes act as filters of the lymph in its course from the various organs and tissues to the point where it is returned to the blood. The lymphatic nodes filter pathogenic bacteria from the lymphatic fluid; if they did not general infection of the blood would be inevitable.

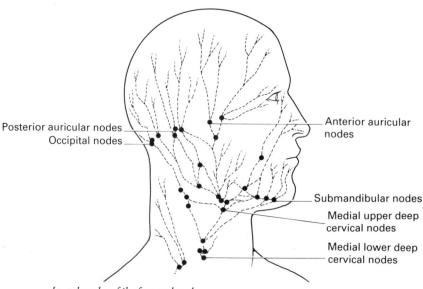

Lymph nodes of the face and neck

Functions of the lymphatic system

The lymphatic system offers a second line of defence against bacterial invasion, the first being the presence of the *leucocytes* in the blood at the site of injury or infection. The lymphatic system is responsible for the production of lymphocytes and, to some degree, blood plasma protein. The lymphocytes are formed in the lymph nodes, and the plasma protein is formed by the disintegration of these same cells into plasma globulin.

The nerves of the face and neck

A basic knowledge of the nerves of the face and neck is necessary for the beauty therapist.

There are twelve pairs of cranial nerves which are associated with the different areas of the head, face and neck. Some of the nerves are *sensory* nerves, some are *motor* nerves and some are bundles of both sensory and motor nerves and are called *mixed* nerves.

Sensory nerves

These are nerves which convey messages of sensation (e.g. touch, pain, heat, cold and pressure) to the central nervous system.

Motor nerves

These are nerves which carry messages from the central nervous system to an organ or muscle in response to a sensation, usually resulting in movement.

Mixed nerves

These are groups of both sensory and motor nerves bundled together.

The Cranial Nerves

No.	Name	Type	Function
1	Olfactory	Sensory	Give a sense of smell. The nerve endings start in the mucous membranes in the upper part of the nose. They continue through the olfactory tract to the temporal lobe of the cerebrum.
2	Optic	Sensory	Convey a sense of sight. They begin in the retina of each eye. They pass through the back of the orbital cavity, through the optic coramin of the sphenoid bone. They join at the optic chiasma where the fibres from each eye cross over to go to the opposite side of the cerebrum.

The Cranial Nerves (cont.)

No.	Name	Type	Function
3	Oculomotor	Motor	Supply the four main muscles that move the eyes: the superior, inferior, and medial recti; the inferior oblique muscles; the iris (which controls the amount of light permitted to enter the eye); the ciliary muscles.
4	Trochlear	Motor	Supply the superior oblique muscles, which move the eyes.
5	Trigeminal	Mixed	Sensory nerves: transmit the sensation of taste, heat and pressure. Motor nerves: stimulate the muscles of mastication. This is the largest of the cranial nerves. The trigeminal (3 pathway) nerve has three branches of sensory nerves:

   i) The ophthalmic branch transmits stimuli from the forehead and anterior aspect of the scalp the upper eyelids; the lacrimal glands and the conjunctiva; and the mucous membranes lining the nose.

   ii) The maxillary branch transmits stimuli from the lower eyelids; the cheeks and side of the nose; the upper lip; gums and teeth.

   iii) The mandibular branch transmits stimuli from the side of the scalp and cheeks, including the upper part of the ear pinna; the chin and the lower lip; gums and teeth; and the tongue.

Trigeminal nerve

No.	Name	Type	Function
6	Abducent	Motor	Supply the lateral rectus muscles which move the eyeballs.
7	Facial	Mixed	Sensory nerves: transmit impulses from the taste buds in the anterior two-thirds of the tongue. Motor nerves: convey impulses to the muscles of facial expression.
8	Auditory	Sensory	There are two branches:

   i) The vestibular branch conveys impulses from the semicircular canals in the inner ear to the cerebellum. It therefore affects the sense of balance and equilibrium.

   ii) The cochlea branch transmits impulses from the inner ear to the cerebral cortex where they are perceived as sound.

No.	Name	Type	Function
9	Glossopharyngeal	Mixed	Sensory nerves: transmit impulses from the tonsils, pharynx and the taste buds in the posterior third of the tongue to the medulla oblongata. Motor nerves: stimulate the muscles of the pharynx and the secretory (saliva) cells of the parotid glands.

The Cranial Nerves (cont.)

No.	Name	Type	Function
10	Vagus	Mixed	This nerve has the largest distribution area of the cranial nerves. Sensory nerves: transmit impulses from the membranes of the heart; blood vessels of the thorax and abdomen; the pharynx, larynx, trachea, oesophagus, stomach, intestines, pancreas, spleen, gall bladder, bile ducts, kidneys and ureters to the medulla oblongata. Motor nerves supply the smooth muscles and secretory glands of the same organs.
11	Accessory	Motor	Supply the sternocleidomastoid and trapezius muscles which move the head and shoulders. It also supplies the muscles of the pharynx and larynx.
12	Hypoglossal	Motor	Supply the muscles of the tongue enabling it to move, and also the muscles surrounding the hyoid bone in the front of the throat.

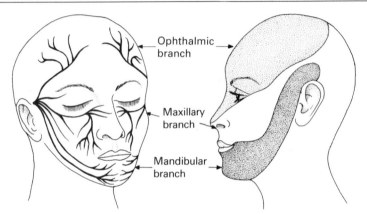

Regions of the trigeminal nerve (see The Cranial Nerves table on page 43)

The skin

The skin is an elastic, flexible organ which has an average surface area of approximately 14 square feet. It consists of a superficial layer of stratified *epithelium* called the *epidermis*, a firm layer of connective tissue called the *dermis* or *corium* and an underlying area of *subcutaneous* tissue.

The epidermis

The stratified epithelial tissue of the epidermis is a continually changing layer. The epidermis can be identified to have five layers. These are:

- *Stratum germinativum.*
- *Stratum spinosum.*
- *Stratum granulosum.*
- *Stratum lucidum.*
- *Stratum corneum.*

The continual process of change starts in the basal layer, or stratum germinativum, of the epidermis where cells are formed. The cells then

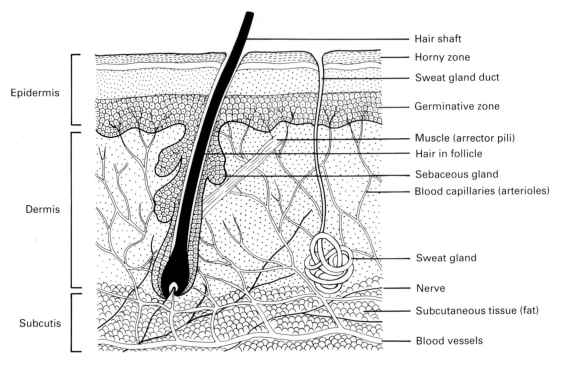

Epidermis

Dermis

Subcutis

Hair shaft
Horny zone
Sweat gland duct
Germinative zone
Muscle (arrector pili)
Hair in follicle
Sebaceous gland
Blood capillaries (arterioles)
Sweat gland
Nerve
Subcutaneous tissue (fat)
Blood vessels

Layers of the skin

journey to the surface of the skin passing through various stages in each layer of the epidermis. They start as moist, living, nucleated cells and end up as dead, flat flakes of *keratin* in the stratum corneum that are worn away with use.

Layers of the epidermis

Stratum germinativum (*basal* layer)

This is the deepest layer of the epidermis; the cells are in close contact with the dermis and it is from here that the basal cells receive their nourishment. *Mitosis* (cell division) takes place in the stratum germinativum and this pushes cells up towards the surface. The cells

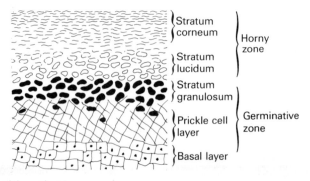

Stratum corneum
Stratum lucidum
Stratum granulosum
Prickle cell layer
Basal layer
Horny zone
Germinative zone

Layers of the epidermis

in this layer are living, moist cells with nuclei. Scattered within these cells are *melanocytes* which are specialised cells that produce the skin pigment, *melanin*. Melanin protects the skin against injury from ultraviolet radiation and is responsible for differing skin colours. It is produced by a complicated chemical reaction involving amino acids and ultraviolet radiation. The melanocytes have *dendrites* (arms) that pass the pigment to the surrounding cells.

Stratum spinosum

This layer is also known as the *prickle cell* layer, because the cells have prickle like threads that join them together. The cells in this layer are polygonal (many sided), contain nuclei and are living. It is difficult to differentiate where the stratum germinativum ends and the stratum spinosum begins. Often the layers are described together as the basal layer.

Stratum granulosum

Moving towards the surface the cells become flattened and grains of *keratohyaline* form – a substance that gives the skin its white appearance. The thickness of the layer varies from area to area. It is thickest on the palms and soles and absent from the lips.

The process of keratinisation begins in this area: this is the change from living, moist, nucleated cells into dead, flat, horny flakes of keratin.

Stratum lucidum

This layer derives its name from its clear, almost transparent appearance. It is only a few cells thick and is believed to be the water barrier zone. The nuclei are now becoming indistinct and the cells are much flatter.

Stratum corneum

The stratum corneum consists of many layers of dead, flat flakes of keratin. The cells have disappeared along with the moisture and the nuclei. The thickness again varies from one part of the body to another, being thickest in areas of wear and pressure. The process of keratinisation is complete. The flakes of keratin come off continually in a process known as *desquamation*.

The epidermis rests upon the dermis. Although the basal layer of the epidermis is mitotically active, and therefore living, it does not have a blood or nerve supply. The lower border of the epidermis is very irregular and has finger-like projections called *papillae* (see the papillary layer, below).

The dermis

This can also be called the true skin. It is a mass of connective tissue, containing blood vessels, lymphatic vessels, nerves, tactile corpuscles, glands and hair follicles. The thickness of the dermis is difficult to measure and varies from area to area. The dermis can be described as two layers, the upper or *papillary* layer and the deeper, *reticular* layer. The reticular layer gives the skin its pliability.

The papillary layer

This is the layer of the dermis lying immediately under the epidermis. It consists of finger-like projections called *papillae* that interlock with the dermis. The papillae increase the surface area of the dermis in contact with the epidermis. The upper portion of the dermis (see below) is very rich in blood and nerves, providing the basal layer with nutrients and sensation. The papillae are, therefore, most numerous in the sensitive areas such as finger tips.

The reticular layer

This is the deeper portion of the dermis. The reticular layer contains fat cells, blood vessels, lymphatic vessels, nerves, sebaceous and sudoriferous glands, hair follicles and fibrous, collagen and elastic tissues.

The subcutaneous layer (subcutis)

This is the underlying layer of the skin. It has no definite boundaries with the dermis and the thickness varies considerably from one area to another. It consists basically of bundles of loosely connected tissue, fat cells, blood vessels, nerves and lymphatic vessels. Very deep hair follicles extend into this area. It acts as a protection layer both from physical blows and heat loss.

Appendages of the skin

An appendage is something attached to an organ; the appendages of the skin are: hair and follicles, nails (see Structure and function of nails in Chapter 11), sebaceous glands and sudoriferous glands.

Hair and follicles

A hair follicle is a tube of epidermal cells that extends into the dermis, receiving nourishment from an adapted capillary, the dermal papilla. The follicle is multi-layered like the epidermis and the length of the follicle continually changes with the hair growth cycle.

Attached to the side of the hair follicle is a small muscle – the *arrector pili* muscle. When contracted the arrector pili causes the hair to stand on end and gives rise to goose pimples.

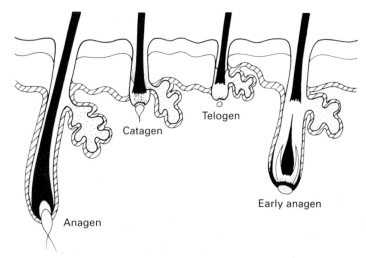

Stages of hair growth

A hair is a dead, keratinised structure that grows from the follicle. It grows in a cycle that is continuous and individual to the follicle. The length of the growth or *anagen* phase varies from one part of the body to another. The hair follicle then has a rest or *telogen* phase. The transition from the anagen to the telogen phase is called the *catagen* phase.

Sebaceous glands

Sebaceous glands are small, lobular glands which are epidermal in origin and situated in the dermis. Most sebaceous glands open inside a hair follicle and secrete sebum into the follicle. Sebaceous glands are largest and most numerous on the scalp, forehead, cheeks and chin – they are found over the entire surface of the body except the palms and soles. Sebum is a fatty substance that lubricates the skin and hair shaft keeping it soft and supple. Sebum consists of oil, water and fatty acids. The secretion of the sebaceous glands is controlled by the endocrine system and becomes very active in puberty. Sebum forms part of the *acid mantle*.

Sudoriferous glands

Eccrine glands

Eccrine or sweat glands excrete water and water soluble substances and are found all over the body apart from on the lips and the sexual organs. The main functions of the eccrine glands are temperature control by evaporation and elimination of waste products. The gland is a coiled mass of tubes and is situated in the dermis; the sweat duct passes up through the layers of the epidermis and opens directly on to the skin surface. These glands respond to the autonomic nervous system, excreting in times of stress, excitement, nervousness, etc.

Apocrine glands

Apocrine glands or *large coil* glands are also situated in the dermis, but their ducts usually open into hair follicles. They are situated in the underarm, breast and genital areas of the body. The apocrine glands are more prone to bacterial attack and therefore give rise to more body odour.

Functions of the skin

The skin is the largest organ in the body. More than just a wrapper, it has seven main functions:

1 Secretion.
2 Temperature regulation.
3 Absorption.
4 Protection.
5 Excretion and elimination.
6 Sensation.
7 Vitamin D production.

1 Secretion

The skin secretes from three glands. The glands and their secretions are described in Table 3.2 below.

Table 3.2

Gland	Secretion	Composition of secretion
Sebaceous	Sebum	Water, oil and fatty acids
Eccrine sweat gland	Sweat	Water and water-based substances
Apocrine sweat gland	Sweat	Water, salts and iron

These secretions help to lubricate the skin and hair, keeping them both soft and supple. The secretions are also involved in protection, as part of the acid mantle (see page 51), and in temperature regulation.

2 Temperature regulation

The skin helps to maintain the body's temperature at 37 °C (98.4 °F) in three ways.

Blood vessels

The superficial capillaries in the skin dilate and contract according to the external temperature. In hot conditions the vessels dilate, diverting blood to the surface. This gives the skin a flushed appearance and helps the body to cool down. In cold conditions the capillaries contract, diverting blood away from the surface deep into the skin. This gives the skin a white, cold appearance and conserves body heat. (The blood vessels also respond under emotional circumstances giving rise to blushing and the 'white as a sheet' appearance.)

Evaporation of sweat

The sweat excreted on to the surface of the skin evaporates and therefore has a cooling effect.

Subcutaneous fat

The fatty deposits in the subcutaneous region serve as an insulator, hence conserving heat. (Generally thin people feel the cold more than fat people.)

3 Absorption

The ability of the skin to absorb substances applied to its surface is a very debatable point. Naturally the skin repels water and other substances in its protective role. However, it has been proved scientifically that some substances can enter the body via the skin.

4 Protection

The skin protects the body in many ways:

Physical protection

- Desquamation – the surface of the skin continually flaking off.
- Continual – the surface of the skin is a complete, unbroken layer over the entire body.
- The subcutaneous layer acts as a cushion against blows.
- Waterproof – the skin repels water.
- Early warning system – due to the large number of nerve endings the skin warns the body about heat, pain, etc.
- Blood supply – blood clots when it comes into contact with air and also carries leucocytes and antibodies to fight infection. If the skin is broken both of the processes help to minimise the damage.

Chemical protection

- Acid mantle – the secretions of the three skin glands produce an acidic substance on the surface of the skin called the acid mantle. This is fungistatic and bacteriostatic.
- Melanin production – the production of melanin helps to protect the body from harmful ultraviolet radiation.

5 Excretion and elimination

In both eccrine and apocrine sweat there are waste products. The body rids itself of small amounts of various waste products via the skin.

6 Sensation

The papillary layer of the dermis contains many nerve endings that make us aware of our surroundings. They act as an early warning system to indicate heat, cold, pain, pressure and other external factors. These lie at various levels in the skin and are most numerous in the sensitive areas, e.g. finger tips, genital areas.

7 Vitamin D production

Vitamin D is also referred to as the sunshine vitamin because it is the ultraviolet radiation in sunlight that converts a substance in sebum to vitamin D.

The skin is a highly complex organ that needs careful and specific attention in order to function correctly and in turn look good. The beauty therapist comes into contact with the skin during **every** treatment. It is therefore vital that in order to carry out a treatment completely, safely and effectively the beauty therapist has a sound knowledge of the skin, its structure and its functions.

Self check

1 List the bones of the skull.
2 Name three muscles of mastication and three muscles of facial expression, stating the origin, insertion and action of each one.
3 List the functions of the blood.
4 Name the main artery supplying the head and give the names of four branches of this main artery.
5 Name the vein that drains the head.
6 What is lymph?
7 What are lymph nodes?
8 Briefly describe the structure and functions of the lymphatic system.
9 How many pairs of cranial nerves are there?
10 Explain the difference between motor and sensory nerves.
11 Name and describe the layers of the epidermis.
12 Explain how the function of the skin is related to its structure.
13 What are the appendages of the skin?
14 Describe the structure and function of the three skin glands.
15 How does the skin protect the body?
16 Why is a knowledge of the skin vital to the beauty specialist?

CHAPTER FOUR

Facial Massage

Facial massage stimulates the skin, improving function, protection and regeneration. It is also extremely relaxing and enjoyable, helping to relieve stress in today's busy world. A healthy skin is well equipped to cope with the demands of everyday life, but a demanding lifestyle and heavy workload can take its toll on the skin. Facial massage increases regeneration and maintains the skin's correct oil and fluid balance.

Massage can be stimulating, relaxing, toning, refining.

Massage routines can be planned which fit the time available and meet exact skin and client need. Within the *basic facial* (15–20 minutes' massage), the *pore treatment* (10 minutes' massage) and the *continental facial* (20–25 minutes' massage) provide a sound framework to meet most skin conditions.

Skilful massage technique, adapted to the minute nature and attachment of the facial muscles, should tone and stimulate the tissues without causing skin distension, irritation or loss of relaxation. For clients suffering from nervous tension, stress or depression, the relaxing aspects of massage should be emphasised.

Indications for massage treatment

- Normal skins requiring deep cleansing, skin balancing and refinement.
- Dry or dehydrated skins, needing stimulation of cellular function.
- Mature skins, where regeneration, deeper stimulation and surface desquamation is needed to delay signs of ageing.
- Younger, blemished or greasy skins, requiring cleansing, toning and refining action to free blocked pores and improve function.
- Delicate, sensitive skin conditions, where gentle stimulation, pH stabilising and oil–fluid balancing are needed.
- Conditions of nervous stress, depression or fatigue where tension is evident, causing muscular pain.

Contra-indications to massage

- Hyper-sensitive skins prone to allergic reaction.
- Extremely vascular skin conditions.

- Any evidence of acute inflammation, bites, stings, etc.
- Skin infection, irritation, or other evidence of sepsis and malfunction requiring medical attention.
- Diabetics (unstable skin conditions and poor healing capacity).
- Asthmatic or sinus disorders.
- Excessively loose skin.

Manual massage movements

The different groups of facial massage movements each have different purposes and effects. These effects are matched against the needs of the client's skin (indications), or may point out that they are not suitable for specific skins (contra-indications).

Effleurage
Light pressure, flowing movements, including stroking and roll-patting.

Petrissage
Compression movements,which include kneading, knuckling, lifting, rolling, pinching frictions and many other techniques involving increased pressure and vascular stimulation.

Tapotement
Percussion movements, covering all light tapping, whipping movements, performed to increase nervous response to stimulation.

Vibrations
Rapid contractions and relaxation of the muscles of the therapist's hands and lower arms, producing the controlled vibratory action.

Effleurage movements

Effleurage, or stroking movements, are performed with light, even pressure, in a rhythmical continuous fashion. The pressure used varies according to the underlying structures and muscle bulk but should never become unduly heavy. Effleurage prepares the tissues for deeper massage, links up movements and completes the sequence. The hand contours to the skin with the maximum palmar surface of the hand in contact, whilst even pressure, rhythm and rate of movement are established.

Effects of superficial effleurage
- A reflex vascular and nervous response from the surface layers of the skin occurs, causing increased skin temperature, warmth and colour.

• Relaxation results as the client becomes accustomed to the therapist's hands, and strain is relieved.

Effects of deeper effleurage
Deeper effleurage is performed when relaxation of muscle tissue has been achieved. A more mechanical response is attained, through increased vascular and lymphatic activity, by constriction and dilation of subcutaneous blood and lymphatic vessels.

Effects of effleurage: Summary

1 Aids venous circulation.
2 Aids arterial circulation by removal of congestion in the veins.
3 Lymphatic circulation is improved and absorption of waste products hastened.
4 Aids desquamation, so cleansing the skin, freeing surface adhesions.
5 Aids relaxation in preparation for further massage.
6 Relaxes contracted, tense muscle fibres.

Petrissage movements

Petrissage movements are only used on relaxed muscle tissue,as the intermittent pressure applied is deeper than effleurage movements. Compressing and relaxing the tissues causes surface reactions (local skin temperature and colour change), and increased vascular and lymphatic response.

The movements are performed slowly and rhythmically with the palmar surface of the fingers, thumb and fingers, or the entire palmar surface of the hands being used to conform to the contour of the area. The increased effect of petrissage movements would make them unnecessary and unsuitable for sensitive skins. Mature or loose skin conditions would need adaptation, perhaps only using frictions rather than kneading movements.

The pressure used in petrissage must relate to the muscle size and degree of tension present. No heavy petrissage movements are applied until the muscle tissue is relaxed. Effleurage movements are used to link compression movements and to maintain or re-establish relaxation.

In the younger client, improved skin function and removal of horny, keratinised cells increases basal layer activity resulting in a fresher, more refined skin texture. Increased lymphatic and vascular flow improves the skin's nutrition and defence against bacteria.

Effects of petrissage: Summary

1 Compression and relaxation of muscles cause blood and lymphatic vessels to be filled and emptied, thus increasing circulation and removal of waste products.
2 The skin, superficial and deeper tissues are all stimulated to further activity, improving cellular functions and regeneration.
3 Desquamation (shedding) removes surface cellular matter and leaves the skin clear, refreshed and refined.
4 Larger contracted muscles are relaxed and muscle tone is improved through compression and relaxation of muscle fibres.

Tapotement movements

Tapotement or percussion movements are performed in a light, brisk and stimulating manner. The rhythm of the strokes is important, as the fingers are continually breaking contact with the skin and the movements could be irritating if performed incorrectly. Where petrissage would not be indicated, tapotement may be used to advantage to achieve a fast vascular reaction without compression of the tissues. This is due to the skin's nervous response to the stimulus.

Tapotement is effective for loose skin problems, where skin distension might result from compression movements, yet stimulation is needed, e.g. around the eyes or loose crepey skin on the neck.

Effects of tapotement : Summary

1 Stimulation of the skin through reflex nervous response.
2 Increased vascular activity. Light tapotement causes blanching of the skin, constriction of the vessels, and, if continued, produces erythema, reddening of the skin, due to the interchange of the blood.
3 Tightening, toning effect on skin and superficial muscle tissue.

Vibrations

Static or running vibrations are performed on delicate skin conditions, or within a general facial sequence, where additional relaxation without over stimulation of surface tissues is required. Vibrations are applied on a nerve centre, or running along the path of a nerve, and they are produced by a rapid contraction and relaxation of the therapist's arm muscles so that a fine trembling or vibration results. The entire palmar surface of the hand may be used or, for an intensive effect, the tips of the first two fingers or the thumbs can produce excellent relaxation results.

Facial massage routines for the fine, sensitive skin can be based on vibratory movements, which combine gentle stimulation with relaxation, whilst avoiding surface irritation or capillary damage.

Effects of vibrations: Summary

1 Relaxation, relief of tension.
2 Gentle stimulation of the deeper skin layers.
3 Stimulation of nerves, relieving fatigue and muscular pain.

Massage technique

The most important requirement for massage is to concentrate on the client, her needs, tensions, etc. and perform the massage with care and awareness of facial anatomy.

Other requirements for massage are to:

- Maintain an even rhythm.
- Establish the correct rate of movement.
- Keep the hands flexible, so that they fit the contour of the area.
- Maintain the correct body posture during facial massage.
- Regulate pressure according to the muscle bulk and specific skin condition observed.
- Choose and apply the movements correctly to meet the needs of the skin.

Client bonding

Developing 'good hands' for massage relies more on client awareness than being proficient with a wide range of massage routines – though these help to build the techniques needed. If hands move attractively and movements flow well, the massage will be enjoyable and relaxing for the client and contribute to a satisfactory relationship between client and therapist.

Correct positioning

Controlled movements of the hands will only be possible if the therapist's body posture is correct, well supported, with a free range of arm movement. Fatigue will be avoided and correct technique maintained if both the client and operator are in a comfortable position for the general facial application. A comfortable chair or facial bed suited to the operator's height is essential to good massage technique.

Developing a sense of touch

Basic technique should be established within cleansing and basic facial routines before proceeding to more advanced massage routines. Flexible hands develop gradually and can be improved by following daily hand mobility exercises.

Developing a sense of touch relies on thinking about what you are doing and having an awareness of the tension or tone present in the muscles and adjusting pressure accordingly. Long and careful practice is the only way to develop this sense of touch which is so vital to the beauty specialist.

Hand mobility exercises

The mobility of the hands can be increased gradually, increasing the range of movement, dexterity and control through daily practice of hand exercises.

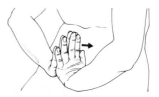

1 Press the fingers back from the palms to their fullest limits, with the fingers held together.

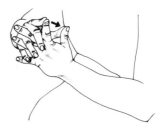

2 Press each finger back separately.

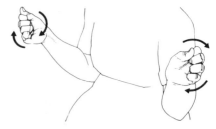

3 Rotate the hands and wrists, with the elbows held close to the sides, and the hands formed into fists. A full rotation should be attempted, with even rhythm, stretching the fingers tendons fully.

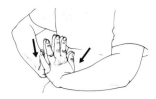

4 Form the hands into a praying position in front of the chest, with palms and fingers in full contact.Press the hands downwards, attempting to keep the palms together, until the action is felt on the wrists and lower arm muscles.

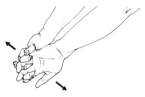

5 With the backs of the hands together, fingers interlocked, press the backs of the wrists together and pull against the fingers.

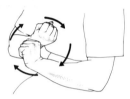

6 With the arms bent at the elbows, wrists held at chest height and the hands formed into fists, revolve the hands around each other.

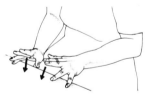

7 Attempt to tap the fingers of both hands in a co-ordinated rhythm, on to a hard surface. Increase the speed, making both hands keep in rhythm. Increased practice of the slower hand will improve its speed and control. Work first index to little finger, then reverse the sequence.

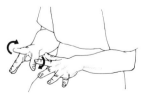

8 Practise making each finger and thumb form rotaries in the air, endeavouring to make each work independently of the others. Attempt full circles to the left and then to the right.

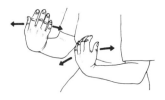

9 Vigorously shake the hands and wrists to increase general mobility and circulation.

The basic facial massage routine

Using the routines of simple massage techniques, effleurage, petrissage, and tapotement will allow natural rhythm, rate, pressure and hand flexibility to develop. Acting as a framework, the 15-minute sequence can be adapted to suit the skin, increasing or decreasing repetitions of movements, or deleting them completely if unsuitable.

The purpose of the individual movements and how they affect skin and underlying muscle must be understood, so that as experience grows, routines can be personally tailored to the client's needs.

Preparation

The client is prepared for general facial treatment. Her skin is cleansed, inspected, a suitable massage medium is chosen and applied with effleurage movements.

Massage routine

1 Deep rollpatting movement (effleurage)
Rollpatting is applied at the established rate of seven inches per second, lifting and moulding the platysma muscle from its origin (fascia of the pectoralis major muscle) to its insertion in the mandible bone. The hands follow each other from the the left clavicle, across the sternum to the right clavicle,and return with a continuous movement. The hands contour to the mandible, follow the path of the left superficial cheek muscles, pass across the chin, cover the right cheek, and the fingers apply detailed strokes to the nostrils and bridge of the nose. The movement concludes on the forehead with lifting of the occipitofrontalis muscles, performed slowly and lightly, without causing the eyes to open. Both hands return to the sternum via the outer border of the face.

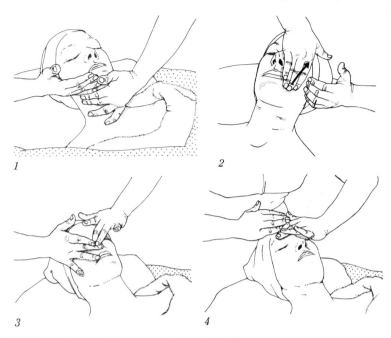

1

2

3

4

2 Throat brace (effleurage and petrissage)

The hands form a relaxed V-shape over the sternum, following the direction of the sternomastoid muscles, with the fingers straight and interlocked at the tips. The movement lifts the platysma and steromastoid muscles and forms a brace along the mandible. Pressure is maintained below and onto the lower jaw, back to the mastoid process, in an upward direction, as the hands divide. Link effleurage returns the hands to the sternum, and the movement is repeated six times.

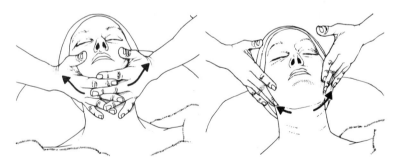

3 Whipping movement (tapotement)

This is a continuous, light percussion movement applied superficially to the platysma and sternomastoid muscles of the neck. A rhythm of one longer and two shorter strokes is used to develop a flicking, whipping effect as technique and speed improves. The hands contour to the throat and the whipping passes from the left to the right side of the mandible and back. The strokes move outwards, flicking off in a fan like movement as they reach the lower jaw. The fingers individually lift and roll the platysma muscle against the mandible, continuing until slight skin reddening is present.

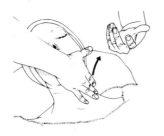
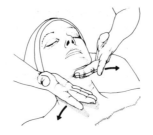
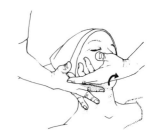

4 Tapping (tapotement)

This is a light, fast tapping movement, applied upwards under the mandible, lifting the muscles against the bone, with the strokes passing backwards and forwards across the jaw. The duration and intensity of this percussion movement will depend on the degree of muscle tone and adipose (fatty) tissue present along the contour. The hands divide at the point of the mandible and return to the mastoid process.

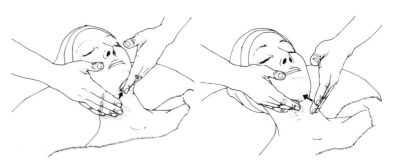

5 Broad sweeping effleurage (linking movement)

A deeper effleurage link movement, to re-establish relaxation and break the activity of the sequence. The movement sweeps down the sternomastoid muscles, over the upper fibres of the pectoralis major, contours around the deltoid and lifts the upper fibres of the trapezius forward to return to the starting position. The hands contour to the area, keeping the maximum palmar surface in contact with the client and using the established rate and an even rhythm to increase relaxation. Pressure must be regulated according to muscle bulk and tension. Repeat six times.

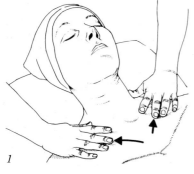

1

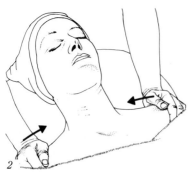

2

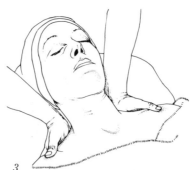

3

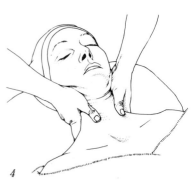

4

6 Knuckling (petrissage)

Knuckling is performed with hands formed into loose fists. The wrists complete half-rotations while the fingers work independently to give circular compression and relaxation movements. The movement is applied slowly and deeply on areas of adequate muscle bulk and superficially on surface tissues. Starting at the mastoid process, the hands form into fists as they move down the sternomastoid muscles, and knuckling commences on the bulk of these muscles. The strokes move to the trapezius muscle, with deeper pressure, and reverse rotations, returning via the sternomastoid to the start position. Repeat three times.

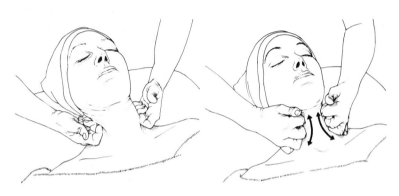

7 Facial lift (effleurage and petrissage)

Linking the neck and facial sections of the routine, the movement starts as an effleurage stroke and changes to a compression movement as it reaches the face. The facial lift begins as in the throat brace, with the hands moulding to the mandible. It changes into the facial lift at the tringularis muscle position, by losing palmar contact, and lifts the superficial cheek muscles with the heel of the hand. Upward pressure is applied at the mandible, and immediately decreased as the hands pass upwards, losing contact with the face. The heels of the hands pick up the occipitofrontalis, whilst retaining contact with the levators of the lips, and the hands move into an effleurage movement of the forehead, decreasing the pressure and speed of the strokes. The hands return to the start position via the outer borders of the face, and the movement is repeated three to six times.

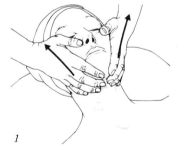

1

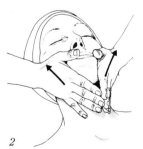

2

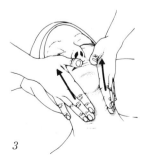

3

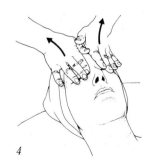

4

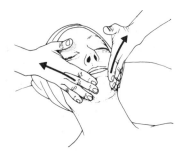

8 Cheek lifting, zygomatic movement (petrissage)

The hands lift from the point of the mandible, drop down and pick up the zygomatic muscles from the corner of the mouth attachments, and lift upward and outward to the zygomatic arch. The face is supported by the hands, and care must be taken to avoid distortion of the eyes or any general discomfort. Repeat six times linking the strokes with effleurage.

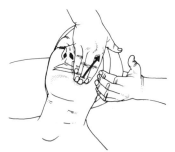

9 Cheek rollpatting (deep effleurage)

The hands follow each other, with the index and second fingers in contact with the superficial cheek muscles. The positions of the zygomatic, risorius and levators are picked out with specific rollpatting strokes in a fan-shaped pattern, from the mouth to the outer borders of the left cheek. The movement crosses the chin rolling deeply into the cleft, and repeats on the right side. The hands divide and finish on the mastoid process. The movement should be performed as one continuous movement.

10 Frictions on the centre panel (petrissage)

The thumbs are used to move the surface tissues over the underlying bony structures, in a circular and brisk manner, to remove surface adhesions and aid desquamation (skin shedding). The thumbs work in opposing rotaries on the chin area, with firm pressure forming between them to create a stimulating effect. The movement is applied around the obicularis oris to the nostrils and bridge of the nose, and completes with effleurage to the temples area. Link effleurage returns the hands to the start position, and the movement is repeated three to six times, depending on skin blockage in the central area and the reaction produced. The last repeat ends on the temples.

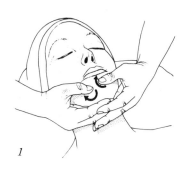

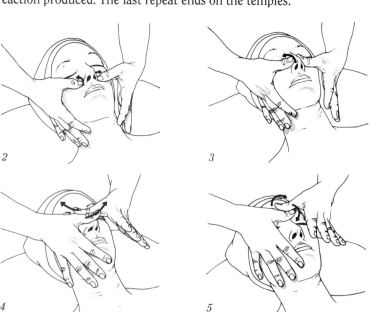

1   *2*   *3*

4   *5*

11 Forehead frictions (petrissage)

Light but brisk friction movements cover the occipitofrontalis area, using the finger tips in semicircular movements against each other. The stimulating action of the movement helps to prevent the formation of permanent expression lines horizontally across the forehead. The duration of the application will depend on the vascular response of the skin and the amount of subcutaneous adipose (fatty) tissue present. Downward pressure must be avoided to prevent client discomfort. The movement concludes at the temples, the hands dividing at the centre brow.

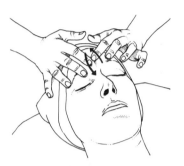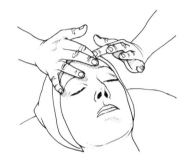

12 Forehead rollpatting (effleurage)

A slow, gentle rollpatting rhythm is established, with the hands moving continuously from the left to the right temple and back, lifting the frontalis and upper fibres of the orbicularis oculi muscles. The strokes are applied at half the established rate and the movement finishes with upward strokes over the corrugator muscle. The hands divide and finish at the temples. It should be executed as one continuous, flowing movement.

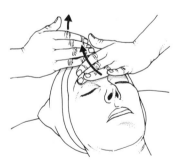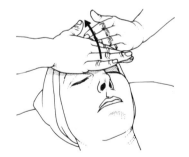

13 Circles around the eyes (effleurage)

With the longest or index fingers bent, the movement sweeps under the eye then inwards towards the nose, following the orbicularis oculi (eye sphincter) muscles. The movement is light on the under-eye tissues, but changes at the nose to lift firmly with the palmar surface of the index finger to raise the inner eye corner, and, changing direction again, lifts the upper fibres of the eye muscle and the frontalis. The lift is maintained as the movement passes along the eyebrows to the temples. The wrists and forearms control the movement, with the lifting and holding elements being applied from the arm positions of the therapist. Repeat six times.

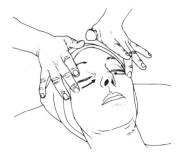
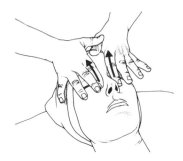
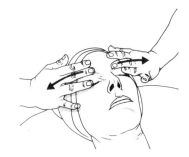

14 Reinforced eye circling (effleurage)

The movement commences as for eye circling described above, but the movement is reinforced at the forehead by all the fingers lifting the orbicularis oculi and occipitofrontalis muscles. The movement is stronger and the eye sphincter more involved.

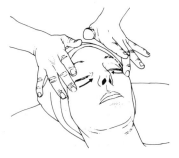
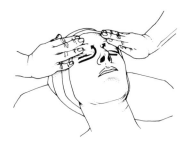

15 Tapping on the cheeks (tapotement)

The hands commence light, sharp tapping above the mandible, with the fingers working in unison. The movement covers the entire cheek area up to the eyes and changes into effleurage to link back to the temples. The taps must be fast and rhythmical. Pressure can be adjusted to the skin's sensitivity and reaction to the application. Repeat three to six times.

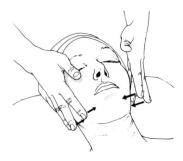

16 Facial lift

As in movement 7. Repeat six times with even pressure and rate of movement.

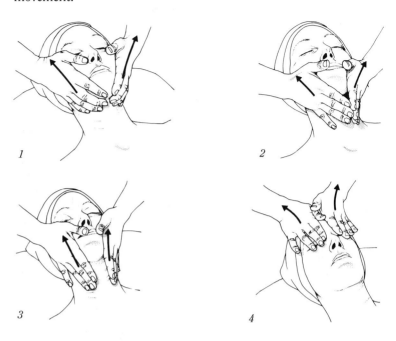

1   *2*

3   *4*

17 General rollpatting

As in movement 1, but now performed more deeply due to the relaxation of muscle fibres caused by the massage. Strokes conclude with gentle upward pressure on the temples.

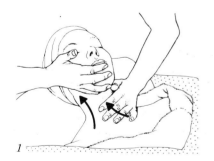

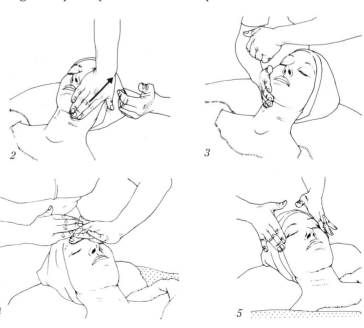

1   *2*   *3*

4   *5*

Completion

The massage cream is removed in the same manner as for the cleansing sequence and the skin inspected to determine further electrical treatment or the mask choice. In a classic facial (based only on manual and cosmetic aspects) the mask stage follows, and the mask is quickly applied over the face area, and the neck if indicated.

The skin may be wiped over with mild tonic solution or refreshed with a vaporiser spray between the massage and mask stages if it appears excessively oily. This is not strictly necessary as the mask removes all surface oil from the skin, but it is pleasant and cooling after the massage. If a mask stage does not follow the massage, toning must be very thorough and performed with the correct toning lotion to settle the skin and free it from massage cream.

Treatment routines are now extremely varied and electrically biased. The classic frame of treatment which used to make up facial therapy is now very diverse. This gives more reason for trying to incorporate some relaxing massage elements into the modern routines.

Pore treatment massage routine

The pore treatment routine is a facial sequence designed to stimulate the skin, improve function, refine the skin and improve its texture. Removal of scar tissue and control of oily secretions can be accomplished with regular treatment.

The pore treatment massage is not designed to be relaxing, but it does provide some light relief for the client within the electrically biased treatment for the oily and blemished skin (see Chapter 9, Electrical Treatment). Its effect is mainly superficial and it is not designed to affect or tone the muscles of facial expression.

Indications for treatment

- Adolescent skin conditions,with over activity of the sebaceous glands causing blocked pores and a coarse skin texture.
- The combination skin with oily centre panel persisting in the 20–30 age range, requiring more refining to reduce scar tissue, and improve uneven texture and colour (from previous acne vulgaris or over exposure).
- Blemished compacted skin with a glassy, oily appearance, coarse texture and uneven colour may be treated once medical permission has been granted. Evidence of skin infection, pustules, irritation, etc. might restrict treatment as manual massage may spread, not restrict the nature of the condition. The massage is combined into a treatment routine of manual and electrical applications.

- Scarred skin conditions.
- Oily skin conditions associated with high humidity conditions, where the skin could tend to unevenness of texture, through increased oil and perspiration flow. Refreshing massage with gel products are very popular.
- Heavily pigmented skins, found in all age groups and nationalities, respond well to this form of stimulating massage. The compacted hyper-keratinisation of the skin benefits both from the refining and regeneration aspects of the massage.
- Within male skin treatment,where deep cleansing and refining effects are needed.

Preparation

The client is prepared for general facial therapy,with hair and clothing well protected against the specialised creams, solutions and masks to be employed. General cleansing may be followed by specialised cleansing in the case of adolescent skin (see Chapter 9, Electrical Treatment) to remove all oily matter.

Suitable creams are applied to the face: herbal, sulphur (medicated), seaweed cream for the oily or blocked areas and bland cream for the neck and other unaffected parts of the face.

Massage routine

1 Pinchment movement (light petrissage)

The thumb and index finger of both hands pick up a small amount of skin and release it sharply. The movement covers the entire neck and face, wherever sufficient skin tissue allows the pinchment to be applied. A rhythmical and planned pattern of strokes increases vascular and lymphatic flow and prepares the face for further massage. The movement ends at the temples and the hands return to the angle of the mandible.

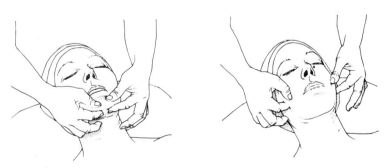

2 General rotaries on the lower face (petrissage)

The subcutaneous tissues and superficial muscles are involved in this compression and relaxation movement. The thumbs of both hands compress and release the tissues of the neck and lower face, causing mechanical constriction and dilation of surface vessels. An immediate reaction is seen and care must be taken to avoid sensitive skin areas, split capillaries, etc. Pressure is applied and released smoothly with skin firmness and sensitivity deciding the amount of pressure used. This circular movement is repeated over suitable areas until the desired result (erythema, skin reddening) has been achieved. The hands finish at the mandible and change to chin frictions.

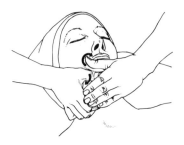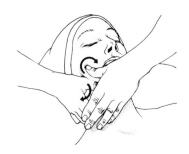

3 Chin frictions (petrissage)

With the fingers loosely placed under the mandible, the thumbs complete small brisk rotaries on the chin, moving the surface layers over the underlying bony structures with the pads of the thumbs. The skin is compressed and released between the thumbs, causing skin desquamation and stimulation. The whole chin is covered with continuous moving rotaries so that the skin does not become irritated, and the movement finishes with a flick up of the thumbs over the oral sphincter. The movement may be repeated according to skin blockage, scar tissue evident and general sensitivity.

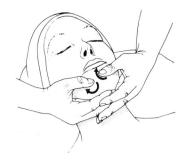

4 Rotaries on the nose (petrissage)

The movement commences on the chin, moves over the orbicularis oris muscle, and works deeply in the nostril area, each thumb working independently with firm rotaries over the surface of the skin. This superficial movement concludes with a sweeping stroke, under the eyes, returning to the chin via the sides of the face.

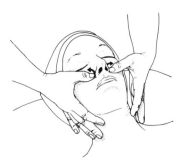

5 Frictions on the nose and centre forehead (petrissage)

With the fingers loosely held under the mandible, the movement commences on the nose tip with firm rotaries, moving up and over the tip to the bridge of the nose. The hands change direction and the thumbs exert pressure towards each other in a criss-crossing motion up to the corrugator muscle between the brows. Firm rotaries recommence on the area, and the movement concludes with effleurage back to the start position.

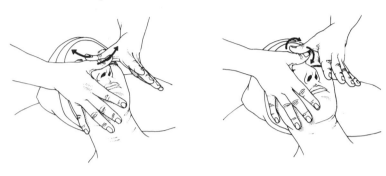

6 Rollpatting and whipping (effleurage and tapotement)

The movement commences at the mandible with deep, rollpatting cheek strokes, then changes to a one-finger whipping movement on the risorius muscle with increased pressure and rate of movement. The fingers roll deeply into the chin fold, passing backwards and forwards several times, and the pattern is repeated on the right cheek. From the risorius position the fingers move to the nose and light, whipping movements are applied over the nostrils, bridge of the nose and the levators of the upper lip. The hands work together, first covering one side of the nose and then the other, concluding with gentle forehead rollpatting, finishing on the temples.

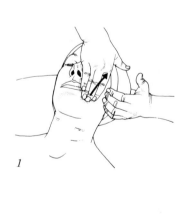

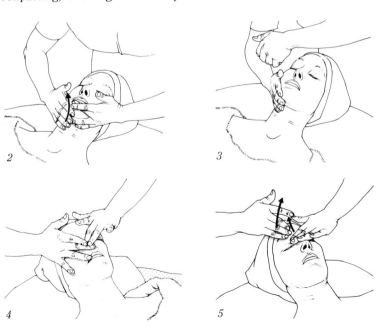

7 Forehead frictions (petrissage, method A)

The hands face each other and friction movements are applied to the entire forehead area. Compression is maintained between the fingers, and care taken to avoid downward pressure on the frontal bone. The left hand moves backwards and forwards, forming a ridge of subcutaneous tissue, which the right hand presses against. When the left hand moves backwards it has to release and contact the skin with smooth and controlled movements, to avoid moving the head and causing discomfort. The right hand moves up and down against the compressed ridge and creates an immediate, stimulating effect. The hands divide at the centre of the forehead and repeat the friction three times.

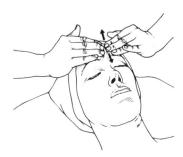

8 Forehead frictions (petrissage, method B)

The movement commences as in 7, but the hands move in opposition to each other, working in close connection to create the friction effect on the occipitofrontalis muscle area.

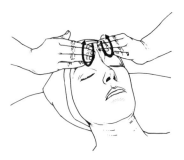

9 Forehead frictions, circular (petrissage)

The movement commences as in 7, but the fingers form opposing circular strokes, to create the stimulating effect.

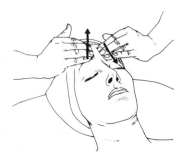

10 Tapping (tapotement)

A tapotement movement covering the entire facial area, commencing at the mandible, progressing up the face to the forehead and concluding at the temples.

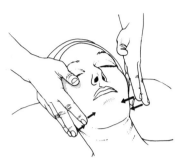

11 Soothing static movement (effleurage)

A soothing contact movement of the cheeks and forehead used to calm sensory nerve endings after the vigorous pore treatment sequence. The hands contour to the mandible, remain static, then progress to the cheeks, and hold the superficial cheek muscles in a relaxed position for a few seconds. The movement is repeated on the forehead area, and the routine concludes with gentle upward pressure on the temples.

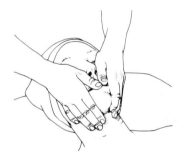
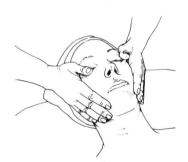
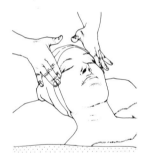

Conclusion

The pore treatment massage movements are extremely stimulating and skin inspection is essential after cream removal to ascertain the degree of sensitivity present, prior to mask choice and application.

The Continental facial massage (face, neck and shoulder girdle)

The Continental facial sequence treats the face, neck and shoulder areas extensively providing a very relaxing and luxurious routine for the mature client (40 years onwards). It works deeply on the muscles of the face, and on the larger muscles of the shoulder girdle. Special attention is given to the eye and neck areas where help is needed to delay ageing signs. By releasing tension in the neck and shoulders the client is able to gain more benefit from the following massage routine, so wherever stress and tension are evident, the Continental facial should be considered.

The massage technique for the Continental facial is more advanced and increased strength, hand control and flexibility are necessary before the Continental massage routine should be attempted by the therapist.

Indications for treatment

- Mature skin conditions with dry, crepey or loose texture and evident expression lines around the mouth and eyes, and between the nose and mouth.
- Premature ageing in the younger client, where neglect, incorrect skin care or exposure to the elements has caused dehydration, lines, etc. to be present.
- Evidence of stress, depression, worry or fatigue, or following a period of ill health, to relax and revive the client.
- As a preventative measure on younger clients to delay the ageing process.

Preparation

Robing prepares the client for more extensive massage, with the towelling or gown passing across the breasts and under the arms, freeing the upper arms, shoulders and upper back for massage. Paper sheeting or towels protect the blankets surrounding the client. This is hygienic practice and inspires confidence.

The face, neck, shoulder, upper arm and back areas must be cleansed thoroughly with an extended form of cleansing which starts the relaxation process and prepares the way for the deeper massage to follow. Removal procedures check that all robing that could become soiled is protected.

Suitable nourishing, hydrating or firming creams are applied with rollpatting strokes.

Massage routine

1 Broad sweeping effleurage
Superficial effleurage followed by deep effleurage over the sterno-mastoid, pectoralis, deltoid and trapezius muscles, up to the occipital cavity at the base of the skull, returning to the angle of the mandible. Repeat six times.

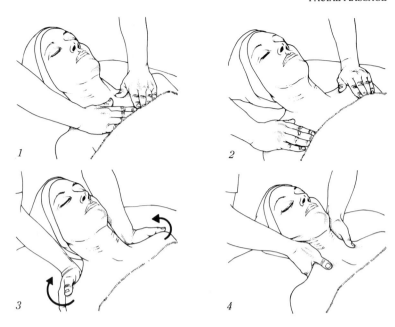

2 Knuckling (petrissage)

The movement starts with link effleurage and progresses to the pectoralis muscle area on either side of the sternum. Deep knuckling is applied from the pectoralis to the deltoid muscles and then changes to thumb-kneading on the deltoid, forming small circles. The movement is completed with effleurage over the trapezius muscle and returns to the occipital cavity. Repeat six times.

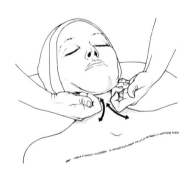
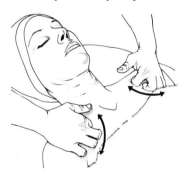
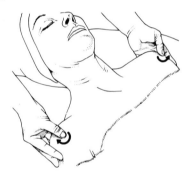

3 Throat brace

As in the basic facial.

4 Trapezius rolling (petrissage, kneading)

With the head placed slightly to the right, both hands alternately lift and knead the trapezius muscles from the shoulder to the occipital cavity on the left side. The right hand commences, completes four to six repetitions and links across to the right side, whilst the left hand follows. The sequence is repeated on the right side, with the head turned to the left and the left hand commencing. On completion both hands return to the mastoid process area, and the head is placed centrally.

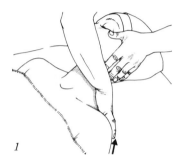

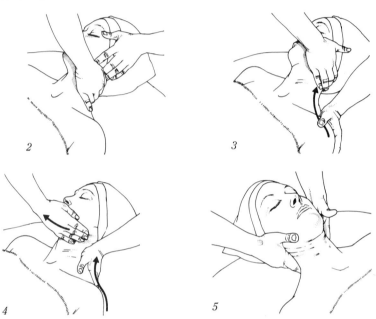

5 Broad sweeping effleurage

As in movement 1, repeated six times.

6 Kneading on the trapezius (petrissage)

The movement begins as in 1, and changes into a firm kneading of the trapezius, with a forward lifting movement, using the palmar surface of the hand, with the thumbs abducted. The entire muscle bulk is covered with varying pressure, right up to its insertion in the occipital cavity. Repeat three times.

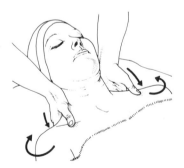

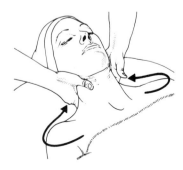

7 Triangular movement (effleurage lifting movement)

Each hand works separately, forming a triangular-shaped movement over the chest and neck. Superficial effleurage moves down the sterno-mastoid muscle changing into broad sweeping over the pectoralis and sternum areas, and contoured lifting effleurage from the origin to the insertion of the platysma, finishing each stroke in a firm upward direction on the point of the mandible. The platysma is held against the lower jaw, and then the movement relaxes, the hand returns to the angle of the mandible, and the alternate hand repeats the movement. Repeat four times slowly on each side.

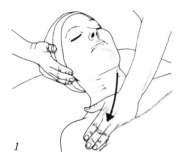

1

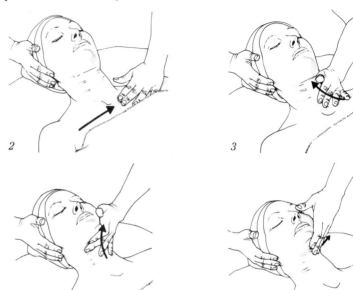

2 *3*

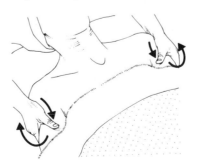

4 *5*

8 Deep kneading on the shoulder girdle muscles (petrissage)

The movement commences with sweeping effleurage, and progresses to deep kneading on the biceps, triceps, deltoid and trapezius muscles. The maximum area of the hand should be in contact, with pressure maintained between the fingers and thumbs wherever possible. The sequence may be applied in three stages with linking effleurage, or as one long active movement as experience of the routine grows.

A relaxed posture, steady breathing rhythm and free arm movements are needed to develop the hand control and sustained strength required to perform this movement without strain.

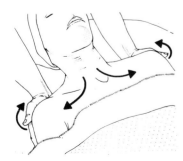

9 Sweeping effleurage and vibration

As in movement 1 with the addition of vibrations in the occipital cavity. Forearm muscles contract and relax, to produce a fine, trembling vibration at the finger tips placed at the base of the skull. The vibration is held for a few seconds, and the movement repeated six times.

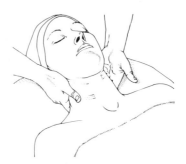

10 Kneading along the mandible (petrissage)

The movement commences with link effleurage, with the mandible passing between the thumb and bent index finger to the point of the chin. The kneading movement progresses back towards the ears, compressing and relaxing along the jaw, with smooth rhythmical strokes, to the angle of the mandible. Repeat six times.

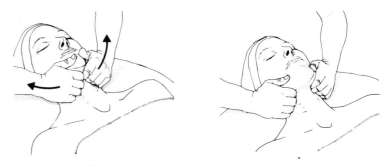

11 Lifting movement under the mandible (petrissage for lymphatic drainage)

A lifting compression movement along the mandible, linked with effleurage using the palmar surface of the fingers with the thumbs abducted. Progresses from the point to the angle of the jaw, with four compression strokes in the direction of the lymphatic nodes.

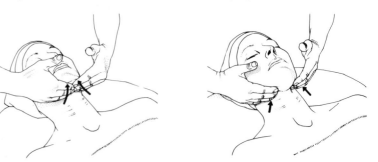

12 Chin crossing movement (effleurage and petrissage)

Both hands commence at the angle of the mandible. The right hand crosses the chin lifting the left superficial cheek muscles, and returns to the right cheek to lift the masseter muscle from the mandible to the zygomatic arch. The left hand replaces the right, continuing and then releasing the compression, to link with effleurage across the chin. The movement is then repeated on the left side. The hands alternate, making and breaking contact smoothly, with the main emphasis being placed at the mandible level, whilst compressing and lifting the masseter muscle with the heel of the hand, moving backwards. To finish the continuous movement, the hands divide at the point of the chin returning to the angle of the jaw. Repeat three times.

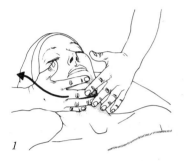

1

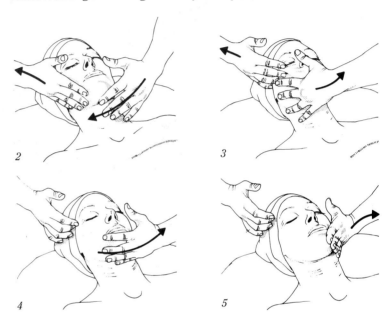

2 *3*

4 *5*

13 Thumb kneading of the chin and lower facial muscles (petrissage)

Compression and relaxation of the lower facial muscles, the triangularis, depressor of the lower lip and platysma, using both thumbs working in opposition in order to form kneading movements along the mandible.

The pressure and rate of application are dictated by the muscle bulk and sensitivity present; a continuous movement.

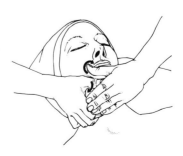

14 Lip bracing movement (effleurage)

The hands form a cradle over the orbicularis oris muscle and lightly follow the shape of the oral sphincter to the corners of the mouth. The index and second fingers of both hands smooth out superficial lines gently and the movement repeats six times.

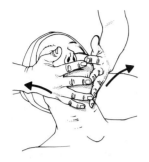
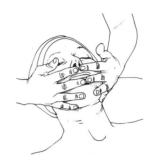
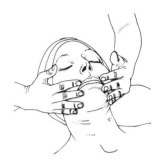

15 Facial lift (effleurage and petrissage)

As in the basic training facial; the facial lift links the lower and upper facial movements, and is repeated six times.

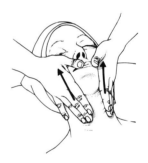

16 Forehead rollpatting (effleurage)

Slow, deep rollpatting, lifting the orbicularis oculi muscles, from the left to the right temples and back, completing 16 rollpatting strokes across the forehead. At the left temple the movement changes to superficial effleurage, first on the crow's feet area, then under the eye and back to the outer eye area, using the index or second finger for four strokes on each section. The movement links across the forehead with slow rollpatting, repeats on the right eye, returns to the central brow, and divides to return to the temples.

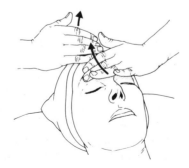
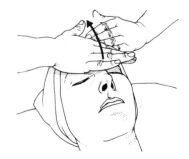

The movement should be performed slowly and carefully to increase the relaxation aspects of the massage sequence. The movement should be adjusted in pressure and speed in relation to underlying bony structures.

17 Eye circling and lifting (effleurage)

From the temples the second fingers perform superficial circles under the eyes, towards the nose, following the orbicularis oculi muscle fibres. The index fingers join the movement at the nose to form a lifting stroke at the corrugator muscle. The hands change direction to lift the upper fibres of the orbicularis oculi and frontalis muscles, along the length of the eyebrow back to the temples. The upwards lifting movement is maintained along the upper fibres of the eye muscles, raising the upper lids, but not opening the eyes. Repeat six times.

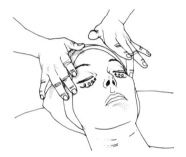 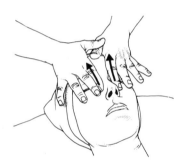 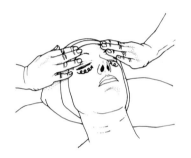

18 Forehead frictions (petrissage)

As in movement 11 of the basic facial.

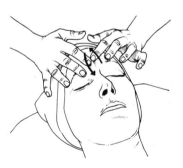 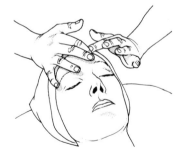

19 Eye lifting movement (effleurage)

Effleurage under the eye progresses to lifting of the corrugator muscle with the index finger. Lifting pressure is maintained by the index finger and then transferred first to the fourth, third, second and index fingers, moving outwards to the temples, keeping the upper lids and eyebrows lifted. Repeat six times.

Finger control and evenness of rhythm are important points of technique in this movement if relaxation is to be maintained.

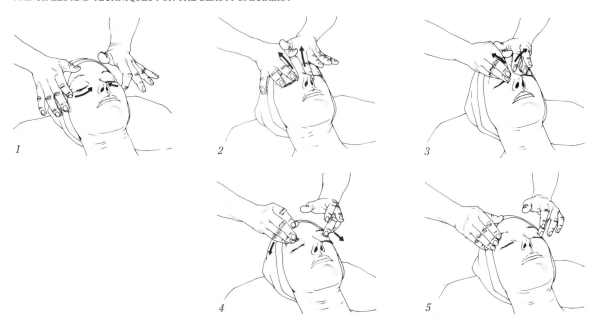

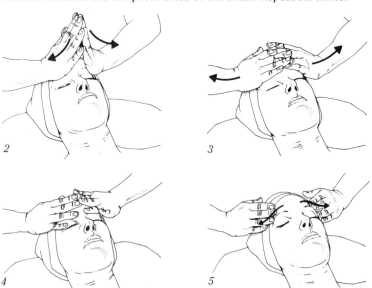

20 Praying movement (effleurage and petrissage)

Effleurage under the eye progresses to a lifting movement of the frontalis muscle, where the hands pivot on the central brow and form a praying position which stretches and lifts the occipitofrontalis muscles towards the temporal areas of the skull. Repeat six times.

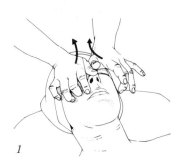

21 Tapotement along the mandible

Effleurage from the temples to the mandible brings the hands into position under the mandible. Tapotement is applied in a tapping sequence, backwards and forwards along the jaw. The intensity of the taps increases, with the fingers forming outward fan-like strokes, concentrating on the central area under the point of the mandible where adipose tissue accumulates. The masseter muscle area may be included in the movement, if muscle tone is poor. The movement is applied until the skin is slightly red and warm.

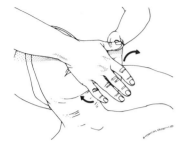 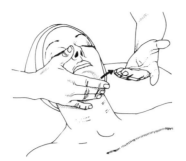 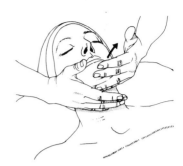

22 Knuckling on the sternomastoid (petrissage)

The movement commences on the clavicle area, with knuckling of the sternomastoid muscle up to the mastoid process. It progresses along the mandible and is linked by effleurage back to the clavicle. Repeat six times.

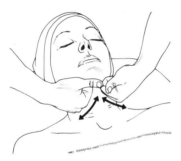 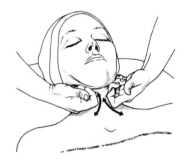

23 Facial lift

As in movement 7 of the basic facial.

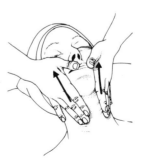

24 Rollpatting (effleurage)

Deep slow rollpatting over the entire shoulder, neck and face areas concludes the massage sequence, finishing with gentle upward pressure on the temples.

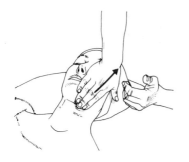 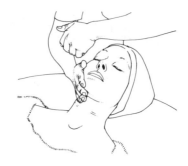 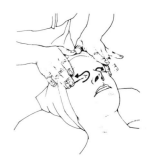

Conclusion

After removal of the massage cream and skin inspection, the appropriate mask may be applied to the face and neck. As an alternative the cream may be left on the neck and a warm throat pad applied for the duration of the facial mask.

These three facial routines cover all general facial conditions and age groups. Specialised skin treatments combining massage and electrical applications for specific conditions will be dealt with in later chapters.

Self check

1 State six contra-indications to a facial massage.
2 Give four reasons why massage is beneficial for a mature skin.
3 What are the most important requirements for a facial massage?
4 Name the four classical massage movements and give the effects of each one.
5 State six indications for facial massage.
6 Describe the properties required for a massage medium.

CHAPTER FIVE

Skin Diseases and Disorders

On magnified inspection very few skins are found to be perfect in texture and general appearance. Recognition of skin disorders and blemishes is important as they may contra-indicate or limit the treatment planned. Medical agreement is necessary in the treatment of certain stages of adolescent skin disturbance and other conditions where sepsis is present. Knowledge of the skin's physiology gives guidance as to the reasons for malfunction and possible causes of imperfections. However, recognition is the most important aspect for the therapist, preventing her from treating cosmetically conditions which require medical attention.

Whilst it is within a beauty specialist's competence to treat minor skin complaints, she must, as a professional person, refer acute and chronic skin disorders to the client's personal physician.

Many minor skin imperfections can be cured or controlled by salon treatment and cosmetic home care sequences, and success in these applications will increase client confidence and the operator's professional status. Acceptance of the limitations in cases which are outside the field of reference will prevent client disappointment. Suspected infectious conditions on the face, hands and feet should be referred for medical attention, and must be noticed prior to treatment. Primary inspection is vital if cross-infection is to be avoided, and due to the exposed position of the therapist, regarding the client's personal circumstances, and the open method of appointment booking, she should take additional care to safeguard herself, her clinic, and her other clients from the risk of infection.

Common sense and a sound knowledge of skin diseases, minor blemishes and pigmentation abnormalities will guide the therapist in her decision regarding the application of salon treatment. Any condition which appears irritated, inflamed or where secondary infection is present should be referred for medical attention. As the client may consult her beauty specialist first, it is the beauty specialist's duty to see not only that she receives the most suitable attention, but also that the treatments should not increase or prolong her complaint.

Dermatological terms

- **Erythema** – redness of the skin, caused by vascular dilation.
- **Pigmentation** – the colour of the skin due to the amount of melanin or carotene produced.
- **Lesion** – any change of the skin, which may be in texture, structure or pigmentation.
- **Oedema** – swelling.
- **Acute** – swift onset, severe.
- **Chronic** – slow onset, lasting a long time.
- **Benign** – mild, non-cancerous.
- **Malignant** – very virulent, cancerous.
- **Macule** – area of discoloration on the skin; it can be seen but not felt. Vary in size and colour.

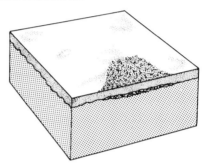

Macule

- **Papule** – a small, firm, raised lump, which does not contain fluid. Vary in size up to 0.5 cm.

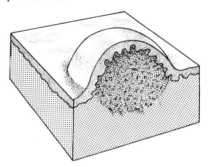

Papule

- **Nodule** – a large papule, usually more deeply seated.

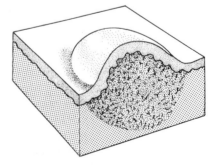

Nodule

- **Vesicle** – a small blister or raised pocket of skin containing fluid.

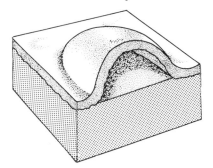

Vesicle

- **Bulla** – a large blister, can be enormous.
- **Pustule** – a raised lesion containing pus, may be any size, can occur in the skin or in hair follicles.
- **Weal** – an elevation of the skin caused by oedema of the dermis. Usually has a whitish centre with red edges. Can vary in size.
- **Scales** – loosened horny cells, often indicates incomplete keratinisation. May be dry or oily.

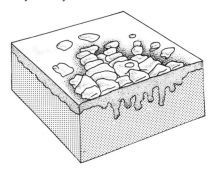

Scale

- **Burrows** – irregular, short lines on the skin, they can be dark or speckled.
- **Plaques** – a raised, thickening of a portion of skin with well defined edges, may be flat or rough on the surface.
- **Cyst** or **wen** – a deeply seated, fluid-filled cavity.
- **Fissure** – a crack or split in the epidermis.

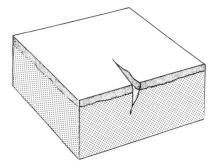

Fissure

- **Ulcer** – an area of total loss of the epidermis; the dermis can also be affected.

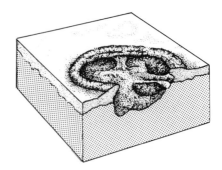

Ulcer

- **Erosion** – a partial loss of the epidermis.

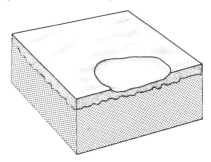

Erosion

- **Atrophy** – a loss or wasting of thickness of the epidermis.
- **Crust** – dried fluid on the skin surface. Red/black crusts: blood. Yellow/green crusts: pus. Horny crusts: serum.

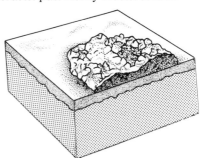

Crust

- **Lichenification** – a thickening of the epidermal layers, giving the skin a mauvish leathery apperance.
- **Comedones** – commonly called blackheads. Usually formed by trapped sebum in a pore. The sebum dries and hardens and forms a plug. The surface becomes black due to oxidation or melanin production. Can occur in a hair follicle.
- **Milia** – commonly called whiteheads. They are formed by trapped sebum under the skin. They have no opening on to the surface and therefore remain white. Very common in dry skin, particularly around the eye area and upper cheeks. Milia formation can often follow damage such as sunburn.
- **Skin tags** – small stalk-shaped tags of loose fibrous tissue often found on the neck and trunk of middle-aged and elderly people.
- **Keloid** – this is a type of scar tissue that becomes thickened and hard. More common in African skin.

Bacterial-based problems

Boils or furuncles

These are usually an infection of a hair follicle caused by staphylococci bacteria. Acute inflammation occurs with pus formation. Multiple boils close together form a *carbuncle*. Boils are a contra-indication to treatment in a salon as they are infectious. Medical treatment must be sought.

Abscess

This is an acute bacterial infection showing redness and localised swelling. An abscess is a contra-indication to salon treatment due to the infectious nature of the lesion and medical advice should be sought.

Impetigo

The lesions of impetigo include vesicles and bullae with erythema. Impetigo usually affects the face, ears and hands and is caused by staphylococcus aureus bacteria. It is common in children and can occur as a secondary infection to other lesions or as a result of poor hygiene. It is highly contagious and therefore is a contra-indication to salon treatments – medical treatment is necessary.

Fungal diseases

Ringworm is a fungal infection producing a superficial infection of the skin, hair and nails. There are many species of the fungus which affect the human body, so it is convenient to describe them according to the site affected. The most common problems associated with ringworm are:

- *Tinea unguium* – ringworm of the nails (see Chapter 11, Treatment of the Arms and Legs).
- *Tinea pedis* – (ringworm of the feet) is a very common infection transmitted via swimming pools, changing rooms, saunas, bathroom floors, etc. The skin between the toes becomes white and soggy; rubbing off infected skin can leave raw areas. It is highly contagious and therefore a contra-indication to beauty treatments, particularly pedicure.
- *Tinea capitis* (ringworm of the scalp): the fungus affects the surface

of the skin and grows in the hair shaft. It appears as round scaly patches with hair broken off in bald patches.

- *Tinea barbae* (ringworm of the beard) shows as scaly patches with partial hair loss; pustules and nodules can occur in some cases. Both Tinea capitis and Tinea barbae can result in alopecia (hair loss)
- *Tinea cruris* (ringworm of the groin) is an acute eruption involving the groin and inside thigh. The lesions are scaly and obviously very irritating.
- *Tinea corporis* (ringworm of the body) causes ring-shaped lesions (hence the name). They can be single or multiple and can be scaly or inflamed. The primary lesion is a small, red macule that spreads outwards and heals in the centre. It is common in children.

The infections show different characteristics according to the area affected. All forms of ringworm infection are contra-indications to salon treatment. Medical treatment is usually needed to clear up the condition.

Viral skin conditions

Herpes simplex (cold sore)

Blisters can form around the mouth or nostril area, usually commencing as an itchy patch of erythema. The vesicles erupt and become crusted – they weep if scratched. Cold sores can accompany a cold and are often recurring. The area should be left alone and salon treatment postponed until the condition has cleared.

Herpes zoster (shingles)

This is an acute, painful disease characterised by linear lesions running along a nerve pathway. It is caused by the chicken pox virus and often affects older people who have had chicken pox as a child. The eruption is usually preceded by pain for up to a week, followed by patchy areas of erythema. Vesicles and papules then erupt which can leave scar tissue. Medical attention is required and salon treatment is contra-indicated.

Warts or verrucae

Warts are localised growths of the epidermis caused by virus. It is the prickle cell layer of the epidermis that is affected. There are a number of different types of verruca, the most common and relevant to beauty therapists are as follows.

Common warts (verruca vulgaris)

These occur most commonly on the hands but can also be found on the face and body. A wart is a firm papule with a rough horny surface. The size varies from less than a millimetre to over a centimetre in diameter. Verruca vulgaris can be coloured and may appear in groups, often around the nail fold.

Flat warts (verruca plana)

This type of lesion is flat topped and occurs mainly on the face and the backs of the hands, appearing as a pearly elevation.

Plantar warts (verruca plantaris)

Plantar warts occur on the soles of the feet and are often referred to simply as 'verrucas'. Plantar warts appear as a yellowish-white area with no lesion above the surface – this is due to the weight of the body. The wart, common in children and adolescents, becomes pressed into the foot and causes a lot of discomfort.

All warts are caused by viral infection and should therefore be regarded as a contra-indication to beauty treatments. There is a certain amount of 'mystery' involved with warts and a lot of legends and myths surround their treatment, but medical advice should be sought for diagnosis and removal.

Parasitic skin problems

Scabies

This is a contagious skin disease caused by a mite that burrows in the horny layer of the skin. In the infected areas, vesicles, papules and burrows are found and intense itching is the main symptom. The mite can effect any areas – common sites are fingers, arms, feet and body folds. The mite is spread by close contact, e.g. children holding hands. There is often an incubation period before itching commences. Medical attention is required and anybody with scabies may not be treated in the salon.

Pediculosis (lice)

This is an infestation of the hair or clothes with wingless insects that suck the blood. Different areas can be affected as follows:

- *Pediculosis capitis* – head lice.
- *Pediculosis corporis* – body lice.
- *Pediculosis pubis* – pubic hair lice.

In any area of the body, infestation causes intense irritation and is spread by contact, e.g. combs, brushes, pillows, public transport. The nits and egg cases can be seen in a good light, particularly on dark hair.

Medical attention is required and anybody with lice may not be treated in the salon.

Allergic skin disorders

Eczema

This is a non-infective inflammatory disorder of the skin. It can have external or internal causes and it is often difficult to determine the origin. It commences with an itching red area with pin-head size vesicles and progresses to scaly dry patches often with more vesicle formation and weeping.

- Internal stimulus via the bloodstream can cause endogenous eczema.
- External contact with a substance can cause exogenous eczema – or contact dermatitis (see later).

Endogenous eczema (eczema)

Endogenous eczema affects the upper dermis and epidermis. Various changes occur in the epidermal cells causing vesicles, redness, flaking and intense itching. Eczema can occur anywhere on the body, and has many different causes and treatments. As for beauty treatments, once a medical diagnosis has been made it is discretionary whether or not to treat someone suffering from eczema. A lot of factors need to be considered, e.g. site, extent of lesions, treatment being considered, etc.

Exogenous eczema dermatitis

This is a reaction to a substance in contact with the skin. It starts as an erythema with itching or irritation. Papules and vesicles may appear, burst and form a crust. Oedema may also be present. Dermatitis is often occupational and is not contagious at all. It can affect both sexes at any age and on any part of the body. There are many substances that can set up the reaction, e.g. plants, drugs, clothing, cosmetics, metals, chemicals, etc. It is often very difficult to determine exactly what has caused the problem – medical patch testing is necessary to pin-point the substance involved.

Beauty treatments are discretionary – really a matter of common sense – discussing with the client the substance(s) involved and the extent of the lesions, etc.

Although both eczema and dermatitis can appear dreadful and be extensive, neither of them are at all contagious.

Urticaria (nettle rash or hives)

An elevation of the skin into weals, usually appearing white in the centre with a red area around the border. They are itchy and may be the size of a pin-head up to a few centimetres across. The weals last between half an hour and twenty four hours – disappearing without trace.

Urticaria has many causes, internal and external: the most common is the introduction of a foreign protein which causes the mast cells to release histamine into the skin. Food allergies, light, heat, drugs, plants (nettles), animals, emotional upsets can all produce urticaria. Urticaria is in no way contagious and only a contra-indication over the weals for a very short period.

Psoriasis

Psoriasis can affect the entire body and facial areas, but is often seen on the limbs, situated on the knees and elbow areas. The lesions of psoriasis commence as dull red papules, the size of pin-heads, and they develop into plaques which are bright red in colour, with sharply defined margins. The patches of psoriasis may have flaky silvery-white scales, overlying the surface, which give the condition a distinct appearance. The cause of the condition is not known, but it does appear to be a recurring complaint, and in some cases may be present in small areas for most of the individual's life. It is possibly hereditary.

Psoriasis may attack the nail fold, or the nail bed, and causes pitting of the nail plate and a build up of cells under the free edge.

All psoriasis conditions of the skin and nails require medical attention, although a small proportion of salon clients may have small areas which appear at times of stress and which may not prohibit treatment as long as the area involved is completely avoided, and the client's doctor is in agreement with the treatment being undertaken.

Soothing salon applications and a feeling of well being achieved through relaxation may be useful in preventing a recurrence of the condition, as it is thought to be connected with the nervous state of the individual.

Pigmentary disorders

Freckles (ephelides)

Small pigmented areas of skin which become more evident on exposure to sunlight and are found in greatest quantity on the face, arms and legs. Fair-skinned, red-haired people often have an abundance of freckles.

Lentigo

Darker areas of pigmentation – more distinct than freckles, with a slightly raised appearance.

Chloasma

Patch pigmentation of the cheeks, forehead and chin, which often occurs in pregnancy and as a side effect of the contraceptive pill. The discolouration usually disappears as the hormone levels return to normal.

Vitiligo

A patchy loss of pigmentation in the skin and hair, which can occur on any area, the face and backs of hands being common sites. It usually commences as small patches which may converge to form fairly large areas.

In winter it may be invisible and it is more obvious in dark-skinned people. The melanocytes are absent and the areas affected must be protected from ultraviolet exposure.

Most beauty treatments can be carried out and cosmetic camouflage can be particularly useful to disguise this condition which often causes anxiety and embarrassment.

Spider naevus (telangiectatic angioma)

The spider naevus consists of a central dilated vessel, with smaller capillaries radiating from it like the legs of a spider. It is often called a broken vein, and may be isolated or in an area of vascular skin such as cheeks. The spider naevus usually develops in adult life, and is commonly found on the face, particularly on the upper cheek and eye areas. It responds well to diathermy (heat) coagulation treatment, performed by a skilled electrologist.

Port wine stain (capillary haemangioma)

The port wine stain consists of a large area of dilated capillaries, causing a pink or dark red skin colour which makes it contrast vividly with surrounding skin. The stain is commonly found on the face and, as the skin texture is normal, application of cosmetic masking camouflage is very successful in alleviating embarrassment and distress. The port wine stain does not usually regress and its treatment is limited.

Strawberry mark (cavernous haemangioma)

A brightly pigmented skin area, seen at birth or developing soon afterwards, which usually disappears before adult life.

Pigmented naevi

Pigmented naevi may occur on any part of the body and are often found on the neck and face, being sometimes associated with strong hair growth (pigmented hairy naevi). They normally vary in size from a pin-head to several centimetres, but in rare cases may be extremely large. The pigmentation present may be light brown to very dark or black. Pigmented naevi, with the exception of the coal black variety, are classed as benign tumours, and their removal is usually for cosmetic reasons. Small pigmented naevi can be removed by an electrologist using diathermy coagulation, if medical agreement is given, or they can be surgically excised with very successful results.

Papilloma (moles)

Moles are a common occurrence on the face and body and are present in several different forms, varying in size, colour and vascular appearance. All raised moles require medical agreement prior to electrology treatment, or they can be removed surgically if they cause distress.

Skin gland disorders

Seborrhoea

Seborrhoea is caused by over-activity of the sebaceous glands, secretion, an excess of sebum and abnormal oiliness of the skin's surface. The situation and density of the sebaceous glands in the scalp, face, centre of chest and back cause the seborrhoea to be most evident in these areas. During puberty the activity of the glands is increased due to hormonal changes,and the sebaceous gland ducts and hair follicles become enlarged, the skin becomes coarser and open pores are evident. The excessive oily secretion blocks the outward flow of sebum to the surface, and it becomes lodged in the follicle and sebaceous duct. The retained sebum increases in amount, and the external area hardens to form a comedone (blackhead). Seborrhoea is the basis for several skin diseases, particularly acne vulgaris.

Acne vulgaris

In acne vulgaris the skin appears greasy, has a dull sallow colour, and blackheads, papules, pustules and scars are often present at the same time. Acne vulgaris is most commonly found in adolescents and it may involve the entire face, chest and shoulder girdle, or be confined in any one of these areas. Seborrhoea is present and forms comedones in varying intensities depending on the influence of the endocrine glands on the sebaceous secretion.

Acne is the most common skin condition. Research continues into the cause and treatment and with medical approval the beauty therapist can successfully assist acne sufferers.

Acne rosacea

Acne rosacea, like acne vulgaris, is an eruption which affects the face and is associated with seborrhoea (excessive oiliness). The cutaneous vessels of the nose and cheeks are the most affected, giving a red flushed appearance, particularly after the intake of food or a change in temperature. The disease may be of long standing, and is disfiguring as the skin becomes lumpy and thickened with papules and pustules. Rosacea is sometimes confused with acne vulgaris, due to its location, but it seldom appears before the age of 30, whilst acne vulgaris has usually regressed by this age.

Hyperhidrosis

The secretion of an excessive amount of sweat, which may have an offensive odour. It particularly affects the feet, axillae and the groin.

Anidrosis

An absence of sweat, due to the breakdown of the sweat glands and congenital factors.

Bromidrosis

A condition in which the sweat has a particularly offensive odour.

Miliaria (prickly heat)

This is caused by sweat-duct blockage induced by temperature changes (tropical heat/humidity). Sweat cannot evaporate and so it penetrates the epidermis causing itching and localised oedema.

Skin cancer

Skin cancer can occur in various forms; the most common are: basal cell carcinoma (rodent ulcer), squamous cell carcinoma and malignant melanoma.

Basal cell carcinoma

A slow growing, locally malignant growth usually found on the face or exposed areas. It is a growth of basal cells that, although slow growing, can be very invasive locally. The lesion has an ulcerated centre with a raised, pearly border and it does not heal. It is easily cured when treated early enough. It is possibly caused by exposure to ultraviolet.

Squamous cell carcinoma

These growths also appear on exposed areas and are thought to be caused by chemicals, sunlight or physical irritants. The lesions consist of columns of cells that pass inwards through the epidermis into surrounding tissue. The carcinoma commences as a small nodule which grows rapidly, forming a raised area. Metastasis can occur.

Malignant melanoma

This type of cancer usually affects middle-aged and elderly people. About 50% of cases may arise from existing moles. The mole may change size or shape or colour, it may become itchy or even painful. Prolonged exposure to ultraviolet light is thought to be the cause.

Any lesion on the skin that changes shape, colour or becomes painful, or does not heal, should be referred for immediate medical attention. It is vital to stress that as beauty therapists we do not diagnose skin conditions, we simply observe very thoroughly in order to determine if a treatment can be carried out or not. Our limited knowledge of dermatology is for recognition purposes only.

Self check

1 Why do beauty therapists need to know about skin diseases and disorders?
2 What is a lesion? Name the common skin lesions.
3 What is the difference between acute and chronic?
4 Name and describe one common skin problem caused by:
   (a) A bacteria.
   (b) A fungus.
   (c) A virus.
   (d) A parasite

5 What is the common name given to each of the following?
   (a) *Tinea pedis*.
   (b) *Verruca vulgaris*.
   (c) *Herpes simplex*.
6 What is eczema?
7 Describe seborrhoea.
8 Name three common pigmentary disorders.
9 Differentiate between vitiligo and chloasma.
10 Name and describe the appearance of three common skin cancers.

CHAPTER SIX

Mask Therapy

Mask applications

Masks have a traditional place in facial therapy and have previously been best known for deep cleansing and refining of the skin. The latest mask therapy offers masks with a wider range of active ingredients and actions. Improved convenience of use has changed the way that masks are used in treatment, greatly increasing their scope and popularity with clients and making them a standard item in home care plans.

Masks come in many forms, some simple like the classic clay mask, others complex, forming complete treatments such as the four-stage mask treatment or thermal mask routines.

Masks can also act as a carrier for an active ingredient such as a plant extract, essential oil, seaweed, etc. Non-setting gels, geloids and emulsions containing liposome carriers are typical of this new type of biological mask which has gained widespread popularity in the industry.

The terms *face mask* and *face pack* are interchangeable. Masks can be applied as a paste or cream that sets directly on to the skin, or in the case of a gel or fruit mask can be applied over gauze for easy removal.

An extremely wide range of masks is available to suit all skin conditions; these include:

- Setting masks (clay type).
- Non-setting masks (natural and plant ingredients).
- Phytotherapy masks (based on plant and herb extracts and essential oils).
- Specialised masks (e.g. peel off masks, thermal masks, warm oil, paraffin wax).

Effects of masks

Masks can:

- Reduce skin irritation.
- Sooth and calm.
- Moisturise.
- Soften the skin.
- Remove excess oil from the skin.
- Deep cleanse and refine the pores.
- Lighten skin colour.

- Refresh the skin.
- Stimulate the circulation.

The application of the mask in the facial sequence can vary, according to its effects and whether it is used in association with electrotherapy. In manual routines the mask will normally be applied after massage, whilst in combined routines its placing will alter according to its effect. Cleansing actions may be placed earlier in the sequence and soothing, moisturising actions closer to the conclusion. Some facial routines may include more than one mask, pack or compress.

Contra-indications to treatment

Mask applications in modern therapy practice are seldom left on the skin for more than 10 minutes unless of a specialised nature.

Masks should not be applied:

- If skin infection is present.
- If the skin is sunburnt.
- Where there are cuts, bites or small wounds.
- On to hypersensitive skin (special anti-inflammatory mask application may be possible, but the skin must be recognised).

Skin preparation

Skin inspection after massage will help to determine the ideal mask choice.

For maximum effect with masks designed to *cleanse*, *refine*, *desquamate* and *stimulate*, the skin must be thoroughly clean before the mask application and free of all traces of massage medium, makeup, etc.

For greatest benefit from masks designed to *nourish*, *moisturise*, *soften* and *calm*, the massage medium remaining on the skin may or may not be removed prior to the mask application depending on the skin's needs. In some instances the active creams or oils used within massage add to the results achieved within the mask stage.

The mask is applied thinly over the skin, the client made warm and comfortable, and eye pads applied if desired. The therapist should stay with the client during the short duration of the mask in case of anxiety or skin reaction which would require the mask be removed at once.

Setting masks

Setting masks include basic clay masks which offer excellent cleansing, toning and stimulation effects. The masks are prepared by mixing clay powders with liquids such as purified water, rose water or witch hazel in varying proportions according to the type of skin being treated. The masks are applied thinly with a brush and are normally left on the skin until they have dried. Once dried, they are removed quickly with tepid water and cotton wool tissues. The low cost and effectiveness of clay masks makes them a popular clinic and college choice.

Basic clay ingredients

- **Calamine** is a pale pink powder containing zinc carbonate, which has a soothing effect on inflamed skin, reducing vascularity. A mild, gentle action is produced.
- **Magnesium carbonate** is a mildly astringent white powder suitable for refining skin with open pores. It also has a stimulating action which can be used to tighten and firm the skin.
- **Kaolin** is a natural creamy white powder which is stronger in effect than magnesium carbonate. It cleanses the skin and helps to remove impurities. It stimulates the circulation, hastens the removal of waste products and improves skin function.
- **Fuller's earth** is a grey–green powder, with a strong action on the circulation. It adheres to dead cells on the skin's surface, giving it excellent desquamating and cleansing actions and making it the ideal mask for seborrhoea.
- **Sulphur** is a fine yellow powder which is rarely used alone but may be added to fuller's earth for use on extremely oily skin.

Active ingredients

- **Rose water** gives a mild toning effect.
- **Orange flower** water gives a stimulating and tonic effect.
- **Witch hazel** is drying and stimulating, with an astringent action.
- **Almond oil** may be added to the basic masks for dry skin to increase hydration of the skin.
- **Glycerol/glycerine**, a humectant which can be added to masks for dry and dehydrated skin to prevent them from drying completely.

Table 6.1 shows some suggested recipes for a variety of skin conditions.

Application and removal of clay masks

The mask should be prepared just prior to use. It should be smoothly mixed, free from lumps and of a consistency that will not run when applied to the face and neck. It should be thinly applied so that the mask stage of the facial does not exceed 10 minutes.

Table 6.1 Mask recipes

Skin type	Powdered ingredients	Liquid ingredients
Normal skin	1 part kaolin 1 part calamine or magnesium carbonate	Purified water or rose-water
Dry skin	1 part calamine 1 part kaolin	Rose-water, a few drops of almond oil
Oily skin	1 part magnesium carbonate 1 part kaolin Depending on severity, a small amount of fuller's earth could be added	Orange flower water, a few drops of witch hazel
Sensititive skin	Calamine	Purified water or rose-water, a few drops of glycerol to prevent setting
Acnefied skin	2 parts fuller's earth 1 part kaolin – small amount of sulphur (optional)	Witch hazel
Oily skin with open pores	1 part magnesium carbonate 1 part fuller's earth	Witch hazel slightly diluted with purified water
Dry/dehydrated skin with open pores	1 part magnesium carbonate 1 part calamine	Rose-water, a few drops of almond oil and glycerol

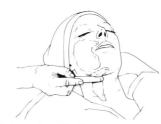

Basic mask application

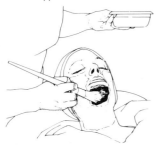

Combined formula mask

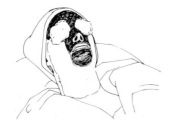

The completed mask setting

When applying the mask:

1 Check that the hairline is covered and that towels and blankets are protected by tissues.
2 Warn the client that the mask is about to be applied and may feel cold initially.
3 Using a brush or disposable spatula, quickly apply a thin film of mask paste evenly over the skin.
4 If two mask mixtures are to be applied on a combined skin type, apply the one with the strongest action first to allow maximum time on the skin.
5 Avoid getting the mask in the eyes, nostrils or mouth and leave the hairline and eyebrows free to keep the client clean and tidy.
6 The client will experience skin reaction, e.g. tightening, tingling, etc, as the mask dries, and the purpose of this should be explained to the client.
7 Apply eye pads soaked in cooling eye lotion, or encourage the client to shut her eyes and relax.
8 When the mask has dried sufficiently it should be removed gently with either warm towels, damp sponges or cotton wool tissues. The mask may be pre-moistened to hasten its removal and to prevent the cleaning up procedure becoming annoying.
9 If the mask concludes the facial sequence, the skin is toned and day protection applied.

Phytotherapy masks

Masks with active phyto or plant derived ingredients, are very advanced in action and convenient and economic in use. Their effect on the skin comes from the particular action of the plant extracts or essential oils they carry. They are mainly of a non-setting type, that is they dry and form a soft film over the skin but do not set hard like clay masks. Some masks (like the liposome types) almost disappear into the skin, appearing to be absorbed.

Phytotherapy or biological masks are very professional in their presentation and are often mixed specially for the client. Their formulas are as individual as the natural product masks that were popular previously (the honey, egg, and fruit-based masks which are still useful for home use). Phytotherapy masks, however, offer a great deal more in the busy clinic than natural product masks, allowing the mask therapy to be tailored exactly to the client's needs and providing an easy and effective mask product for home use.

Mask medium

For ease of application the ingredients of a phytotherapy mask are combined into a jelly, geloid or creamy emulsion base medium (or a liposome carrier may be used). The biological ingredients act through the vascular network of the dermal layers of the skin, where the trace elements of the ingredients create increased activity in the basal layer of the skin. Refinement of skin texture is a result of increased skin function (improvement in respiration and elimination).

Liposome mask carrier

The latest liposomes act as hollowed-out carriers which can penetrate the protective layer of the skin (epidermis) and travel to the deeper (dermal) layers. Encapsulated within the tiny liposome spheres are active ingredients (plant extracts, essential oils) to stimulate, regenerate or correct the oil–hydric balance of the skin. Active ingredients carried by the liposomes into the dermal layers of the skin can also calm, sooth and settle the sensitive and couperose affected skin.

Liposome masks with active gels are mixed by the therapist just prior to use, providing an ideal means of introducing these popular biological elements into the skin. The actions of the different plant extracts and essential oils must be studied so that the correct effect is created. Ready mixed masks are also available, and once again the ingredients need careful consideration prior to use. Reactions noted after application will help to develop knowledge of the mask's special uses in the clinic.

Some of the active biological gels may also be used within ionisation routines (galvanic current) as an economic alternative to ampoules. This extends their application even further, making clinic treatment varied and effective for the client.

Application

A very small quantity of mask is prepared (either mixed for the client or ready made) and applied thinly over the face, and throat if necessary. The mask is allowed to dry for !0 minutes or until sufficient activity is felt by the client. It is removed thoroughly and gently with tepid water, making sure that with transparent masks, which appear to disappear into the skin, all the product is actually removed.

Table 6.2 shows some of the common phyto ingredients used. There are literally hundreds of ready made masks, so choice of product must be made according to its active ingredients, and their known effects on the skin.

Table 6.2 Phytotherapy and biological masks

Skin type	Active phyto ingredients	Carrier base	Natural product masks for home use
Normal skin	Sweet basil, lavender, sandalwood, camomile, rosemary, rose	Emulsion or gel	Oatmeal packs (mixed with water, rose-water, lemon juice). Fruit-based packs mixed with cream, applied on gauze
Combination/oily skin	Fenugreek, menthol, thyme, rosemary	Emulsion, gel or clay base	Egg white and lemon juice, beaten and applied all over oily areas. Cucumber pack – crushed cucumber mixed with cream and a few drops of tincture of benzoin applied on gauze
Seborrhoea/acneic skin	Seaweed extract, bio-sulphur, Irish moss, squalene	Emulsion, gel or clay base	Yeast packs (brewers' yeast)
Dry/dehydrated skin	Royal jelly, patchouli, camomile, geranium, sandalwood	Emulsion, gel or liposome carrier	Dry skin egg mask – egg yolk, honey, almond oil mixed and applied for 15–20 minutes
Mature skin	Royal jelly, ginseng, sandalwood, lavender	Emulsion, gel or liposome carrier	Honey mask – honey plus a few drops of orange or lemon juice warmed and applied for 15–20 minutes
Sensitive skin	Camomile (azulene), lavender, calendula (marigold), St John's wort	Emulsion, gel or liposome carrier	Avocado pack – mashed fruit applied on gauze or directly to the skin
Couperose skin	Horse chestnut	Emulsion, gel or liposome carrier	Wheat germ mask – natural wheat germ and water mixed to a stiff paste applied on gauze for 15–20 minutes

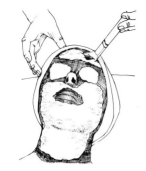

Fruit mask on gauze

Natural product masks

Though largely replaced by the more advanced phyto masks, the natural masks are useful in certain cases and add variety in the clinic. They are now used more within home plans as they give good results at very low cost.

Natural ingredients are used as fresh as possible and the mask applied immediately. Ingredients for natural masks include eggs, honey, fruit juices, cream and pulp from fruits and vegetables such as raspberries, strawberries, paw paw, avocado, carrots, cucumbers, etc.

Application

The ingredients are either applied directly on to the skin, or on to gauze for ease of application and removal and to contain the ingredients. The mask/pack can be left on the skin for 15–20 minutes (at home), removed and the skin wiped gently with tepid water.

Natural ingredients

- Most soft fruits have an acid reaction on the skin (they can be mixed with yoghurt, cream or egg white to lessen the acidic reaction).
- Egg white has a toning and tightening effect on the skin (the addition of lemon juice increases skin refining action).
- Egg yolk is nourishing to the skin (the addition of honey and almond oil increases the effect).
- Honey with the addition of citrus fruit juice softens and nourishes the skin, delaying the formation of lines.
- Cucumber gently stimulates the skin, and with the addition of cream and a few drops of tincture of benzoin may be applied even on sensitive skin.
- Avocado fruit is full of natural oil, so suitable for dry and mature skin.

Specialised masks: peel-off masks

The ease of application and removal and their novelty makes peel-off masks popular. The masks are available in a ready mixed gel form and in pellets which need warming prior to application. The mask is applied with a brush or spatula in an even layer over the face and neck. It forms a flexible film after 10 minutes, and, after loosening the edges of the mask, it is peeled off in one piece for a fast removal.

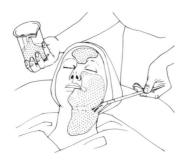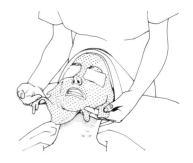

Most of the mask's effect is in relation to the creams, ampoules or gels applied prior to the masks application. The mask hastens the absorption of these products, induces sweating in the skin and tightens the skin as it shrinks and dries. Cleansing, stimulating and refining effects make the peel-off masks suitable for dry, dehydrated and mature skins.

Specialised masks: thermal/mineral masks

Any thermal /mineral mask that remains in the mixing bowl or jug after application should be allowed to harden and be disposed as a solid piece into a waste bin. Do not rinse the creamy paste down a sink: it will block the pipe as it hardens.

Thermal masks come in many different forms, so manufacturers' instructions must be followed. A chemical reaction between the ingredients produces the thermal or heat reaction for all these masks, so electrical equipment is not required.

The heat produced increases the absorption of the creams, etc. applied prior to the mask's application. The routine is extremely relaxing and the skin is stimulated. The effect on the skin varies according to the specific products chosen for use, and the routine is often developed into a four-part sequence of one hour's duration, as the mask can take 45 minutes for the full effect to take place. This makes the mineral/thermal mask a complete treatment in itself.

Application

1 Cleanse the face with a suitable cleansing milk for the skin type (sensitive, dry, oily, dehydrated, etc.) and inspect it carefully to determine an accurate skin assessment.
2 Apply an ampoule suited to the skin type, manually or with galvanic ionisation.
3 Apply a cream suited to skin type and apply massage to the face and neck. Leave the cream on the skin.
4 Apply an even layer of specific cream to work in association with the thermal/mineral mask. The eyes, nostrils (and mouth in some cases) should be left free.
5 The thermal/mineral mask is mixed exactly to manufacturers' instructions and quickly applied in a thick layer to the face and

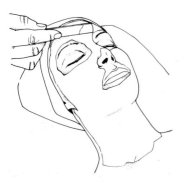

Underlying cream application

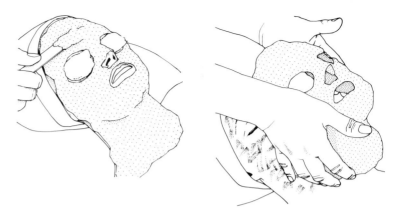

neck, avoiding the eyes and nostrils (and lips if the client is inclined to be claustrophobic).

6 Check that the mask is evenly and thickly applied to ensure even heat distribution and penetration action.

7 Cover the eyes with cotton wool pads and check that the client is comfortable and not anxious. Stay in contact with the client over the 25–30 minute period.

8 The heat effect starts to develop gradually and reaches a comfortable level to aid penetration and stimulate the skin.

9 The mask begins to feel heavy as it hardens and cools into a solid piece.

10 After removal of the eye pads the mask is lifted off in one piece and the skin cleared of remaining cream. If the mask has gone on well, it comes off well and does not break over the narrow areas, such as the sides of the eyes, above the lip, etc.

11 The skin is toned and will be found to look relaxed, hydrated and with fine lines eased from the heat produced within the mask.

Specialised masks: paraffin wax masks

Paraffin wax treatment:

- Increases local skin temperature.
- Induces perspiration.
- Increases the skin's capacity to absorb oils and creams.
- Improves skin respiration.
- Cleanses the skin, freeing surface adhesions and correcting pH balance.
- Softens the skin, improving elasticity and smoothness of texture.
- Improves skin colour and tone.
- Delays ageing signs and eases fine lines.
- Helps release and replace surface horny cells from basal layers to produce a younger finer skin texture.

Indications for paraffin wax treatment

- Dry, dehydrated skin requiring stimulation and correction of oil and moisture balance.
- Mature skins needing regeneration.
- Crepey, finely lined skin where gentle stimulation is needed.
- Uneven textured skin – deep cleanse, refine and correct the pH balance.
- Seborrhoea conditions – to remove surface adhesions, oily skin blockage and promote desquamation.
- Preventative treatment against ageing signs.

Contra-indications

- Highly nervous, tense clients.
- Extremely vascular complexions.
- Sepsis, skin infection and irritation.
- High temperature for any reason.

Preparation

Equipment

A small quantity of clean, sterilised paraffin wax is prepared in a small wax heater or larger wax bath. Thermostatic controls maintain the wax at a constant temperature 49 °C (120°F) ready for use. Brushes are used for the application, allowing swift and controlled work. The usual safety precautions for using electrical equipment are taken (see Chapter 9, Electrical Treatment).

Client preparation

A semi-reclining chair position is chosen to allow a safe and easy wax application and to avoid any risk of warm wax falling on the client. Gowns, towels, etc. are protected from the wax with disposable paper towels in the case of accident.

Facial cleansing is gently applied (to avoid over stimulation) and the skin is inspected to determine sensitivity and any imperfections that would alter the length or intensity of treatment.

Application

1 Massage may be applied with suitable creams or oils.
2 Additional cream may be applied to ease removal and enhance the effectiveness of the treatment.
3 Eye pads must be applied for safety reasons and to aid relaxation.
4 Wax is quickly applied at a temperature as warm as can be comfortably tolerated by the client to form a fine layer over the face and neck.

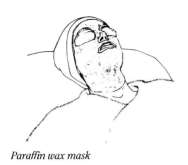

Paraffin wax mask

5 Next, a firm layer of wax is built up over the throat, cheeks, chin, nose and forehead forming a complete mask, but avoiding the lips, nostrils, eyebrows and hairline.

6 Heat builds up initially within the mask, then as it cools and sets the features become immobilised.

7 The client should be encouraged to relax until all the therapeutic effects of the heat are gone, but the mask is still pliable and just warm to the touch. The therapist stays in contact with the client during this time.

8 Application time varies from 10–20 minutes, depending on skin temperature and reaction and tolerance to heat.

9 Waxing fits within the one-hour facial sequence as a setting mask is not used and makeup is not applied (since the skin is unsettled for a time after the routine).

Removal

The mask is released around its edges, the eye pads are removed and the mask is eased off gently in one piece, with the hands lifting it first from the throat. Skin toning and moisture protection complete the routine.

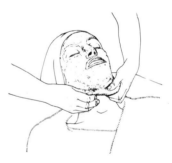

Specialised masks: warm oil masks (using infra-red or radiant heat irradiation)

The warm oil mask treatment combines the therapeutic effects of infra-red and radiant heat rays with a fine oil application. The dry, dehydrated and mature skin gains immediate benefit from treatment through improved elasticity, smoothness and softness of texture. Improved colour and skin tone are clearly evident to the client over a course of treatment.

Effects of local application of infra-red rays

- A rise in temperature.
- Erythema (an increase in colour due to vasodilation).

- A calming effect on sensory nerve endings.
- Increased activity of sweat glands.
- Sedative effect, enhanced by the general relaxation of the client, due to both the heat application and skilful client preparation and handling.

Infra-red and radiant heat

Infra-red rays are electromagnetic waves with wavelengths between 7000 Å and 4 000 000 Å (700 nm and 400 000 nm approximately). When infra-red rays are absorbed by the tissues of the body, heat is produced at the point where they are absorbed. This heat is conducted to the deeper tissues by the blood circulation.

Heat generators available

In non-luminous generators, infra-red is produced by a heating element embedded in a fire clay material and few visible rays are produced. The infra-red rays produced have wavelengths between 7700 Å and 150 000 Å. Although less penetrating than infra-red from luminous generators, the infra-red produced is less irritating and therefore non-luminous generators are more frequently used within beauty therapy applications.

Luminous generators produce radiant (visible) heat. The element is apparent and visible rays are produced in addition to infra-red rays. The coiled filament surrounds a fire clay emitter which produces infra-red and visible rays with wavelengths between 6000 Å and 40 000 Å when it reaches maximum output. Many of the radiant heat rays have wavelengths in the region of 10 000 Å. These rays are more penetrating, but have greater irritant properties than infra-red on the surface tissues.

Shorter wavelength infra-red rays penetrate to the deeper parts of the dermis or the subcutaneous tissues, while the longer wavelength rays are absorbed in the superficial epidermis.

Indications for oil mask treatment

- Crepey, finely lined, mature skin.
- Premature ageing of the skin.
- Dehydration of skin tissue.
- Preventative treatment on the younger 'dry' skin.

Contra-indications to oil mask treatment

- Extremely vascular complexions.
- Hypersensitive skins.
- Very nervous, highly strung clients.
- Areas of dilated capillaries must be excluded from the exposure by covering them with damp cotton wool pads to prevent heat penetration.

Preparation

Equipment

The ray lamp and emitter are prepared and checked to ensure that they are in good working order, i.e. undented reflector, firmly clamped arms, etc. The infra-red lamp takes 10–15 minutes to reach maximum *emission* (output). So the lamp should be positioned safely and left to warm up ready to bring into position. The usual safety precautions for using electrical equipment are taken (see Chapter 9, Electrical Treatment).

Warm oil, gauze, scissors, bowls, etc. must also be prepared

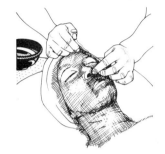

Preparation of gauze mask

Client Preparation

The client's skin is cleansed and inspected for areas of sensitivity and imperfections which could alter treatment, and any necessary action is taken.

A piece of gauze should be cut to the shape of the face and neck with holes for nostrils and mouth if required.

Application

1 The gauze is soaked in warm oil (almond) and placed over the face using eye pads for protection.
2 Check that prominent areas such as the nose tip are not left exposed.
3 The timing and distance of the lamp is decided (with regard to the inverse square law, see Chapter 10, page 180) and brought into position (this distance is usually between 50 cm and 1 m (18 in–3 feet) according to the intensity of the lamp, the sensitivity of the skin, and its reaction to the heat, if known).
4 The lamp position should be checked to ensure to that it cannot fall on the client.
5 The therapist should stay in close attendance, checking the skin reaction at intervals until the required result is achieved (8–20 minutes).
6 The lamp is removed.
7 The gauze mask is removed and excess oil massaged into the skin. Remaining oil can then be removed with soft, slightly damp tissues.
8 As the respiration of the skin is increased, oil will continue to be present in the superficial tissues for some time and the skin will appear unsettled and stimulated for a considerable period. The effects and benefits will be seen more clearly a day after treatment.
9 A mild, refreshing lotion may be sprayed over the skin if desired and moisturiser applied as a final protective step.

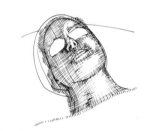

Oil mask treatment

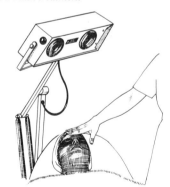

Lamp in position

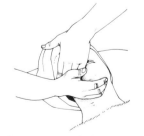

Gentle massage to aid oil absorption

Self check

1 State the effect and skin type that each of the following mask ingredients would be used for:
   (a) Calamine.
   (b) Almond oil.
   (c) Honey.
   (d) Oatmeal.
   (e) Rose-water.
   (f) Glycerol.

2 Give two reasons why a mature skin would benefit from a peeling mask.

3 Explain how you decide upon the mask ingredients for your client's skin.

4 What are the contra-indications to the use of face masks?

5 Give the formula for a clay based mask for each of the following skin types:
   (a) Oily skin with comedones.
   (b) Dry, wrinkled skin.
   (c) Sensitive skin.
   (d) Dehydrated skin.

6 Name three different ingredients which have the following effects when used in natural masks:
   (a) Stimulating.
   (b) Emollient.
   (c) Refining.
   (d) Soothing.

CHAPTER SEVEN # Lash and Brow Treatments

Minor facial treatments

Many small grooming and glamour treatments are combined into the facial routine for convenience and time saving for the client. All slightly irritating or uncomfortable small treatments, i.e. waxing, tinting, brow plucking, are completed after cleansing prior to the more relaxing aspects of treatment. Applied in combination, very little additional preparation is required specifically for the extra service.

Small treatments may also be applied quickly and profitably on their own. The client remains fully clothed and is prepared in a semi-upright facial chair and protected with disposable tissues.

Eyebrow shaping

Well shaped eyebrows give definition to the face and form a frame to accentuate the eyes. Plucking the eyebrow hairs is a minor treatment which fits well within a facial routine when applied after cleansing. As a grooming service, it combines well with eyelash and brow tinting or waxing of the lip or chin to form a profitable routine (see Chapter 12, Depilatory Treatments).

Deciding eyebrow shape

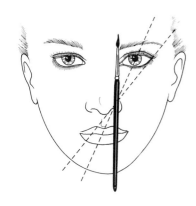

There are three main guidelines to determine the correct shape and length for eyebrows:

1 Place a fine tapered brush beside the nose and inner aspect of the eye. Any hairs on the inner side of the brush should be removed.
2 Place a fine brush in a line from the nose to the outer aspect of the eye. Remove any hair lying outside this line.
3 Placing the brush in a line from the nose to the centre of the pupil of the eye will indicate where the highest point of the arch should be.

Normally only hairs growing under the eyebrows are removed. Occasionally a few stray hairs may be removed from above to tidy the line. Eyebrow shape is partly governed by shape of face and partly by present fashion. The thin, stencilled lines of the 1940s are light years away from the natural 'Brooke Shields' style eyebrows of the 1990s. Eyebrows that are too thin look very unnatural and can affect the total look of someone's face. If the brows are too wide apart it causes the eyes to look surprised. If they are thick and bushy and meet in the centre it creates a stern or heavy expression.

The client's personal preference is of most importance. The beauty therapist's suggestion can be explained using a mirror. Changes to the shape of the brows must be discussed with the client and guidance given on the basis of their natural shape and the client's facial proportions.

Corrective eyebrow shapes

The eyebrows can be used to create an angular or rounded appearance on different facial contours. A well-shaped brow is essential for all makeup work, but it can be made to change, refine, or improve a facial shape. Tinting can be used to emphasise, lengthen or slightly change the eyebrow shape to accentuate a particular effect.

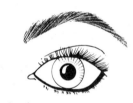

Angular shape

Angular shape
An angular shape can be used to give flat planes to a rounded face. The angle of the brow can be reflected in the makeup shading and contouring to give an elegant appearance. The angular eyebrow can be used to create many looks and can reflect an appearance of harshness, elegance and sophistication.

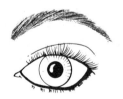

Rounded shape

Rounded shape
The more natural line of the rounded brow can give an innocent, fresh appearance, and blends well if a general makeup is worn. The line should follow the prominence of the frontal bone and be shaped into a tapered end, encompassing the rounded shape of the eye itself. Clients with large eyes or very wide foreheads should be given a rounded shape to show their eyes to the best advantage.

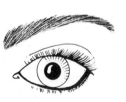

Sweeping shape

Sweeping shape
A sweeping eyebrow shape is very flattering to the majority of clients, giving width and expression to the eye area of the face. The sweeping eyebrow shape frees a large expanse of upper lid skin for eye makeup and allows full artistry in this area. The sweeping line of the brow opens the eyes, gives interest to a narrow face, and can help to balance an over-large mouth or nose shape. This shape of brow can be used to create many different illusions from the romantic to the very natural look, depending on the rest of the makeup.

Equipment required

The equipment required should become part of the normal trolley preparations, i.e. ordinary or automatic tweezers, antiseptic solution, soothing lotion, cotton wool, small bowls, a hand mirror, an eyebrow brush. Natural daylight or illuminated magnification is essential to produce a neat, fast shaping with the minimum discomfort and operator strain.

Method

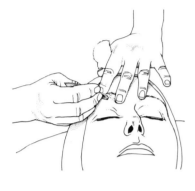

With all the makeup removed, the plucking commences between the brows, removing stray hairs and spacing the inner corners. Wiping over the brows with a damp, antiseptic pad between pluckings removes the loose hairs, cools the skin and gives protection against infection. The shape of the brows is formed by removing hairs below the brow, plucking in the direction of the growth,and supporting and stretching with the other hand.

Stray hairs above the brow and at the temple area should be removed, as long as they do not form part of the eyebrow itself. Strong, individual coarse hairs within the eyebrow may be removed if they detract from the finished line and do not leave uncovered skin areas. The finished shape of the eyebrows should not be determined, if major reshaping is undertaken, until the client has agreed to both brows in their approximate form. Final shaping can then be concluded to the client's satisfaction.

Extremely heavy brows can be gradually reduced over two or three shapings. This reduces client discomfort and allows her to get accustomed to her new image slowly.

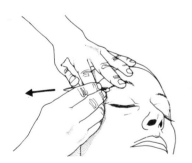

Overplucked brows must be allowed to grow and be kept tidy until sufficient hair is available to form a new line. Eyebrow tinting can be used to advantage to increase the apparent bulk of insignificant brows.

Although classed as a minor treatment, eyebrow shaping can be an extremely important part of the client's overall grooming routine. Care should be taken initially to develop the best shape possible, one which flatters the client's face and with which she feels comfortable. This shape can then be followed subsequently.

Matching the brows

To get the brows to appear even it is important to stand away from the client periodically whilst shaping the brows to assess the overall effect, to check whether the brows are even, and at the same time level and not becoming too thin. Brows that are not matched naturally, for curve or position of the face, can be made to appear similar by skilful shaping and removal of unwanted hairs. Tinting can be used to form brows out of almost nothing — to the great joy of the client. White hairs and tough, spiky hairs can be removed if they are spoiling the overall shape and their removal does not make the brows uneven.

The finished brow should be smoothed into shape and soothing lotion applied to prevent infection resulting from treatment and reduce skin redness.

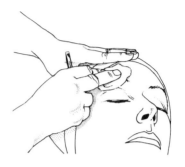

Eyebrow and lash tinting

The cosmetic effect of brow and lash tinting is to enhance the general appearance, define or correct brow shapes and emphasise the lashes with intensified colour. The convenience of permanent colour makes tinting a very popular and profitable salon treatment. If tinting is combined with a facial treatment, it is applied after cleansing and prior to massage.

Equipment required

Different forms of permanent eyelash and brow tint include cream, jelly and liquid formulas, all of which require combination with 10 volume peroxide to activate them prior to application. The colour choice of blue, grey, brown and black permits many shades and colour tones to be produced, individually suited to the client. The base colour of the hairs affects the density of the finished result and care must be taken not to over tint or a strong harsh effect will be created.

The items required for tinting are the chosen type of tint, 10 volume peroxide, water, an eye dropper, a small brush, orange stick, cotton wool and mixing palette. Soothing eye solution should also be available in case of irritation resulting from the tint.

While gaining experience in shaping brows, consult frequently with the client so that she is happy with the finished effect. Constant checking and an overall idea of the finished shape to be created should guard against disasters. Once plucked, the hair cannot be replaced, although it will grow back in time. Taking the trouble to consult with the client, apart from being a fundamental courtesy, is good business sense. On small treatments such as eyebrow shaping, a client will try out the therapist's ability to perform the task quickly and efficiently and also their willingness to work in accord with the client's wishes. Satisfaction on such a relatively minor treatment could result in further clinic treatment of a much more profitable type.

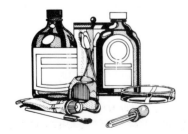

Contra-indications to brow and lash tinting

Although modern tints are mainly of vegetable origin, they are still activated by a peroxide solution and will occasionally cause skin irritation. Even patch testing does not rule out completely the possibility of eye irritation if the tint substance comes into contact with the delicate skin of the eye itself.

To avoid problems, contra-indications must be checked with the client:

- Any history of sensitivity or allergy to eye makeup.
- Conjunctivitis.
- Eczema in the brow or lash hairs. The increased skin proliferation (shedding) seen in eczema and dermatitis conditions leaves the skin exposed and open to bacterial invasion and a reaction and swelling could result.
- Psoriasis in the eye area.
- Excessively dry, flaky skin should be treated with caution, whether it has resulted from neglect or through systemic causes such as thyroid abnormality.
- Difficult skin prone to cosmetic reactions and a tendency to an unstable skin texture should be patch tested before each application to check changes occurring in the client's system.
- Very highly strung, nervous clients with periods of high and low sensitivity must be patch tested each time.
- Clients who normally wear glasses, with hypersensitive skin around the eyes, should be treated gently and cream tints used for greater control.
- Skin irritation from any source which affects the area is classed as a contra-indication to tinting at that time.
- Clients unable to keep their eyes still, either from some nervous problem, old age or from a dislike of having their eyes touched, could prove difficult to treat. Success in this situation depends largely on the therapist's client-handling abilities and steadiness of hand.

Certain points must be followed to minimise the risk of this popular treatment:

- Patch testing.
- Performing the tint meticulously, with attention to protection of the skin and scrupulous removal of the tint on conclusion.

The therapist must use her own judgement as to who is suitable for tinting – not a great many clients are contra-indicated. The therapist must have the confidence to say when it is not advisable, as the risks to the clinic's reputation are considerable if the client suffers pain or distress from an eye infection.

The legal position regarding tinting and the clinic's liability would be that every reasonable care had been seen to be taken to safeguard the client's well being. Keeping client's records, checking contra-indications, patch testing and performing the treatment only if suitable would appear to meet these criteria.

Patch testing

Patch testing is performed on an occasion previous to the tinting. The interval between testing and tinting should ideally be at least 48 hours and not longer than a week. The patch can be applied when the initial enquiry is made, or within an eyebrow shaping where it has been suggested by the therapist, or during a normal regular facial treatment as an extension into related treatments. If the therapist suggests and completes the preparation for the tint, a subsequent booking for the treatment is assured.

A small quantity of tint is mixed and painted or rubbed on to the skin with a brush or cotton wool bud in an area immediately behind the ear so that it is unobtrusive. If no irritation results after 48 hours, it may be washed off and the client can be considered suitable for tinting. Only an area the size of a small coin need be covered. If irritation does result the tint should be washed off and soothing antiseptic cream used to calm the skin. Once the offending tint is removed, the irritation normally disappears.

The importance of patch testing reasonably close to the actual time of tinting is due to changes occurring in the body, particularly if medication is taken or the client is on hormone therapy. For the same reason, the patch testing should be repeated if the lashes and brows have not been tested for a long time. Pregnant clients often produce strange reactions to tinting procedures even if they normally have regular tinting with no problems. A client's lack of sensitivity a year before is no guide to her immediate reaction, nor is regular hair tinting, as the tints employed in hairdressing are differently formulated from lash tints. Also, the skin around the eyes is considerably more sensitive than the scalp.

Reaction to tinting, if it occurs even after careful checking, can include swelling of the eye skin, irritation and inflammation of the eyeball itself causing weeping, and conjunctivitis if severe. Although tinting is freely available in salons and stores, sometimes with scant regard to safety or procedure, therapists have a professional duty to safeguard their clients and must follow sensible guide lines to ensure a satisfactory level of proficiency.

Application: cream tints

Brows

The cream tints are the most manageable and so are ideal for delicate or mature skins where the risks of skin irritation or staining are highest. The softer colour combinations it is possible to achieve with cream tints suit the mature or fair-skinned individual and avoid an artificial appearance being produced.

If the brows and lashes are to be tinted, the whole area should be cleansed thoroughly to remove any oil, adhesions, etc. and the brows shaped if necessary.

Although ideally the brows should be shaped on a previous occasion, in commercial practice this is seldom the case and they are plucked just prior to tinting. As long as the skin is completely covered with protective cream in the areas not to be tinted, no tint will be able to penetrate the open hair follicles and cause skin irritation. Major

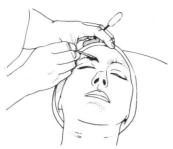
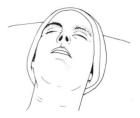

Preparation and application of tint

reshaping likely to cause skin irritation should naturally not be combined with the tinting sequence.

The brows and lashes are surrounded by a light film of cream or oil applied with a cotton wool tipped orange stick, to prevent skin staining. A small amount of tint is mixed with two drops of 10 volume peroxide to form an even coloured emulsion of smooth texture. This is applied first to the underneath brow hairs to ensure complete coverage, working towards the centre brow and then to the surface eyebrow, smoothing and shaping the finished line. The second brow is completed and a visual and time check kept on the first brow to determine colour formation. Removal of the tint after 3–5 minutes is accomplished by firm wiping strokes with a damp pad to ensure that no tint remains on the brows or skin.

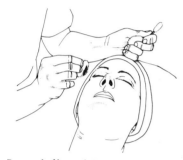

Removal of brow tint

Fine blond hair colours easily and should be checked at regular intervals to prevent over-coloration. The inner eye corner tint can be removed for checking purposes and reapplied if insufficient colour is present.

Red hair is very resistant to tinting, and may require double the exposure time to achieve a satisfactory result.

Dark brows may only require definition at the outer corners, or to blend in white hairs, and so a natural shade can be used to give a uniform tone to the whole brow and produce a more distinct profile aspect to the brow.

Lashes

The lashes should be tinted after the brows in a combined sequence as the timing is not so critical due to the deeper colours preferred for lash tints. Any tint remaining from the brows may be used for the lashes with the addition, if necessary, of a small amount of a darker tone.

The under eye skin should be protected by applying a thin coat of petroleum jelly and then damp cotton wool pieces shaped to fit snugly under the lower lashes. Once the upper and lower lashes are in place, the client must be advised not to open her eyes, to reduce the risks of irritation resulting from tint entering the eye. Once the lower pads are in place, more petroleum jelly can be applied to the upper lid to prevent staining.

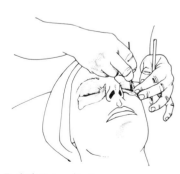

Eyelash tint application

The tint mixture is applied carefully, and coats and encloses the lashes right down to the skin of the lids. Any tint which does touch the skin must be removed promptly to avoid skin staining (which can occur even through the protective film of cream or petroleum jelly).

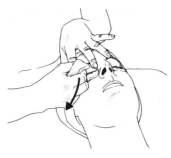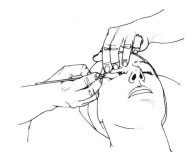

Tint removal

The second eye is completed and 5–8 minutes' development time is allowed, depending on natural colouring and the finished tone required. The tint is removed with downward strokes on to the protective pad, and care must be taken not to open the eyes until all the tint substance has been removed. The procedure is repeated gently until the lashes are clean and no tint remains to be a source of irritation.

A final check with the eyes open will reveal any tint present in the roots of the lashes, and this must be removed gently with a cotton wool tip with the eye skin supported with the other hand. The eyes may be bathed with a soothing Optrex solution to relieve any discomfort or irritation.

Jelly tints

The method of use for jelly tints is identical to cream tints, but greater care is necessary to avoid skin staining as the more fluid consistency is liable to seep into the skin and cause irritation. The jelly tints are ideal for younger clients with firm unwrinkled skins who require a fashion effect and do not need the subtle colour blending possible with cream tints. Jelly tints are increasing in popularity due to their economy of use and speed of application. Both creams and jellies have fairly long-lasting effects and normally require repeating every 6–8 weeks as the natural growth cycle of the hairs and general sunlight exposure gradually reduces the colour intensity.

Liquid tints

Liquid tints are composed of two solutions which are applied, one after the other, to produce a colour change. The limited range of colour and the dangers of seepage restricts their professional use and places them on the retail market for home use. The results achieved with liquid tints are not sufficiently reliable for them to be offered as a salon treat-ment, but as many customers may have used them at some time it is necessary for the therapist to have a knowledge of their action.

General points on tinting

Neat, fast and careful application is necessary in tinting to achieve complete coverage without causing client discomfort or skin staining. A half-hour period should be sufficient for shaping the brows and tinting both the brows and lashes.

The time taken to tint lashes separately should not exceed 15 minutes once proficiency has been reached.

At the time of booking a tint, a client can be asked to reduce the amount of eye makeup worn when coming for treatment. This saves the time that would otherwise be wasted removing heavy mascara applications before the tinting can commence. It also reduces aggravation to the area, skin reddening and skin irritation within the tinting sequence.

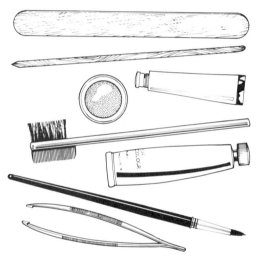

Lash tinting accessories

Application of semi-permanent individual lashes

The individual lash application is classed as a treatment due to the time involved and the semi-permanent nature of the lashes. The more recent natural makeup fashions have increased the demand for a more personal, less obvious form of lash emphasis. Personally tailored top and bottom lashes are attached individually, and have to be replaced regularly to maintain the full effect. It is a successful salon treatment, needing regular application and associated sale of lashes to complete the routine.

Equipment

The lash kit comprises the different-sized lashes and adhesive specifically formulated to maintain attachment without causing irritation. Tweezers and scissors are also needed to fix and shape the lashes. All other items should be present as part of the normal trolley preparation.

Contra-indications

Sensitive and delicate skin around the eyes will be found to be irritated by any artificial form of lash, especially semi-permanent forms. Some clients can tolerate individual lashes, however, whilst normal false lashes on a backing strip prove irritating due to the weight involved. These clients might be candidates for permanent eyeline treatment (see below).

Application

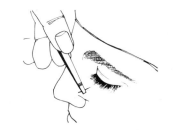

Application of semi-permanent lashes

With the client in a relaxed, semi-reclining position, the eyes are cleansed and all traces of oil, makeup, etc. removed. The individual lashes are shaped and attached with special adhesive to the roots of the natural lashes, not to the skin itself. A natural sweep, filling out and lengthening of the lash line is achieved by constant checking with the eyes open and then closed, until first the top and then the bottom set of lashes is finished.

The individual lashes must follow the curve of the natural lashes, and if these are very straight they should be curled slightly with eyelash curling tools before attachment commences. The lashes may be cut if necessary to give a personalised finish, but careful choice of the correct-sized lash from the kit should prevent a lot of unnecessary shaping.

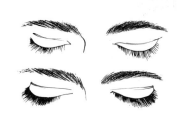

Treated and untreated eyes

The use of mascara should not be necessary after the lash applications as the client should be advised to handle the lashes as little as possible to minimise natural displacement. Even without mascara application and removal, the normal wear and tear on the lashes will demand that they receive attention every two to three weeks, depending on the effect desired. Since these are a glamour item, clients are very willing to spend to maintain the flattering appearance of the lashes.

Permanent eyeline and eyebrow colour

The new treatment gaining popularity is permanent lash line, which gives permanent colour along the base of the lashes to provide an

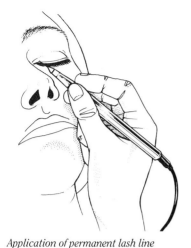

Application of permanent lash line

intensified eye line to flatter and define the eyes. It is applied in a similar way on the brows to give permanent colour and shape.

Added permanent eyeline and eyebrow colour is an electrical process which works in a similar way to a tattoo, using indelible inks which become imprinted into the skin. It is a delicate and skilful process, as the work is close to the eyes and has to be completed gradually. It is an expensive treatment, but highly profitable to the clinic.

As the application is permanent, counselling must be undertaken to ensure that clients understand that it is a process that cannot be reversed. It is very popular with dark-haired clients, especially Asiatic or Indian women who particularly enjoy wearing a defined eye line as it suits their features and eye shape and is part of their cultural background. Their black hair and dark brows and lashes are unlikely to change to the whim of fashion.

Self check

1 If a client required both a brow tint and a shape, in what order would you do it? Give reasons for your answer.
2 With the aid of a diagram, show the correct way to measure the eyebrows before a reshape.
3 Explain how and why a patch test must be carried out prior to a lash tint.
4 Describe the appearance of an adverse skin reaction to a patch test.
5 Give five contra-indications to lash tinting and five indications.
6 Explain why razors and depilatory creams should not be used for eyebrow shaping.
7 Explain why, during eyebrow shaping:
    (a) Hairs are plucked mainly from under the brow.
    (b) Brows must be brushed frequently.
    (c) Hairs are plucked only in the direction of the growth.
8 If a client finds plucking of the eyebrows very uncomfortable, how could you make it more bearable for her?
9 What are the advantages of using semi-permanent or individual lashes in preference to strip lashes?
10 Describe the procedure for applying false lashes.

CHAPTER EIGHT Makeup

Makeup techniques

Modern makeup is an art form, able to create different images to reflect mood or personality. The role of the makeup should be known to follow fashion trends and can be adapted to suit the time of year, or created for a special occasion.

The makeup artist has access to the latest and best cosmetics and styles to introduce to her clients, and can apply basic techniques of colour blending to produce attractive and flattering makeups.

Day makeup is the most difficult type to apply as it is seen in both natural and artificial light, and poor technique shows clearly at close range. Mastering basic techniques through day makeup allows full concentration to be given to the artistic side of photographic and fashion makeup.

Makeup based on correction of facial shapes is outdated for the modern makeup artist, who uses colour, texture and natural contouring to enhance attractive features and minimise faults.

Makeup products: moisturisers, foundations

Pre-makeup base (moisturisers)

Moisturisers applied prior to makeup will help to retain moisture and keep the skin smooth and supple. As the skin loses a lot of its natural moisture through evaporation, it is particularly affected by extremes of temperature, sun exposure and drying (low humidity) conditions found in centrally heated buildings. Dehydration soon becomes evident if a suitable barrier product is not used regularly to safeguard the skin.

Advanced moisturisers work as day treatment products and support nightly skin care. They also act as sun screens and protection against environmental pollution.

Moisture creams, emulsions and liquids have different proportions of water to oil in their formulations, providing products to suit all skins:

- Moisture creams give greatest day protection for the dry, mature skins to support nightly skin care.
- Moisture emulsions containing varying active ingredients may be applied on many different skin conditions to good effect (e.g. dry, combination, sensitive skin).
- Liquid hydro-emulsions provide a non-greasy protective film for the oily skin which carries on the corrective action of night products.
- Tinted pre-makeup bases correct or improve skin colour, reducing high colour, brightening sallow complexions or giving a glow to the tanned face.
- Sports bases – combined moisturiser and lightly textured tinted foundation – are ideal for suntanned and coloured skins.
- Moisturising ampoules contain concentrated, fast-acting products to rectify and control dehydration problems.

Application

Thinly applied over the face and throat with flowing movements, the moisturiser should settle into a slightly tacky film before foundation is applied. A well chosen and correctly applied moisture base helps to prolong the perfect finish of makeup and prevent colour change.

Tinted foundation/base

The choice of tinted foundation or base depends on:

- Colour – it should match or improve the natural skin tone and be fashionable.
- Texture – matt or more oily/soft textured either to flatten and disguise poor texture or enhance a clear complexion.
- Covering properties – opaqueness, ability to cover small imperfections, high colour, uneven skin colour, etc.
- Lasting properties – durability, ability to stay perfect for as long as possible.
- Suitability for the skin condition – dry, oily, sensitive, etc.

Foundation consistency acts as a rough guide to application:

Skin type	Choice of foundation/base
Dry and mature	Cream or moisturised emulsion
Dry and sensitive	Cream or oil-based
Combination skin (oily centre panel area)	Liquid, semi-liquid all-in-one foundation (fluid and powder combined)
Oily	Non-oily, astringent or water based (combined). Cake or block type, suspended liquid (combined)
Blemished, acne	Medicated liquid or block (drying and germicidal)
Allergic/hypersensitive	Hypoallergenic (with all known irritants screened out)

Foundations for special purposes

1 Tinted foundations for improving facial colouring, i.e. green, mauve, apricot, which are components in custom blended foundations (foundations specially blended for the client by the clinic).
2 Treatment foundations combining tinted preparations and additional nutrient elements, for the mature, crepey or lined skin.
3 Concealing foundations, to disguise and heal facial blemishes, scars, acne, etc., which are applied directly over the blemish, prior to the medicated foundation application or replacing it. The products are opaque, firm textured with excellent covering properties.
4 Sports base, sun screened, tinted emulsions which act as an ultraviolet screen and provide a natural looking day makeup.
5 Cosmetic camouflage products which disguise disfigurements, birth marks, etc. and include covering creams and a variety of foundation items.
6 Theatrical foundations, with a wide colour range to suit stage, photographic and fashion/modelling work.

Foundation colours and uses

The foundation acts as a basic canvas on which to build the makeup and with careful choice can minimise skin faults, smooth out texture problems and improve the skin colour.

Foundations come in a wide range of shades, or can be custom blended to meet individual need. Colours in the medium range, mid-beige, rose beige, tawny peach, cool and medium beige/tan will be most popular and will be used more frequently than others in a range. These useful colours can look quite different depending on the natural skin tone.

The client's wishes and hopes should be listened to, to produce a makeup which matches her needs and includes some of her suggestions. The makeup should reflect her life style and personality and be suited to its purpose, e.g. a new look, improvement or up-dating, makeup for a special event. If a client is not happy with her makeup, however beautifully applied, it is a failure and perhaps spoils her overall pleasure of the treatment.

Colour suggestions

Skin tones	Foundation colours
Light and pale skins	Light warm beige; soft peach.
Translucent skins	Creamy pink beige.
Medium skin tones	Cool beige; rose beige; warm peach; soft beige (tan); pink/tan; sun bronze.
Dark skin tones	Dark beige; deep peach (corrective); sun bronze (to accentuate a tan); luminous light olive (also suitable for coloured skins).

Corrective Foundation Colours

Complexion	Colour tone
Highly coloured, vascular complexion	Flat beige or olive, to tone down the colour, may be used as a correction on affected areas prior to general foundation application.
Uneven, blotchy or veined complexions	Medium beige and tawny tones may be used to regulate the basic colour and minimise irregularities. Covering cream in medium beige may be applied over particularly prominent veins or areas of discoloration.
Sallow, discoloured or pigmented complexions	Medium pink/beige or pink/tawny tones may be used depending on general colouring. The darker the base skin tone, the more colour-lifting effect is required. Vivid areas of pigmentation may be covered with masking creams prior to the general foundation application.

Foundation application

With the client in a semi-upright position, the chosen foundation may be applied according to consistency using fingers or sterilised small sponges.

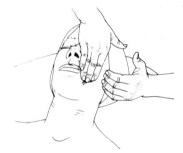

Foundation application: finger method

Creamy foundations
Cream products may be applied with light effleurage movements keeping the finger tips in contact and the residue of the makeup in the palm of the hand, commencing at the throat and working swiftly over the face and eye areas, to form an even film.

Semi-liquid foundations
Semi-liquid and all-in-one combined foundations are the most popular. To speed the application, small dots of foundation are put on the chin, cheeks, and forehead areas before general blending starts. These foundations do not require fixing with powder, so their finish is dryer and checking is necessary to avoid harsh lines or streaking occurring.

To avoid colour build-up on vellus hairs, around the hairline, etc., the tinted base can be brought close to, but not onto, the soft hairs, and the foundation blended very finely with a damp sponge over the area.

Liquid foundations
Liquid foundations are more difficult to control and cosmetic sponges may be used to achieve good coverage and prevent accidental soiling.

Setting to a matt film, the skin texture then needs to be re-established by hand contact with the face to bring back natural gloss and life. Liquid foundations provide the ideal coverage for oily and blemished complexions, camouflaging and protecting without aggravating the existing conditions. Excessive oil secretions can cause tinted foundations to change colour, so oil-free preparations are preferable for the oily skin.

Cake or block foundations

Cake or block foundations are applied with a clean cosmetic sponge and water to achieve good coverage and a matt texture. Block foundations are similar in effect to liquids, but are available in a wider ranges of colour and application. Skin cover can be increased by altering the thickness of the application. Compact blocks are a popular choice for younger clients, combining convenience and low cost.

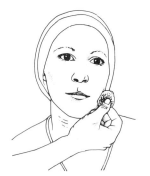

Foundation application: sponge method

Medicated foundations

Medicated foundations are available in liquid, semi-liquid, all-in-one and block forms which cover the skin effectively yet are anti-bacterial in action, helping to dry and heal the skin.

Clients with blemished skin should be encouraged to leave their skin free from makeup whenever possible, but the demoralising effect of an acne skin on the client should be weighed against this advice and a compromise sought.

Cheek colour (rouge, blushers, shaders, highlighters, concealers)

Cheek shapers, shaders and highlighters may be applied either at this stage of the routine (prior to the loose powder), or concluding the makeup (powder blushers, etc.).

All cream-textured products (cheek colour, eye shadow, highlighters, etc.) need setting with loose powder to have long-lasting properties and to avoid colour loss and creasing into facial lines. The powder application also softens the appearance, if applied correctly, and makes the cheek colour appear less obvious.

Types of rouge/blusher

- Cheek gloss, semi-transparent or softly pearlised, in a range of natural tones.
- Powder blushers in compressed palettes with a wide choice of fashion-related colours and matt, softly pearlised or gold dusted effects.
- Cream rouge – softer in effect for the dry and mature skins.
- Golden/earth-toned/sun-toned/desert dust blush powder for a warm and glamorous glow on sun-bronzed skin.

Colour choice

All colours from pink, tawny rose and bright red through to russet brown, sun bronze and yellow are available in rouges and blushers.

Facial shaders/highlighters

Shaders and highlighters are used to accentuate and develop the principle of illuminating and diminishing the facial features. There is a lot of overlap between facial shapers and blusher products now that the range of cheek colours has increased considerably.

Colour choice

Available in colour tones ranging from blank or pearlised white, cream and beige through to darkest brown.

Concealers

Concealers are opaque, beige-coloured, matt-textured products useful for diminishing small imperfections of the skin such as marks, old scars, small areas of dilated capillaries and skin discoloration. They are also used widely to disguise shadows under the eyes, from tiredness, etc. They are used directly over the foundation to blend out any small problems still evident.

Use of concealers can allow a lighter makeup or sports base to be worn rather than a more covering type of foundation.

Application

In day makeup, a soft accentuation of facial contours with shaders and or blusher is all that is needed. Colour should be applied sparingly to prevent colour build-up or an unnatural appearance. Facial contouring can be used to effect on younger clients – just simple cheek contouring with shading, highlighter and a final touch of blush.

A soft blush of colour on the older client is flattering, sweeping around the eyes, upper cheeks and along the jawline to soften the contour.

Most skin tones, apart from florid complexions, are flattered by additional colour which gives lift and vitality to the face. It should not be overdone, especially in the older client, where it just looks unattractive and obvious.

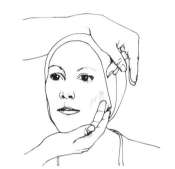

Cream blusher

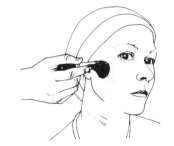

Powder blusher

Makeup products: eye makeup

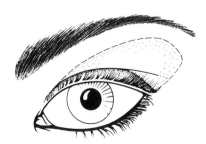

Basic eye makeup

Eye makeup may be used to correct faults, accentuate the eyes, and, by bringing colour to the face, can detract from other poor features. The texture of the products used must be flattering to the eye and suitable for the client's age and skin condition.

The classic eye makeup sequence is first to shape and colour the brows, providing a frame for the eye, then to apply eye shadow, eyeliner and false lashes (if worn) and, lastly, mascara. The diversity of makeup available will alter this routine for fashion work, but the basic sequence remains a convenient guideline for general applications.

Types of eye makeup

Eyebrow makeup

Pencils and crayons are available in a wide range of colours, and brow powders are available in loose powder or compressed block form.

Well-shaped brows can be tinted if necessary to reduce the task of drawing them in even further, or permanent brow colours can be considered.

Eye shadow

- Cream shadows are easy to apply, but tend to crease, so are set with loose powder; mainly used in photographic, fashion and stage makeup.
- Compact powder shadows in palettes come in matt and softly pearlised versions in a range of fashion colours and neutral tones (for the no-makeup look).
- Powder creams have the texture of a cream product but set into a fine matt film, retaining a soft texture and good colour effects.
- Eye pencils and crayons with soft consistency are ideal for detailed and exciting eye makeup work, as they are available in hundreds of fashion colours. They can be used as both shadows and liners.
- Transparent tints give gloss to the brow bone, etc.
- Semi-liquid shadows in tubes or wand applicators with soft textures, attractive colours and good staying power are very convenient and popular with clients.

Eye emphasis

Eye liner

Lining the eyes is a fashion effect which swings in and out of favour depending on the fashion scene at the time. Heavy eye accentuation is coming back into fashion with the revival of the 60s-influenced fashions that are currently enjoying popularity.

In some cultures (e.g. Eastern and Asian), outlining the eyes will always remain popular as it is traditional and intrinsically connected with the concept of female beauty. These are potential clients for permanent eyeline and brow colour.

A fine line of deeper eye shadow colour or dark liner applied close to the roots of the lashes can emphasise the eyes. The liner can appear to open, lengthen or emphasise the eyes according to the way in which it is applied.

If false lashes are applied they are attached over a fine lash line, and mascara and liner retouched as necessary.

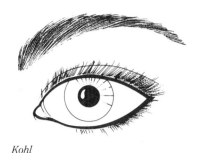

Kohl

Kohl

Accentuating the eyes with a soft, black kohl eye makeup is popular with younger clients, applied in a softly defined fashion right around the inner eye rim and smudged through the lashes to create a romantic, rather Eastern effect. Similar in consistency to the traditional kohl worn by Indian women, it is applied in a similar manner with a brush or blunt-ended stick. A soft pencil version is also available.

To apply the product the therapist must face the client. The client has to keep her eyes open and steady during the procedure. A steady hand is needed to prevent the kohl touching the eyeball itself. Some clients may prefer to apply this final step of the eye makeup themselves. If they wear it all the time, as in the case of Indian women, they have a very exact idea of how they wish it to look.

Although very attractive and in keeping with Eastern features and costume, such evident outlining requires a makeup that will balance its dramatic effect, so is more suited to younger women. Large, clear eyes, strong makeup tones and defined lip colours are necessary to exploit the effect to the full.

Mascara

Block, spiral and liquid forms of mascara provide a large variety of products. Mascara wands offer the most convenient, but expensive, form of eyelash emphasis and, due to the liquid formulation, use is restricted in the case of sensitive or allergy-prone eye conditions. Both contact lens wearers and clients with sensitive eyes should be advised to use hypoallergenic mascara, or tint their eyelashes to prevent the need for heavy mascara applications. Clear mascara is now available for sports wear and to suit the natural makeup look.

Eye makeup application

The basic sequence for day makeup should be followed:

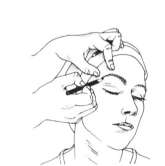

Eyebrow pencil

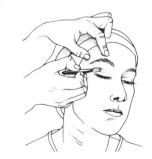

Eye shadow application

- The eyebrows are formed into a natural shape with pencils or eyebrow powder, using short, light strokes to improve the shape and to even up the sparse areas of the brow.
- Shadow is applied to the skin with a small brush or foam-tipped stick, where it is blended using fingers and brushes over the middle and outer part of the lid, extending out towards the eyebrow arch.
- Highlighting can be used to lighten the area under the brow to give the illusion of larger, more brilliant eyes (ivory-toned highlighters).
- Socket emphasis, with deeper toned products, can be applied on clients with large eyes and full smooth lids. It is not suitable on deep-set, small or crepey-skinned eyes.
- Highlighting can be reflected below the eyes on the cheekbone area to show the cheek angles to advantage and balance the eye makeup.
- Eyeliner can be used to give emphasis to the lashes to provide more contrast between the eye and the shadow. A fine, soft line is applied with a tapered brush close to the roots of the lashes, not extending beyond them.

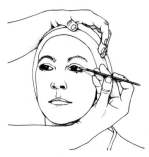

Eye liner

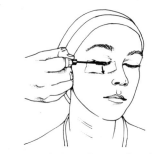

Mascara application: downward strokes

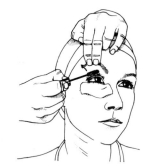

Mascara application: upward sweeping strokes

- A coloured shadow can be applied close to or instead of the dark line, to soften it and give additional colour brilliance.
- Additional lash emphasis or careful fragmented liner application is usually required on the lower lashes to balance the effect and prevent a top-heavy appearance.
- Mascara is applied first downwards over the upper lashes, coating them evenly, then lifting and sweeping them outwards and upwards to give an attractive curve. This is repeated until the desired effect is achieved.
- The lower lashes are covered next, keeping the lashes separate and avoiding touching and staining the skin.

Unsteady eyes should be made up with care and tissues should be used to prevent under-eye skin becoming coated with mascara when the client blinks. Insignificant, sparse or very straight lashes should be tinted in preference to heavy mascara applications as a more natural effect will be achieved. Mascara will then only be needed to curl the lashes, not to coat them.

Fashion trends

Mascara and false or individual lashes also have periods of popularity and decline, but the flattering effect of emphasising and lengthening the natural lash retains mascara as a very popular client product from which they will not be easily parted.

Subtle lash emphasis will always be popular, whether heavy outlining is currently in or out of fashion, as it accentuates the most expressive features of the face and is very flattering. Makeup differs so much around the world that a makeup artist has to be able to complete any effect required. Eyeliner is a standard eye makeup item for many overseas clients, to the extent of having a permanent lash line applied.

Makeup products: lipstick

Lipstick choice and application

The lipstick is a vital part of the entire makeup, giving the effect of pulling the whole face together and harmonising eye, cheek and foundation colours whilst giving vitality and life to the expression. The makeup looks incomplete until the mouth is coloured, and then the balance in the face may need adjustment. More colour, gloss or highlighting may be needed to bring the face to perfection.

Lipstick colour and texture are of equal importance, and choice will depend on whether correction or improvement is needed:

- Softer, creamy textured lipsticks, though not long lasting, are very attractive and pleasant to wear.
- Matt lipsticks are more dry on the mouth, but hold their colour longer.

• Lip gloss and liquid lip tints give an almost transparent film of colour on the mouth and need constant reapplication.

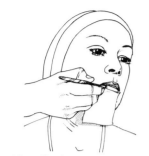

Lipstick application

Application

First the lip line is evenly and cleanly applied, and then the lips filled in evenly with colour. The lips may be blotted and fresh colour applied for a long-lasting effect. Creamy lipsticks and transparent lip tints with their softer texture are only applied once and are not blotted as reapplication is unavoidable.

Full lips should be toned down with soft colours, with their natural shape being sufficient emphasis. Irregular or narrow lips can be disguised with brighter or more pearlised/glossy lipstick used to fill out, diminish or bring areas of the lips forward.

Basic makeup conclusion

Makeup of the face must be approached as a total effect to flatter the features and reflect the personality. Attractive facial expressions can bring beauty into a face comprised of few redeeming features, and the makeup must bring this attractiveness forward, whilst disguising faults.

Looking at the finished makeup will reveal any final touches needed to give it balance. A need for more colour or texture on the eyes, cheeks or the face generally may be apparent after the headband is removed, and the contrast of the hair colour against the makeup is seen. These touches are then applied prior to the client's inspection.

Makeup completion means ensuring that the client looks neat and well groomed before she looks in the mirror. Tidying the client's hair after removal of the headband, robes, etc. and generally seeing that she looks her best and is not disappointed with the final effect are all part of the basic makeup conclusion.

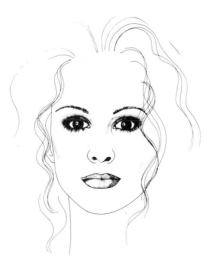

The finished effect

Photographic, evening and high-fashion makeup

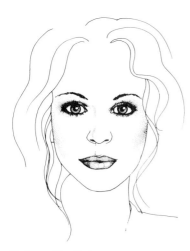

High fashion effect

Before starting the makeup, its purpose should be determined so that it matches the effect required. The lighting under which the makeup will be viewed will indicate the colours and textures that can be used.

Daytime high-fashion effects require great subtlety of technique as the makeup may have to be seen close to and at a distance, i.e. demonstration and modelling applications.

Evening or photographic makeup permits greater contrast of colour and texture to be used, as the artificial lighting throws the face into relief – an effect which can be emphasised by facial contouring and reflective makeup.

Analysis of the face

The modern makeup artist can create flattering makeups based on the individuality of the client's facial features and no longer has to attempt to fit them into an accepted mould. No particular face shape is considered the best; rather with any face interesting contours and individual features are emphasised and faults minimised to create an attractive appearance.

The face should be viewed in profile and full-face, and natural contouring decided. Interesting cheek bones can be emphasised and any faults such as a double chin or over-hanging lids minimised. The areas of shading should be definite with the edges softened and blended in to prevent harsh lines.

Eyebrows can be judged for their effect on the face and corrected if necessary. Irregularly shaped eyes or lips can be made to appear less noticeable by drawing attention away from them to other more distinctive features.

Photographic effect

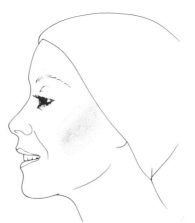

Facial contouring in profile

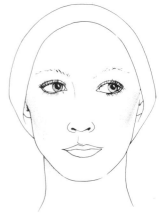

Frontal view shading

134

Facial contouring and correcting

Contouring
The primary contouring and highlighting should be applied prior to the tinted foundation. Its effect is softened by the overall colour, and it becomes fixed into position by it. Photographic makeup permits a wider contrast of colours to be used for shading and highlighting.

Shading the nose
Fleshy or irregularly shaped noses can be refined or straightened by shading, or an illusion of a narrower nasal bridge can be created. The tip of the nose should not be shaded as this will always appear as a smudge.

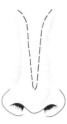

Nose shading

Jaw contouring
Jaw contouring, with light and dark foundations, can appear to firm the jawline, reducing a double chin. It can also lengthen and slim an ageing neck.

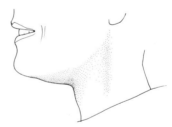

Jaw contouring

Eye accentuation
Eyes may be emphasised, enlarged and opened with cream or ivory-coloured highlighter for evening or fashion effects, and with white shader for photographic work. Overhead lighting throws the eyes into shadow, making it useful to lighten the area.

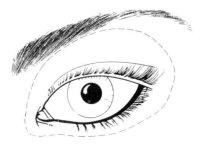

Eye enlarging with highlight

Brow improvement

The brows can be shaped to create the illusion of extra width in a long face, or to soften the contours if the face is very angular (see Chapter 7, Lash and Brow Treatments). Tinting to improve the profile view of the brows is also useful. The brows should be brushed into shape forming a frame for the eye makeup.

Foundations for fashion, evening and photographic makeup

- The texture of the foundation base should be even, matt and give good coverage without appearing heavy.
- For a natural texture, a cosmetic sponge may be used to apply and settle the foundation.
- Different tones of tinted foundation may be used to reflect the underlying shading, but they must be well blended or they will be obvious.
- The finish at this stage is important as the face is being prepared for its final, more flattering makeup and poor preparation will prevent a long-lasting or perfect finished effect.
- The foundation should cover the face and neck, and may also be applied over the eye and lip areas, depending on the subsequent makeup products to be used.
- More vivid and intense colours than those normally worn will be needed for evening and photographic work, due to the draining effect of the artificial lighting.

Blushers and additional colour

Cream and liquid blushers may be used at this stage to emphasise the shading, care being taken not to create colour build-up, which could look artificial for day wear. The colour should not dominate the face, but bring life and vitality to it, accentuating the eyes.

Face powder

Loose powder is not widely used in day makeup. For high-fashion day makeup, evening and photographic makeup it is important as it merges together all the detailed layers of the makeup and sets the final result. The glare reflecting from the face from spotlights and background lighting used in photographic work would spoil the effect if it were not diminished by thorough powdering.

The powder is chosen to harmonise with, not change, the foundation shade. The powder is applied carefully but liberally over all the face, neck, eyes and lips with a rolling movement of the puff. The residue can then be brushed from the face with a soft powder puff or brush, following the skin's natural hair growth direction. All parts of the face should be inspected for loose powder, and the brows especially brushed and retouched.

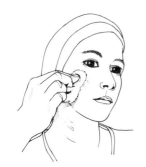

Loose powder application

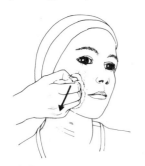

Removal of excess powder

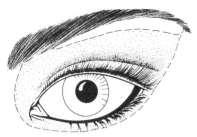

High fashion eye makeup

Eye makeup

As the underlying work has prepared an even-coloured and highlighted matt base, only final colour touches and lash emphasis are required to give extra drama to the eye. Day fashion effects may include:

- Basic colour toned shadows.
- Socket emphasis (on the fuller eye).
- Additional brow reflective highlighting.
- Eye liner.
- Full or partial false lashes (if required).
- Mascara.

The amount of makeup worn will depend on the effect or illusion to be created, and the direction of lighting used to illuminate the face in photographic work. Socket emphasis should be modified for evening and photographic work, otherwise the eye will appear deeply shadowed due to effects of overhead lighting.

The wishes of the photographer really decide the type of makeup that is required, and so the finished effect is a joint effort with the makeup artist working under direction.

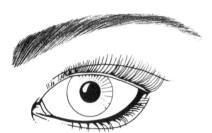

Fine lashes: top

False lashes

False lashes form a standard part of photographic and fashion makeup and in modelling give dramatic effect from a distance. If integrated as part of a total look and chosen and applied with care, false lashes can give a very elegant and attractive appearance to the face. In the same way as eyeliners, false lashes follow fashion trends, losing and regaining favour, but remaining popular at all times with the younger client.

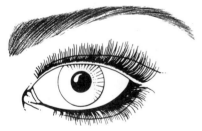

Heavy lashes: top and bottom

Choice

The variety of false lashes available gives a wide range of possible effects for enhancing or correcting the eye.

- Very fine false lashes produce a natural appearance, emphasising the density of the existing lashes without seeming artificial.
- Heavier lashes attached to a more solid base require a more exaggerated makeup to complement them, and should be kept for distance and photographic work.
- Partial lashes to extend width, give uplift or general emphasis to the eye can be very useful in correcting eye faults. They balance the eyes and improve the profile appearance.

The decision to use false lashes will depend on the client's ability to cope with them and the general sensitivity of the eye area. They must suit the overall makeup and be able to be worn confidently by the client.

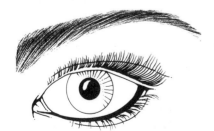

Partial lashes: outer eyes

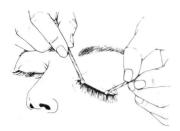

Attachment of false lashes

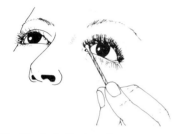

Checking lash attachment

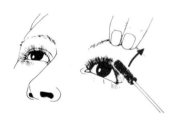

Blending false and natural lashes

Application

- The lashes should be clean, naturally curled and shaped to suit the client's eye. Choice of the correct lashes initially reduces the need for excessive trimming and shaping.
- The eye makeup should be completed up to the eye liner stage.
- False lashes may be applied to the roots of the natural lashes to form a firm attachment. Adhesive is applied directly on to the base strip of the lashes, or with an orange stick in the case of very lightweight varieties.
- The client must remain with her eyes closed for a few seconds to permit the adhesive to set and to prevent the preparation entering the eye and causing irritation.
- The lash should be firmly but gently pressed into position with the orange stick.
- The finished line can be inspected and the inner and outer corners checked for firm attachment.
- The lashes should blend with the natural lashes to form a thicker, longer, more flattering appearance.
- When the adhesive has set and become transparent, the eye makeup may be finished by attachment of lower lashes, if used.
- The lower lashes are attached with the eyes open, and emphasis should be placed on the outer area of the eye to prevent an artificial effect.
- Eyeliner and shadow can be retouched to achieve a perfect finish.
- The lashes may be brushed into a natural shape with the minimum of mascara or a clean brush to combine the false and natural lashes, and to ensure separation of the top and bottom sets.

Correction and emphasis of eye shapes

The principle of emphasising, bringing forward into prominence, and diminishing or regressing with light and dark tones can be used to advantage to improve difficult or irregularly shaped eyes. Use of vibrant colours, tones of the shades picked, and contrasting textures enable the skilful makeup artist to correct or deflect interest away from the eye fault.

No rules can apply to corrective makeup as it is not only the feature that has to be considered, but its relationship to the rest of the face. The profile and frontal view of the eye should always be considered, and difficult eyes not seen as a fault, rather as a challenge to present to their best advantage.

Deep-set eyes

1 The eyes may be brought forward with pale or pearlised colours blended in an oval around the upper and lower lids.
2 The overhanging brow bone should be shaded as a fine line spreading to wing along the crease.
3 The arch of the brow can be emphasised with a white or cream-coloured pearl shadow, also repeated in the centre of the lid.

No eye liner, but fine pointed upper and lower lashes may be applied, for increased definition in the younger client.

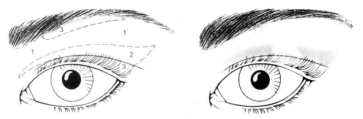

Colour suggestions
(1) Violet   (2) Pearl white   (3) Grape for shading
(1) Pale pink   (2) Pearl pink/white   (3) Burgundy
(1) Pale yellow   (2) Cream   (3) Gold/bronze

Round eyes

1 The entire upper lid may be highlighted with a pale tone.
2 In a full lid socket emphasis may be softly applied to form a sweeping curve, echoing the brow line.
3 A fine dark line, or a more brightly coloured shadow line, can be applied close to the lashes.
4 The arched line of the brow can be accentuated with a pearl white or ivory toned highlighter.
5 A medium tone of the general shade may be applied at the outer corner to lengthen the eye shape and give an attractive profile appearance.
   Individual or false lashes to lengthen and thicken the lash line may be used, with the emphasis placed from the centre lids outwards.

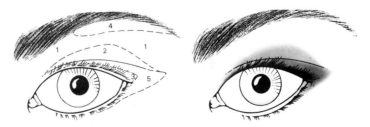

Colour suggestions
(1) Ivory   (2) Dark gold   (3) Gold/brown shadow or brown liner
(4) White or cream highlighter   (5) Cream/gold
(1) Pale pink   (2) Dark burgundy   (3) Grape shadow or liner
(4) White/pink pearl highlight   (5) Medium grape

Small eyes

1 Colour the entire lid with a bright but soft tone to enlarge the eye.
2 Accentuate the centre lid area with a more definite and slightly contrasting shade, blending in to give fullness to the lid.
3 Echo the brow line with a soft sweep of colour in a deeper but harmonising shade.

The outer lashes may be emphasised with mascara, and for the younger client false lashes may be applied at the outer corners.

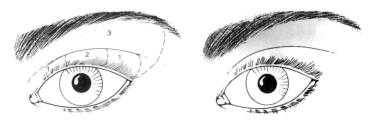

Colour suggestions
(1) White/pale blue (2) Violet (3) Blue/dove grey
(1) Soft yellow (2) Lime green (3) Greeny bronze

Overhanging lids

1 The inner eye corner may be highlighted with soft light colour, which can be repeated under the lower lashes.
2 The overhanging lid area can be subtly shaded to diminish its prominence with a matt-textured, deeper-toned shadow.
3 The under brow area may be highlighted to deflect interest from the overhanging lid.
4 A stronger line of colour close to the roots of the lashes may be applied to add vitality and definition to the eye.

Lashes may be emphasised with mascara to form a natural appearance.

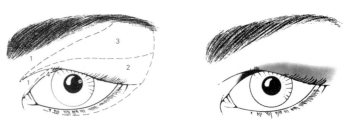

Colour suggestions
(1) Beige (2) Goldy/bronze (3) Ivory (4) Dark gold
(1) Pale aquamarine (2) Soft grey (3) White/grey
(4) Aquamarine

Close-set eyes

1 The entire orbital cavity area should be brought forward with a pale-coloured, soft-textured shadow, in a slightly oval shape.
2 A winging sweep of slightly darker, brighter shadow may be applied, commencing as a fine line, broadening into a wider curve.
3 The under-arch area of the brow may be highlighted with a light, bright, iridescent shadow to give a contrast of textures.

The sweeping brow line can be reinforced with fine, long individual false lashes applied to the outer third of the eye.

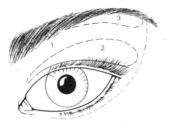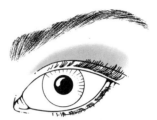

Colour suggestions
(1) Pale cream   (2) Russet brown   (3) Ivory/soft pearl highlighter
(1) Pale avocado green   (2) Brown/green
(3) Pale moss green highlighter

Prominent or heavy-lidded eyes

1 A sombre but rich shade of shadow should be applied to the upper lid to diminish the prominence of the eye.
2 The shape of the eye may be redefined by illuminating the brow bone area to deflect interest from the protruding lids. This colour may be reflected under the lower lashes, depending on the overall fullness of the eye in profile.

Natural lash emphasis is sufficient definition as over-heavy or curled lashes increase the rounded and prominent appearance of the eye.

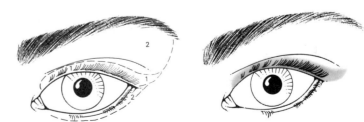

Colour suggestions
(1) Plum   (2) Medium pink
(1) Green/bronze   (2) Pale creamy green
(1) Grape/grey   (2) Pale grey

Lipstick choice and application for fashion, evening and photographic makeup

The intensity of lip colour must balance and be in harmony with the rest of the makeup. Artificial lighting tends to drain colour from the face, so sufficient brilliance is necessary to avoid an unfinished appearance. Working with soft but bright tones permits more improvement in mouth shape and gives definition to the lips.

Using variations in the texture of the lipstick can help to reduce or increase the apparent size of the mouth or improve the proportions of the lips to each other.

An over-large mouth

An over-large mouth should be made up with soft colours and a fairly matt lipstick consistency, otherwise it will tend to dominate the face. The lip line should be even, but not too hard, and kept well within the natural borders of the mouth. Every effort should be made to make up the face to deflect interest to the eyes or cheek bones, diminishing the importance of the lips in the overall effect.

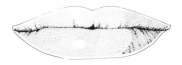

Uneven or small lips

Uneven or small lips can use matt and pearlised/glossy lipstick textures to give apparent fullness to central areas, or to regulate the different lip shapes. It is impossible to make a small mouth appear larger by painting the borders without it appearing obvious, but skilful use of colour can considerably improve the general appearance.

Lighter and darker tones, creamy and matt textures, lip gloss and outlining with lip pencils are all elements of technique available to the makeup artist to produce a more attractive lip appearance.

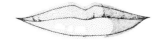

What makes a good makeup artist

All forms of cosmetic makeup can only be learnt by practice, experimentation and development of a good eye for colour and texture. Working with skilled photographic and makeup artists is the finest way to increase personal makeup talents, by first watching their interpretation and then developing personal techniques.

Within general therapy makeup is very important, as it shows the therapist's work to its best advantage to the client. The therapist needs to be a skilled makeup artist: the most immediate benefit of a facial is the improvement in appearance seen by the client, which comes from the makeup.

Makeup for the dark and non-European skin

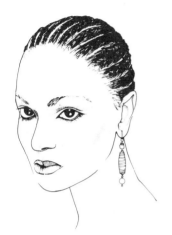

Makeup for dark skin

The varied nationality of clients coming for makeup presents a challenge to the makeup artist, where artistic ability is needed to produce flattering makeups that show the ethnic characteristics to best advantage. Although basic technique is similar, stronger colours and different textures will be needed to correct or enhance the darker skin tones.

Clients of African, Asian or Afro–Asian origin have different head and facial shapes as well as darker skin tones, and these form part of the total look. Concepts of beauty differ widely according to nationality, and through tactful questioning and observation an idea can be gained of the way a client would like to look, which shows her natural beauty to best advantage. Features such as a beautifully shaped head, attractive profile and large, brilliant eyes can then be emphasised.

Some clients will still strive to look European, preferring a lighter complexion and eye and lip colours more suited to a paler skin. Devising a makeup that combines the client's ethnic beauty with the sophisticated image she desires is a challenge for the makeup artist.

Ethnic characteristics

Points that should be considered include:

- Facial shapes.
- Bone structure.
- Shape of the head.
- Hair colour and texture.
- Skin colour, primary tones and shading needed.
- Skin sensitivity.
- Religious and cultural considerations affecting appearance.

Facial shapes/bone structure/shape of the head

- Diversity of facial shapes in the Afro–Asian races makes it impossible to record them as round, oval, square, etc.; rather the head shape should be noted (whether well shaped, etc.).
- The positioning of facial bones is different from that of European women, providing beautiful cheek contours, tilted back to above the eyes, which gives excellent opportunities for emphasis of the upper cheek and eye area.

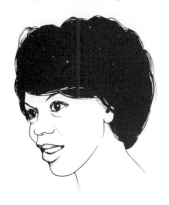

- The jaw bones may be more prominent in the African face, emphasising the larger mouth shape and giving a flatter nasal bridge.
- The Asian face is more oval, sometimes rather long and angular, with flatter planes across the cheek bones requiring a makeup to soften the contours.
- The Asian face has expressive features where the eyes dominate, being emphasised with kohl which adds to the exotic appearance.
- The Eastern face has an overhanging eye fold, flatter facial planes and a small nasal bridge to the nose.

Hair colour and texture

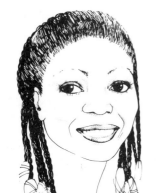

How the hair is worn and its physical appearance makes a lot of difference to makeup. Many Asian and Afro–Asian women have beautiful hair, which retains its sheen and colour well into middle age, and does not appear to go white as early as their European counterpart's. The deep blue–black colouring of the hair forms a dense contrast to the face, allowing richer makeup colours to be used without appearing brash or harsh.

Even when the hair is tightly curled or frizzy as in the negro woman, there is less inclination now to adopt European fashions by torturing the hair into smooth straightened styles. The natural shape of the head is shown or emphasised with beading, or plaiting.

Skin colours

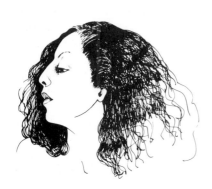

The colour range of African and Asian skins is vast and will be found to contain many primary tones when colour matching is attempted:

- Pale olive.
- Yellow.
- Greeny olive.
- Warm russet.
- Warm red/brown.
- Brown.
- Grey brown.
- Blue–black.

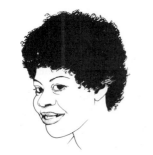

Although just as varied as paler skins, the deeper tones of the skin can act as a basic canvas, not needing to be covered but merely enhanced with makeup. Imperfections can appear less obvious in the darker skin. Where variations of tone do exist they normally show as patches of lighter pigmentation and different texture from the surrounding skin.

Vitiligo (loss of pigment) and patches of very dark pigmentation (of a satiny grey–black even blue–black appearance) can be seen on some African skins and require camouflage makeup to disguise them.

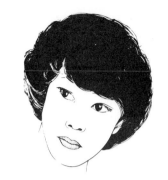

Melanin formation

Changes in the skin colour relate to the presence of melanin-forming (pigment) cells in the superficial skin tissues and irregularities in their behaviour (see Layers of the epidermis, Chapter 3). The number of melanin-forming cells, the melanocytes, is not thought to be more abundant in the coloured skin, but their production of melanin for protection is increased. So there are not more cells, but they are more efficient in providing protection against the ageing effects of sunlight.

Skin sensitivity

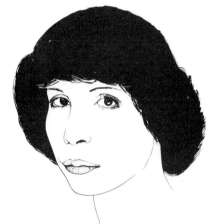

The darker skin often has a higher skin temperature and seems to produce more fluid oils on to its surface. It is often sensitive and liable to injury in treatment because the deeper skin colour disguises the fact that the skin is becoming irritated. Small temperature changes have to be noted through the hands and treatment adjusted. Routines that increase skin shedding should be applied with care (e.g. biological peeling or abrasive masks designed to remove the dead and scarred surface tissue).

Scarring can also occur as a response to injury or from deep-seated infection. Grazing can result in keloid scarring, which forms slowly and becomes apparent some time after the injury has healed superficially. Keloids can form sinewy cords of scar tissue around a damaged area and are extremely disfiguring and difficult to disguise by camouflage methods.

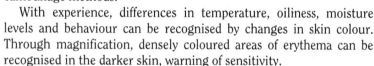

With experience, differences in temperature, oiliness, moisture levels and behaviour can be recognised by changes in skin colour. Through magnification, densely coloured areas of erythema can be recognised in the darker skin, warning of sensitivity.

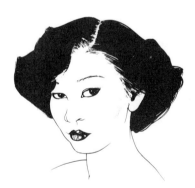

Stretch marks or lines show as changes in texture and elasticity, assuming a silvery and soft skin appearance. These may be visible on the upper breasts and other areas of the body.

Higher skin temperature and oiliness can result in blemishes or a dull, sallow skin colour. In very dark skins this gives the face an ashen, dull look as if the skin were coated. Careful and thorough skin cleansing is needed to refine the skin and corrective makeup should be applied.

Religious and cultural considerations

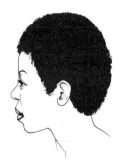

Many of the aspects of facial adornment have a religious significance, particularly in Asian women, and some knowledge of this should prove useful. Adornment of the face and body is a very old art and has a history in many cultures far more ancient than our own.

Makeup choice

Foundations

A wider range of darker colours is gradually becoming available, with useful products being found amongst custom-blended foundations, cosmetic camouflage products and stage makeup ranges. Foundations should be finely textured, suited to skin type and chosen to enhance natural skin colour. Some considerations are:

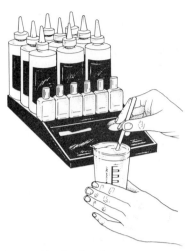

Custom blending foundation

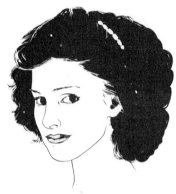

Foundations look quite different on the skin from in the container, as the darker base colour of the skin alters the shade actually seen within makeup. So always try the product on the client. Even transparent/translucent products do not always produce the expected results, being primarily designed to be applied over a pale skin. Some disappear into the skin without trace, others look very obvious and unattractive on the darker skin. Bronzing powders like golden dust, earth dust, etc. can look very attractive brushed lightly over a finished makeup to give texture and life.

- If the skin has yellow undertones, beige-tinted foundation can be used to enhance these whilst reducing red or warm tones in the skin.
- Grey, ashen skin with a purplish sheen which makes an individual look old and drained can be brightened and the colour corrected with warm beige, rose beige foundation or use of a tinted moisture base in apricot or peach.
- Creamy skin tones with just a hint of greeny yellow (Japanese and Chinese skin colours) are difficult to match, but often prefer to look lighter than they are, so porcelain and creamy beige foundations can be used.
- Blue–black skins which really need colours of the plum and magenta type to show off their richness and beauty are also difficult to match and transparent products should be used.
- Afro–Asian skins often need no tinted foundation or powder, as they have an even base tone. Yellow, red, russet, olive or grey undertones may need correcting, to brighten the complexion and even out colour differences around the face.
- If foundation is even slightly too pale, or too thickly applied on the darker skin, it will appear to stand away from the face.
- Where the skin has even colour naturally, no foundation need be applied and translucent shaders, shapers and highlighters can be used to emphasise the beauty of the bone structure.
- Unevenness of skin colour around the face, darker or lighter patches and shadowing around the eyes can be camouflaged at the primary stage of the makeup. A light touch is needed, otherwise attention is drawn to the fault rather than away from it.
- Reddish purple darkening around the eyes (seen in older Asian women) can be concealed effectively with lighter foundation (or concealer) and by deflecting interest away from the eye skin area.
- Transparent products show off and enhance the colour rather than hide it. They are ideal on the darker skin if it is clear and free from scars.

If used, face powder should be neutral in colour and of the loose type, fluffed very lightly over the face. It tends to flatten the effect of foundation used and can give a dull lifeless look to the face.

Highlighters and shaders

The basic principle of light shades bringing a feature forward and darker tones making it appear less obvious still apply on a dark skin, though different colours have to be used to achieve the effects. More

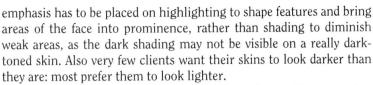

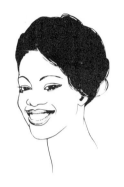

emphasis has to be placed on highlighting to shape features and bring areas of the face into prominence, rather than shading to diminish weak areas, as the dark shading may not be visible on a really dark-toned skin. Also very few clients want their skins to look darker than they are: most prefer them to look lighter.

Slimming the nose is useful in the negro face, with contouring cream or darker foundation applied down the sides of the face, and a paler shade or highlighter used to straighten and slim the centre of the nose. This gives elegance and diminishes the broadness of the nostrils.

For day makeup, correction of the features is rather limited, as much of the correction would be obvious on close scrutiny, but for photographic makeup or modelling, a lot of correction is possible and effective.

Slimming the round or heavy-jawed face requires darker contouring creams applied down the sides of the lower cheek and jawline and highlighting of the upper cheek bone area.

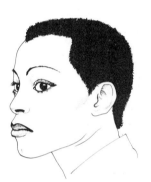

Blushers

The blusher needs to be non-greasy, a creamy gel/fluid, or finely textured powder, otherwise it will appear to 'sit' on top of the skin. The peachy, pink colours most widely available are not really useful on the darker skin and deeper colours have to be sought, e.g. wine, plum, deep soft rose, etc. These may be found amongst lip glosses (in pots), from facial or eye makeup pencils or from stage makeup lines. As all makeup these days is very interchangeable in application, this is acceptable. Gradually colour ranges are growing to accommodate the darker-skinned client.

Lip colour

Deep lip tones, sometimes almost purple on the negro mouth, need correction and clear yellow-toned shades picked to make the mouth appear less large and dark lipped. Transparent lip tints are very useful but should not be too glossy and liquid or the mouth becomes too prominent in the face.

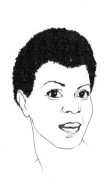

Flattering colours for darker-skinned clients include subtle rose reds, dusky pinks, plums and muted red golds. All look delightful with the darker skin contrast. Harsh, over-vivid or pale colours should be avoided if a natural effect is to be maintained. If the mouth colour and shape is attractive as it is, then lip gloss may be all that is required.

Eye makeup

All the normal crayons, eye pencils, powder shadows and eye glosses can be used to shade the eye and give it prominence.

- The deeper toned the skin is, the richer can be the eye makeup worn. Intense, deep, glowing colours rather than light, vivid ones should be chosen.
- Often the eye is prominent enough without a lot of added colour, but needs definition and lash emphasis to exaggerate the contrast of the eyes against the dark skin.

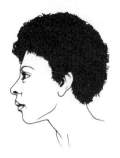

- Ivory and creamy gold are useful neutral colours which show up well on the darker client.
- Translucent tints of pink and plum are also effective, apart from when the skin tends towards this colour naturally, when it should be avoided.
- Younger coloured and negro women can wear primary colours very effectively to create fashion fantasies, but this must be balanced by the rest of the makeup.
- Eye emphasis around the lashes can be from kohl, or a liner dark enough to show against the skin colour – possibly in dark blue, deep green, etc. Lashes can be emphasised in the normal way and are often a feature of the face.

Cosmetic camouflage

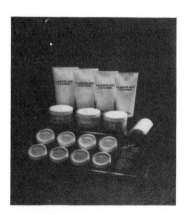

Special cosmetic products are available to the beauty therapist for camouflage work. Faces can be changed, moles, birthmarks and pigmentation abnormalities disguised, and scarring from acne and skin grafts improved with camouflage. Badly damaged faces can be restored after accidents and burns and surgical treatment is completed by skilful application of cosmetic camouflage from a camouflage expert. Blemishes on all parts of the body that cause distress, such as split capillaries, naevi, etc., can be treated in the same way to good effect.

The cosmetic camouflage expert is a beauty therapist who has had special training and experience in the art of masking skin imperfections of all kinds. A sound knowledge of skin conditions and the ranges of camouflage products available is needed. The price and value of the items will be important as, although remedial in effect, the cosmetic masking may have to be purchased by the patient as it is not necessarily covered by medical insurance. In the United Kingdom camouflage cosmetics are available on the National Health Service through prescription, but at the discretion of the individual hospital authorities.

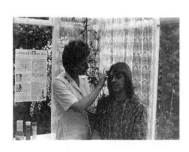

Special training is necessary within the hospital situation to develop the techniques of camouflage procedures. The techniques use the minimum of ordinary makeup combined with masking products to achieve a natural skin colour and texture, completely disguising the imperfection. The effect of the blemish on the patient may also have resulted in a condition of severe psychological stress, making instruction and co-operation difficult.

Application

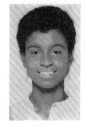

The camouflage technique uses a number of differently coloured, opaque covering creams, which are non-irritant and have a matt finish.

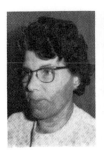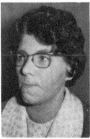

They are durable and allow the skin to perspire normally, permitting extended periods of wear without ill effect.

These masking agents are blended on to the skin to achieve a perfect match with the surrounding area and then set with a special untinted, unperfumed finishing powder. A wide range of colours can be mixed to achieve perfect colour results on all skin colours, including dark skins.

Men can match their complexions, changing the colour blend as the natural skin deepens in the sun. Natural shadows, freckles, and beard growth can be balanced.

Once the correct blend of preparations has been determined by the camouflage expert, the patient is taught the sequence. Application at home should not take more than a few minutes, after practice, and it should last all day as the majority of products are waterproof.

A successful change in appearance can sometimes be a starting point for a new approach to life for many patients, and has great psychological benefit .

Self check

1 State the factors that should be considered when selecting makeup for the following:
   (a) A mature client, day and evening makeup.
   (b) A greasy skin, day and evening makeup.
   (c) A black skin, day and evening makeup.
   (d) A hypersensitive skin, day and evening makeup.

2 With the aid of diagrams, describe how to apply corrective makeup for the following:
   (a) Round eyes.
   (b) Close set eyes.
   (c) Overhanging lids.
   (d) A long, narrow nose.
   (e) A double chin.
   (f) Uneven lips.

3 What considerations should be given when choosing colours for an evening makeup?

4 Why is it advisable to apply lipstick with a lip brush?

5 Explain how cross infection can be avoided when using:
   (a) Lipsticks.
   (b) Eye pencils.
   (c) Eye shadows.
   (d) Mascara.

6 What special considerations must be observed when carrying out makeup on the following:
   (a) A client who wears glasses?
   (b) A client who wears contact lenses?

CHAPTER NINE

Electrical Treatment

Indications for electrical treatment

The decision to use electrical equipment in the facial sequence will be based on:

- The existing skin condition.
- The effect of the specific electrical treatment.
- The skin's response to previous manual or electrical treatment.
- The temperament and wishes of the client.

Electrical treatment speeds the rate at which skin improvement or correction of existing problems can be accomplished. It adds variety to treatment and provides effects that cannot be duplicated manually or cosmetically, such as:

- Fast stimulation of circulation.
- Toning of skin and muscles.
- Chemical reactions on the skin.
- Germicidal, drying and healing actions.
- Deep skin cleansing.
- Changes in skin colour (tanning).
- Changes in the skin's pH.

Equipment may be used at any convenient stage of the routine, according to its effect and the result required. To save time, a logical sequence is followed.

Equipment with cleansing and stimulation effects should be applied early in the routine, prior to the mask, and may replace the manual massage.

Toning, refining, drying or germicidal effects are most beneficial after, or instead of, a mask when the skin is really clean and calm.

Equipment with a two-fold action, i.e. cleansing and germicidal, may be placed with convenience and time considerations in mind. The skin reaction to treatment – which rules what may be applied – will dictate the most suitable stage within the facial routine.

Choice of electrical treatment

Electrical equipment can be applied in a wide range of treatment combinations, and these will be considered in Chapter 10, Treatment

Plans. Here we will look at the actions, contra-indications and applications of the main systems of equipment:

- Steaming/ozone steaming.
- Vibratory treatment.
- Brush massage.
- Vacuum/suction massage.
- Muscle toning.
- High frequency.
- Ultraviolet treatment.
- Galvanic treatment.

All equipment has some specific contra-indications which limit its application, and these have to be known. They are matched against the client's details by tactful questioning and observation of the skin.

There are also some general contra-indications that limit the use of equipment, or require it to be adapted in the treatment. These common sense considerations are for the client's safety and well being, which should be explained when checking her personal/health details.

General contra-indications to electrical treatment

1 Clients of an extremely nervous disposition.
2 Hypersensitive skin, prone to allergic reaction.
3 Diabetic clients, due to the skin's instability and poor healing abilities (medical approval may allow adapted treatment to be possible to balance and maintain skin texture).
4 Skin infection, sepsis and inflammation (adolescent skin conditions may be treated with medical approval).
5 Sinus conditions, where treatment could cause discomfort.
6 A large number of fillings in the teeth or bridge work in dentures would alter or prohibit many electrical applications in the area of the mouth.
7 Extremely vascular skin conditions, where the capillaries have dilated and ruptured to form a widespread varicose appearance.
8 When the client is undergoing medical treatment for a general condition, approval must be sought prior to therapy applications, e.g. high blood pressure, asthmatic conditions.
9 The latter stages of pregnancy.
10 Epileptics. Mild controlled forms (*petit mal*) may have superficial forms of treatment, i.e. vibrators, wax masks, etc., but are contra-indicated for treatments involving current flowing through the skin's surface, or where discomfort is present, as this could precipitate an attack.
11 Migraine sufferers should be treated with caution.
12 Clients who have a heart pacemaker should not have any treatment which imparts an electrical current into the body.

Safety points in the application of electrical treatment

The protection and safety of the client is the primary concern of the facial therapist. Following the correct safety precautions will eliminate accidents, increase efficiency and assure greater client satisfaction.

Location of equipment

1 Equipment should be conveniently placed for safe application on the right or left side of the therapist, according to her natural dexterity.
2 The therapist should be able to perform the treatment satisfactorily with an adequate range of movement and support to ensure client safety and achieve results.
3 Lead connections to the mains supply must be positioned so that they do not become overstretched or disconnected from the sockets. Long trailing leads must be avoided to prevent accidents from clients or therapists tripping.
4 Leads from equipment should not be allowed to trail along metal parts of couches, facial chairs, lounges, etc. Static electricity can build up and discharge unexpectedly on contact causing discomfort or an accident.

Choice, maintenance and use of equipment

1 Well-made, sturdy equipment should be chosen, as the therapist is very dependent on their constant performance and repairing these sophisticated machines is a specialist task.
2 The performance required from the equipment needs to be considered prior to purchase. Heavy-duty clinic models should be chosen to avoid overheating or strain being placed on motors unsuited for the task.
3 The equipment should be well maintained and correctly wired with a proper earth connection. If there is no earth connection, it should be double insulated and this is symbolised by ▣ on the rating plate. Equipment should be ready for use before starting the facial routine, and tested for intermittent performance prior to the client's arrival. Equipment may differ in its wiring and earthing, depending on the safety/quality standards of the country of origin. It should be checked by a qualified electrician if there is any doubt as to its safety, or to avoid it causing interference to other electrical fittings in the proximity,i.e. display lights, etc.
4 The therapist must be familiar with the treatment application, the safety routine and special points relating to the specific method to be applied.

5 The machine should be left ready for the next treatment after the conclusion of the routine, with controls at zero and mains connections off (unless the machine is required again immediately).

6 The machines should be moved as little as possible to prolong their working life and to prevent intermittent performance due to loose or worn connections. Home visiting or mobile beauty specialists should obtain robust equipment especially designed for being transported.

Steaming

Steaming (without ozone) can form part of a facial treatment. It is normally applied for 10 minutes at an early stage of the routine, in association with cleansing. Ozone steaming is corrective in action and plays an important role in the treatment of acne, seborrhoea and oily skin (see Chapter 10, Treatment Plans).

Equipment

Equipment normally provides for both steaming with purified water and ozone steaming. Ozone is produced in the head of the equipment by a reaction between ultraviolet light and water. Water passes over an ultraviolet lamp and becomes ionised to form ozone. The ultraviolet light is produced by a quartz tube high-pressure mercury lamp.

General effects of steaming

- Relaxing.
- Skin softening.
- Cleansing/desquamating.
- Induces perspiration.
- Increases local skin temperature/colour.
- Gently stimulating.

Effects of ozone steaming

- Drying.
- Healing action on blemished skin.
- Anti-bacterial.
- Oxygen formation on the skin.
- Balances pH of skin.
- Stimulating.
- Irritating.

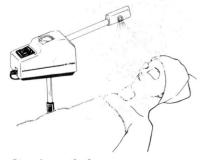

Steaming on the face

Ozone, and the active oxygen produced by its decomposition, destroy organic substances and bacteria. Ozone steaming is a means of activating the circulation of the subcutaneous vessels and providing them with oxygen. The increased blood circulation caused permits the effects of the ozone to act not only on the surface of the epidermis but also in the cutaneous tissues. The physiological actions include:

- The heating action of the ionised water vapour.
- The action of the ozone and its derivatives.
- The action of the ultraviolet radiation arising from decomposition of the ozone.

Indications for steaming

1 Normal skin conditions, to maintain skin texture (application 10 minutes at approx. 30 cm (12 inches).
2 Dehydrated/dry skin conditions, to stimulate the skin (application 5 minutes on the neck and 3–4 on the face, at approx. 38 cm (15 inches).
3 Mature skin conditions for gentle stimulation (application 3–6 minutes at approx. 38 cm (15 inches).

Contra-indications to steaming

- Skin infection.
- Vascular or hypersensitive skin.
- Sunburn.
- Sinus blockage.

Indications for ozone steaming

1 Normal/combination skin, maintenance and correction of pH balance (application 10 minutes at approx. 38 cm (15 inches).
2 Seborrhoea and blemished skin conditions, to heal and disinfect the skin (application 15–25 minutes at approx. 25 cm (10 inches).

Contra-indications to ozone steaming

- Hypersensitive skin.
- Extremely vascular complexions.
- Acne rosacea.
- Sunburn or previous ultraviolet exposure.
- Skin irritation, abrasions, etc.

Application

Equipment preparation

Position the steamer close to the client chair, prior to her arrival, and check the water container for sufficient purified water to complete the treatment, and fill up if necessary.

Check the connections and switch on 10 minutes before the steaming is needed. The vapour switch only is required at this stage in steamers which also have the ozone facility. Check that the unit is actually heating and position the steamer ready to use, but with its applicator arm turned away from the client.

When vapour starts discharging from the head of the equipment, ozone production may be added to the process by switching on the ozone control. A blue light becomes evident in the head of the steamer and the steam becomes ionised, cloud-like and very fine in appearance.

Client preparation

- Allow the steamer to heat whilst preparing the client, i.e. cleansing the skin, etc. When it starts to steam, switch it off until needed.
- The client is placed in a semi-reclining position and eyes and sensitive skin areas are protected with cotton wool pads. The head is covered to protect it from moisture.
- The sensation that the client will experience should be explained, especially if ozone steam is the chosen method, as it has an unusual smell.
- The steamer is switched back on and positioned so that the steam flows over the face or neck.
- Apply the steam for the required period according to skin condition, adjusting it as necessary to cover different parts of the neck and face. Watch the skin for reaction, checking periodically.
- If ozone steaming is the chosen method, it may be switched on at this point. Ozone is produced and oxygen forms on the skin's surface.
- When the required action has been achieved, the steamer may be turned off and turned away from the client, ready for removal after treatment finishes. The client's eye pads are removed.
- Surface skin moisture may be blotted off and the appropriate cream or mask applied.
- With the skin wet from the steaming, vacuum suction may be applied as part of the deep cleansing pore treatment, using the moisture as the massage medium.

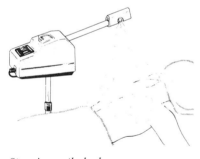

Steaming on the back

Treatment points

- Younger clients may have ozone steaming at frequent intervals to control and heal blemished areas of the face and back. The multi-positioning possible with modern steamers means that steam can be directed at an angle, allowing the back to be treated without risk of scalding or drips.

- Steaming is incorporated into many facial routines and ozone steaming forms part of ozone therapy (see Chapter 10, Treatment Plans).
- Vapour should always be flowing over the ultraviolet lamp whilst it is on, as this prolongs the lamp's life.
- Casual use of ozone steaming should be avoided. It has very beneficial effects on the right skin condition, but is destructive in action and can irritate the skin if wrongly applied.
- The operator should avoid exposing her own eyes to the ozone steam whilst applying treatment. Although the beauty therapist should remain in close proximity to the client, it is not necessary to remain close to the steam itself. Irritation of the cornea of the eye could result from continuous exposure to ozone.
- Ordinary steaming is applied only for short periods in the modern facial, for, though relaxing, its effects of skin softening, etc., can easily be duplicated within facial routines. It is unnecessary and impractical to allocate 15–20 minutes to steaming out of a one-hour facial routine.
- Ozone equipment is prohibited in some countries, due to the carcinogenic risk to the therapist resulting from the positively ionised air. Although medical authorities regard ozone steaming as a health risk for the therapist, it is still one of the most widely used treatments in the beauty industry. Therapists must check their position with local public health authorities.

Vibratory treatment

Facial vibrators produce a succession of mechanical manipulations or vibrations which copy or replace the effects of manual massage. Vibratory treatments are useful to bring fast stimulation to an area, gives variety to routines and is popular with clients.

Equipment

Percussion and audio-sonic vibrators
Percussion vibrations produce simple mechanical vibrations of low penetration and audio-sonic vibrations produce vibrations in the same sound field on the soft tissues of the body. Audio-sonic vibrations have a deeper effect on the tissues, associated with reduced sensation on the skin's surface. This extends their use to mature and delicate skin without causing discomfort or irritation. It also allows them to be applied on muscular tension where pain is present.

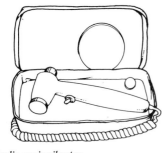

Audio-sonic vibrator

General effects

- Stimulating effect on vascular and lymphatic circulation.
- Superficial effect, low penetration power on subcutaneous tissues (percussion).

- Increases local skin temperature and colour (erythema).
- Does not obtain a muscular contraction, although relaxed muscles could be considered increased in tone or condition.
- No chemical formation on the skin's surface.
- Relaxation of tense muscle fibres (audio-sonic).

Indications for vibratory treatment

Percussion vibrators
1 Dry, dehydrated skin conditions (general stimulation).
2 Normal skins (maintenance purposes).
3 Mature skin (regeneration).
4 General relaxation, on the face, shoulders, upper back and limbs, and to prevent formation of fibrous thickenings and tension/pain developing.

Audio-sonic vibrators
1 Delicate, sensitive skins (gentle stimulation without irritation).
2 Mature skin with vascularity or loose skin texture (gentle stimulation/regeneration action).
3 Stiffness, discomfort or tension in the upper back and neck, where the slight impairment of sensation produced by audio-sonic allows it to be applied to relax the muscles, without causing discomfort to the client.

Contra-indications for vibratory treatment

- Extremely vascular skin conditions.
- Inflammation, sepsis, skin irritation.
- Recent scar tissue.
- Skin infection.
- Sinus blockage (which causes discomfort).
- Extremely bony facial areas should be avoided, especially with audio-sonic.
- Severe muscular pain or inflammation should be directed for medical attention.

Application

Equipment preparation
The chosen system of vibrations is made with the correct applicator head:

- Sponge heads (percussion) and flat disc (audio-sonic) for general facial and neck massage.
- Hard surface discs (percussion) and round, hard applicators (audio-sonic) where intensified action is required (around joints or where muscular tension is present).

- Hedgehog-type applicators (percussion and audio-sonic) are used mainly for scalp massage or where an extreme desquamating effect is needed (rough skin texture or post-acne scarring on the back).

Client preparation

The client's skin is cleansed and brought to the massage stage. According to the effect required, either cream or talc is used as a medium for the massage and the routine applied in the pattern of strokes shown. The application follows the facial contours, avoiding bony areas (these areas can be treated indirectly with the vibrator used

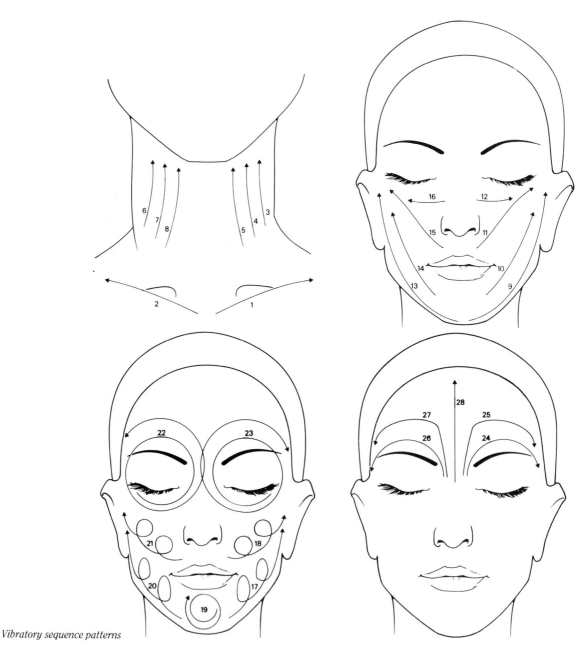

Vibratory sequence patterns

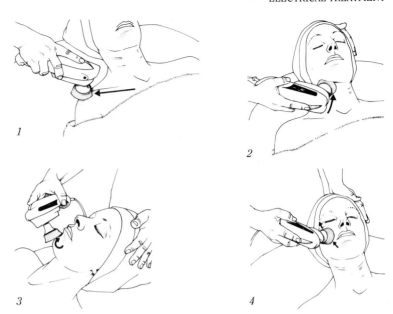

Vibratory treatment: direct application

over the back of the hand). Strokes should be applied smoothly, with minimal breaks in skin contact at the established rate for general massage. Straight and circular movements may be alternated.

Skin warmth and erythema should be watched for on every occasion, as their occurrence can depend on internal and external factors. Only gentle stimulation is needed, and this will be possible within 5–15 minutes, as vibrations provide a faster response than manual methods.

The routine can be adjusted to skin need, and at conclusion the cream or talc is removed and the treatment progresses to the next stage in the facial.

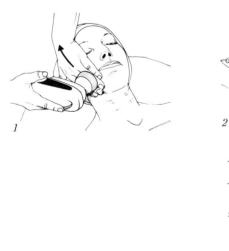

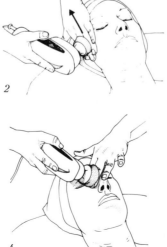

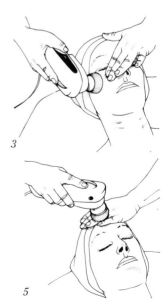

Vibratory treatment: indirect application

Treatment points

- Small, motor-driven vibrators (where the motor is in the head of the equipment) should not be used continuously for more than 20 minutes or overheating will result and the life of the unit will be shortened.
- The applicator heads should be cleaned (washed) and sterilised after use using cold water methods (such as Savlon concentrate, diluted to suitable proportions) and then kept in a sterile container until required.
- Sponge applicators need to be washed and dried very thoroughly, and can be lightly powdered to keep them in good condition. Ideally they should only be used with talcum powder as the massage medium.
- All preparations must be removed from the rubber applicators or they will perish, or shed, as well as be a source of cross infection in the clinic.
- Applicators cannot be sterilised by the autoclave method, due to the high temperatures involved, which would destroy them.

Brush massage

Brush massage is a more stimulating form of massage which provides for variation within facial treatment. Although better known as a cleansing system it can be combined within a range of facial applications or built up into a complete massage treatment, replacing manual massage.

General effects

- Fast stimulation of vascular circulation.
- Increased desquamation (skin shedding).
- Increased skin temperature and colour (erythema).

Indications for brush massage

1 Normal, dry, dehydrated and mature skin conditions.
2 Removal of abrasive masks.

Contra-indications for brush massage

- Sensitive/vascular skins.
- Skin infection.
- Skin irritation.
- Sunburn.
- Loose skin conditions.

Application

Equipment preparation

The applicator head is chosen to meet the skin condition and task:

- Soft bristle brushes are used for general facial and back applications.
- Sponge applicators (where available) provide a gentle alternative to soft brushes.
- Firmer bristle brushes are used for stimulating massage and abrasive mask work.
- Pumice blocks are used for abrasive mask removal on the post-acne scarred skin.

The equipment is checked for performance and the chosen brush firmly connected to the applicator head. The brush equipment is placed in readiness and should be accessible to the working position, so that the application can be given without leads trailing over the client in the course of the routine.

Client preparation

The skin is cleansed with brush or manually according to sensitivity, and treatment proceeds to the massage stage of the facial. Brush massage can be combined with manual massage or replace it. A generous amount of cream suited to the skin type should be applied to the treatment area. The massage may also be applied using talc as a medium, if the skin is of the more oily/combination type.

- The application is applied to the pattern of vibratory strokes, using flowing and circular strokes.
- The therapist keeps a sponge in her other hand to protect eye and mouth areas, etc.
- The brush is lightly held against the skin and parallel to it, avoiding jarring on the bones.
- The brush revolves lightly over the skin, no pressure is needed. Some equipment can revolve clockwise and anticlockwise.
- The speed can be adjusted on the equipment, and should be chosen to suit the skin type and its firmness. Drag should be avoided.
- The colour and the warmth of the skin should be watched as treatment proceeds to avoid over-stimulation.

Abrasive peeling treatment

The foam applicator, special firm brushes or a pumice stone applicator are used to remove the abrasive or peeling mask. Used on the scarred, horny, post-acne skin condition, the action can be varied by removing the mask whilst still moist or allowing the mask to set before removal. Changing the applicator used from the soft sponges or moist brushes to the firmer brushes or pumice blocks, allows the treatment to increase progressively in effect, avoiding overreaction.

Indications for treatment

1 Uneven skin texture on the face, back and upper arms.
2 Discoloured skin areas.
3 Scar tissue.
4 Sallow, blocked and seborrhoea skin conditions.

Contra-indications

- Sensitive skins, dehydrated and mature skins.
- Skin infection.

Application

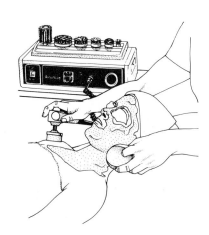

- After the cleansing stage, the abrasive powder is mixed into a fine paste with water and applied as a mask over the entire face or affected areas only.
- For normal skins the paste may be thin in consistency and removed whilst still damp using a moistened sponge applicator, applied at medium speed.
- For thickened oily skin, the mask should be permitted to dry, and removal completed the same way.
- Scar tissue may require more extensive treatment, the second or third mask removal accomplished using the pumice block or firm brush applicator to replace the sponge applicator for greater effect.
- No pressure should be used during the removal; the rotating head provides all the action needed.
- Skin reaction should be watched carefully and will depend on the skin type and the method of removal used. Caution is needed to avoid grazing.
- A moistened sponge guards the eyes and lips from the mask, and then is used to removed the residue of the mask from the skin.
- Hydrating and regenerating products are then applied in the form of masks or creams.
- No makeup should be worn after the abrasive mask treatment.

Treatment points

The applicator brushes and sponge heads should be washed and dried carefully after use and stored in a sterilising cabinet. All cream, oil, etc. must be removed thoroughly with liquid soap solution prior to the sterilisation sequence. Twenty minutes in a vapour sterilising cabinet will prepare the brushes for further use.

In a busy clinic situation, spare brush sets are a great convenience, allowing time for washing and sterilisation procedures.

Facial vacuum/suction treatment

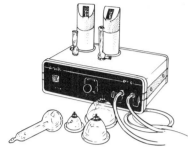

Vacuum unit

Vacuum massage increases the lymphatic and vascular circulation, and is applied following the pattern of the lymphatic nodes of the face. Straight strokes are used in a light, upward lifting manner to encourage lymphatic drainage.

The improvement in skin function and elimination created is used in a range of skin conditions, from the oily blemished skin to the mature skin needing regeneration. Vacuum suction is both cleansing and stimulating in action so is normally applied after cleansing (and steaming/galvanic desincrustation on the oily skin) or is applied as part of the massage stage.

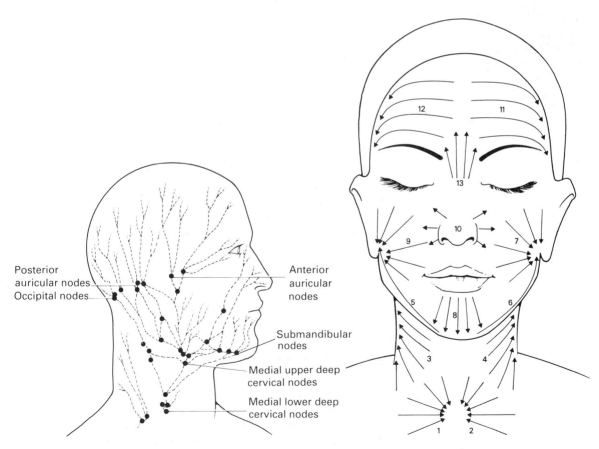

Lymphatic nodes of the face and neck   *Pattern of facial vacuum strokes*

General effects

The fluid in the minute lymph spaces drains quickly, because the small ducts are emptied under pressure and blockages are released. This evokes a vigorous response from the circulation and increased skin temperature and colour (erythema).

Dead skin cells on the surface are released, the skin texture is refined and fine lines are temporarily eased.

Indications for treatment

1 Normal skins, for deep cleansing and gentle stimulation purposes.
2 Oily and blemished skin, providing specialised cleansing when used in combination with ozone steaming and galvanic desincrustation.
3 Dry, dehydrated skins to stimulate the circulation, improve cellular regeneration, delaying ageing signs.
4 Mature skins, used carefully to maintain skin firmness and delay the formation of lines.
5 On ageing skin, to help to prevent the slowing down of skin shedding that can lead to thickened menopausal skin problems around the mouth and chin.

Contra-indications for treatment

Vacuum is sometimes used within treatment of the vascular skin but in a very specific way (see Chapter 10, Treatment Plans).

- Hypersensitive skin, due to the danger of overstimulation and possible capillary damage (bruising).
- Crepey, loose skin conditions, where folds of skin exist.
- Infected acne conditions where secondary infection of the follicle is present, due both to the discomfort caused and the risk of spreading the problem.
- Very fine areas of skin texture around the eyes, where bruising could occur.
- Dilated capillaries on the upper cheeks.

Application

Equipment preparation
Applicators come in a range of sizes and apertures (openings) to create different effects in treatment. Reduced pressure is formed within the glass or plastic cups (*ventouses*) when they are in complete contact with the skin. This lifts and stimulates the skin tissue throughout the stroke applied. The vacuum intensity must be adjusted to the skin reaction and should not exceed a 10% lift into the cup, otherwise capillary damage and bruising could occur. The natural elasticity of the skin alters the amount of resistance the skin presents, and alters the manner in which treatment is applied.

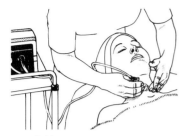

General skin treatment

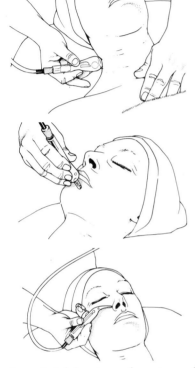

Adjusting the effect

Before applying the vacuum treatment on the client's skin, its degree of pressure should be carefully checked on a soft area of the therapist's skin and adjustments made. A reduction in effect can be made by:

- Decreasing the control on the equipment (reduces vacuum).
- Choosing an applicator with a smaller aperture (opening).
- Applying the strokes more swiftly, restricting the vacuum build-up in the cups.

Choice of applicator

The small applicators/ventouses can be used for a variety of different conditions, according to the lift into the cup produced on the skin. As guidance:

- Applicators with 5 cm openings are suitable for the neck and firm skin on the face (with very low levels of vacuum).
- Shaped, narrow applicators with very small openings are suitable for work on blocked pores, fine lines and sensitive skin areas (using higher levels of vacuum).
- Flattened shaped applicators with narrow openings are used for lines, flexure folds, etc. to ease lines temporarily.
- Larger diameter cups with wider openings (10 cm and above) are used on the upper chest and back areas where adequate subcutaneous tissue is present. Low levels of vacuum are used.

Concentrated cleansing on the centre panel

Client preparation

- The vacuum or suction massage is applied on a clean skin previously prepared with a fine tissue oil, to allow easy flowing strokes without skin drag. Alternatively it is applied on a film of steam, within oily skin treatment plans (see Chapter 10, Treatment Plans).
- The pattern commences at the neck, with the speed and vacuum adjusted to the skin reaction observed. Avoid overlapping strokes or bruising will result.
- The routine progresses up the face, following the pattern shown, concluding between the eyebrows if a general sequence only is to be applied.
- Specialised work with small aperture applicators can follow on the centre panel to help release trapped sebum (previously softened and released by steaming and galvanic routines). Higher levels of vacuum/lift into the cup can be used.
- Work on the flexure/expression lines can be applied on the forehead, from the nose to the mouth, and around the lips themselves. The small, flattened applicators are used carefully, just two to three strokes on each line, with low vacuum/lift into the cup.
- Once the vacuum treatment concludes, the oil is removed and treatment progresses to the next stage within the facial.

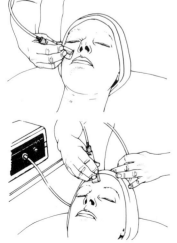

Lifting vacuum massage on wrinkles

Treatment points

Only lifting, not downwards pressure, is used to apply the vacuum massage. Skin contact is broken at the end of the stroke by either releasing the pressure by removing the finger covering the small hole in the cup, or quickly breaking contact with a neat, flicking movement of the wrist.

Small shaped applicators should be protected by cotton wool inside to prevent oil travelling up the tubes into the equipment. This must be removed prior to washing and replaced just prior to use. Some cups have filters incorporated into their design to prevent this occurrence.

Pulsed air – vacuum massage

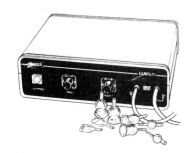

Pulsed air/tapping massage equipment

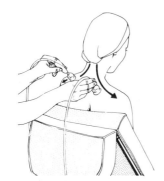

Back treatment

Equipment

Vacuum massage is also available in a pulsed or tapping form, where vacuum alternates with gentle air pressure against the skin.

- Two applicators are used in unison to create gentle stimulation of the skin.
- The treatment is applied towards the lymphatic nodes to encourage lymphatic drainage.
- The pulsed air effect makes the routine easy to apply, with less risk of skin distension or bruising occurring from poor technique. This allows the sensitive and mature skins to be treated at less risk.
- Treatment is normally developed into a routine incorporating the upper back and neck, and is applied after cleansing, prior to, or replacing part of, the massage.

The rhythm of the pressure and vacuum impulses can be infinitely varied. Treatment can start with vigorous tapping massage, with a rhythm of 4–5 impulses per second on skin needing a stimulating and toning effect, and then change gradually to a gentle massage effect on the face.

Application

- Treatment should ideally commence on the upper back, working downwards from the occipital cavity at the base of the skull to the shoulders.
- Strokes are applied using the large ventouses, following the trapezius muscle fibres, using smooth unbroken strokes alternated with circular strokes, following the same path.
- When sufficient skin reaction has been achieved, the client is re-positioned, rests back in the chair and treatment moves to the

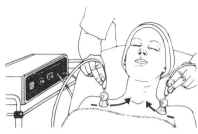

Decolletage

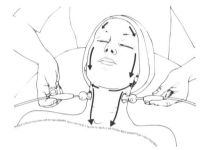

General lymphatic drainage method

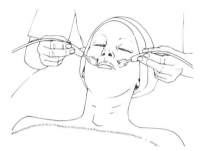

Special treatment of wrinkles and flexure lines

decolletage (upper breast and neck area). If the upper back cannot be included in the routine, this is where treatment will commence.

- Changing to a lower intensity (reducing the vacuum), the upper breast and sternum area is treated with alternating smooth and circular movements.
- The sternomastoid muscle area comes next, using a smaller pair of ventouses, and regulating the vacuum as necessary. The movements work downwards from behind the ears, towards the natural indentation at the base of the throat. Care must be taken to avoid pressure on the trachea (windpipe).
- The area under the mandible follows, with the hands working in unison or alternately. The movement works from the point of the mandible bone to behind the ear and then down to the clavicle following the previous pattern on the neck. This is easier to apply one hand at a time initially, blocking the pressure of the unused applicator with a thumb or fingers, allowing the working applicator to make full contact and build vacuum.
- Treatment moves to the borders of the face, starting at the temples, passing in front of the ears, and down to the clavicle as before. A slight change in the stroke pattern allows the upper cheeks to be avoided if contra-indicated. The size of the ventouses may need changing at this stage, depending on the size of the client's features and skin condition.
- Forehead strokes are applied following the pattern of lymphatic drainage established down to the clavicle. With the broad surfaces of the skin completed, the ventouses are again altered to treat the chin, upper lip, laughter lines and under-eye skin areas more specifically if required. Blocked pores can be treated in the same concentrated way.

Treatment points

Initial treatments with pulsed air–vacuum should be applied with caution until skin reaction is known. The vacuum and duration of the first treatment should be moderated to avoid capillary damage.

Weals and blood spots can be caused on the skin if treatment is concentrated too long on any one area. This is the skin's natural response to injury.

The best way to become proficient with vacuum massage is simply to practise until a natural rhythm and control develops.

Muscle toning (passive muscle contraction)

Muscle toning is passive muscle exercise using a faradic type current to produce contraction of facial muscles without conscious effort on the

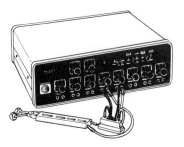

Muscle toning equipment

part of the client. It is an extremely effective way of delaying signs of ageing in the dry and dehydrated skins and is applied within mature skin treatments, normally at the conclusion of the routine after the mask.

Physiological effects of faradic type currents

The name 'faradism' was originally given to the current obtained from a faradic cell, which produced muscular contractions. This early form was an induced alternating current that produced fierce, spasmodic contractions used medically on damaged or denervated muscles.

Modern equipment uses a combination of currents, which whilst providing similar physiological effects do so without discomfort. They are termed faradic type currents and are surged so that the contraction produced closely resembles natural movement and is acceptable to the client. Between each surge of current (pulse) there is a rest, during which no current flows and the muscle relaxes.

The primary sensation is a stimulation of sensory nerves, prickling, slight irritation and colour (erythema) in the area of the applicator. When sufficient intensity of current is applied and the applicator is placed accurately over a motor point, muscle contraction takes place. The surging (pulsing) of the current produces relaxation and prevents muscle fatigue or discomfort. The affected muscles exert a pumping action on blood and lymphatic vessels in the immediate area, improving circulation and elimination in subcutaneous tissues.

Indications for muscle toning

1 Ageing skins with atrophic, withered appearance.
2 Loss of firm facial contours.
3 Evidence of oedema (swelling), due to loss of muscle tone, particularly around the eyes. (Medical approval is required to check the cause of the swelling in case it is associated with a physical condition such as a heart complaint.)
4 As a preventative measure, to delay the effects of ageing and promote a healthy and firm skin appearance.

Contra-indications to muscle toning

- Hypersensitive skins, due to irritation of sensory nerves.
- Highly coloured vascular complexions.
- High blood pressure.
- Very highly strung, nervous clients, due to the need for client co-operation.
- Skin abrasions, due to the discomfort caused.

- A large number of fillings in the teeth, or metal bridge-work in dentures, requires adaptation of exercise positions to avoid discomfort.
- Any area of the face where severe discomfort is experienced within treatment, such as the frontalis muscle area of the forehead.
- The muscles should not be worked if they become fatigued. Any sign of fatigue, tremors, unwillingness to continue contracting, must halt treatment.
- Sinus congestion, due to discomfort.
- Migraine sufferers, as an attack could be brought on by the specific action on the facial nerves.

Application

Equipment preparation
The contraction is applied with a facial unit with active electrodes built in to the surface of the applicator. Applicators can take many forms such as conductive rubber applicators or metal electrodes, each of which calls for a slightly different application procedure. The electrodes are attached to the equipment by leads. All applicators need accurate placing on the muscle motor points for clear and comfortable contractions. The intensity of the current and its timing (pulsing) are altered with the controls on the equipment.

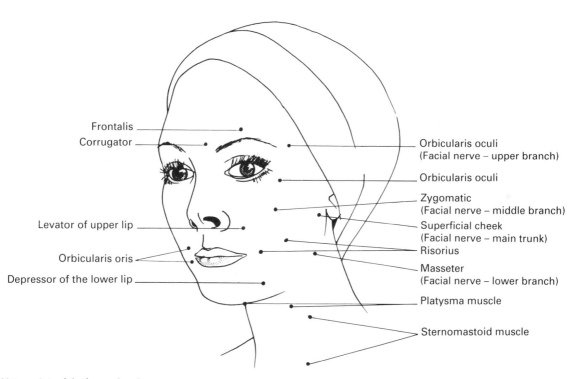

Motor points of the face and neck

Muscle toning systems may be part of a combined facial treatment machine or available as an independent unit. It is important to become familiar with the equipment chosen – get to know the levels at which the current produces a contraction and the ideal rate of pulse (speed of contractions) – then treatment can be applied with confidence. Muscle contraction treatments need to be given with care and with the therapist positioned in such a way that she can control her equipment to make the minute intensity adjustments required for successful treatment.

Client preparation and application

- The client is brought into a semi-upright position, so that her muscles adopt a natural posture with gravity. The therapist sits on a stool facing the client and the equipment to apply the muscle toning.
- The skin should be clean and free from creams, masks, etc. Muscle toning is usually applied after the mask stage of a facial when the skin is very receptive, but it can be applied independently for weak muscle conditions.
- The motor points of the muscles should be determined in relation to muscle size, position and bony attachments (if any), and contractions obtained with the minimum of client discomfort.
- The skin and the electrode are moistened or covered with conductive gel to improve conductivity, reduce skin irritation and improve the muscle point response. The gel is applied prior to contracting each motor point.
- The more accurately the electrode applicator is placed, the faster will be the contraction, with the least primary irritation. Both electrodes must be in firm skin contact for a contraction to occur.
- Application commences on the neck, on the sternomastoid muscles, with 6–8 contractions on each muscle. The therapist can feel the muscle attempting to respond if she places her fingers gently on the area.
- The intensity is kept at a low level until the client becomes familiar with the sensation and relaxes. Careful repositioning to improve the accuracy of the electrode placing will limit the intensity of current needed to obtain a clear muscle movement. Intensity is increased

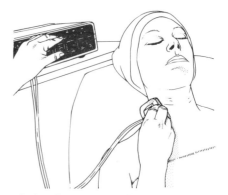

Facial electrode method on the sternomastoid muscle

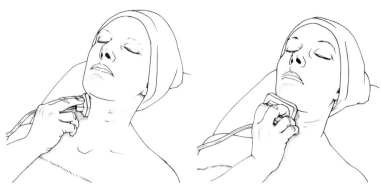

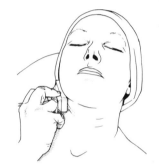

Contraction on the platysma muscle

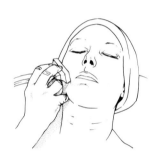

Jawline area and masseter muscle

Superficial cheek muscles

gradually until a comfortable contraction is obtained; this is repeated 6–8 times, and then the intensity is reduced.

- Muscle toning progresses up to the mandible, cheeks and eye areas, applying 6–8 contractions on each motor point.

For a general firming action the sequence should follow from the sternomastoid, via the platysma, masseter, zygomatic, risorius, orbicularis oris and the levators of the lip, to the eye area and the orbicularis oculi sphincter, to conclude on the forehead with the corrugator and frontalis muscles (if not contra-indicated).

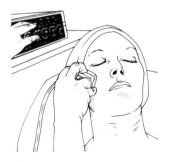

Orbicularis oculi

Treatment points

Muscle toning is most effective and comfortable when applied around the outer borders of the face. In this way, pain from metal fillings or dentures and areas of sensitivity on the upper cheeks can be avoided. By following the main facial nerve branches, most areas of the face can be stimulated into action from outer border positions.

If specific treatment is required on the lip area (for downward lines, caused by weight loss or poorly fitting dentures) the intensity must be carefully regulated to prevent discomfort and subsequent toothache.

When a contraction is completed on a motor point, the current intensity is reduced before moving to the next area. It is then increased gradually to the intensity that will produce a contraction. This improves client acceptance, as the current is not felt until it is in the correct place.

Continual adjustment of the intensity requires that the therapist should be able to see the controls and reach them easily. The therapist can then alter treatment according to the verbal feedback received from the client.

Accurate muscle toning application relies on certain principles:

- Knowledge of the position of the muscles of facial expression, and their action.
- The nerve supply and motor points of the muscles.
- Careful intensity control to provide comfortable, clear contractions.
- Working knowledge of the equipment, its effects and performance.
- Skilful client handling and verbal exchange to gain essential feedback to guide the application and prevent discomfort.

As many of the muscles interlink, and many are served by the facial nerve, it will be difficult to isolate the action of one muscle specifically. This is not important, as muscle toning hopes to copy natural movements and that is how the muscles of facial expression naturally work. Only uncomfortable or unnatural movements should be avoided by repositioning.

High-frequency treatment

The high-frequency current alternates so rapidly that it does not stimulate motor or sensory nerves. It has a frequency of 20 000 Hz (cycles per second) or more and is termed an *oscillating* current.

The high-frequency current (HF) may be applied indirectly (Viennese massage) and directly (for germicidal effect).

Indirect HF passes through the surface of the body and produces a stimulating, anti-congestive effect with no chemical formation on the skin's surface.

Direct HF is an external application, which dries, refines and heals the skin. It produces a germicidal effect, through ozone formation at the skin's surface via the glass electrodes. Direct HF produces an irritating noise, so every attempt should be made to put the client at ease prior to the application so that she is not nervous of the treatment.

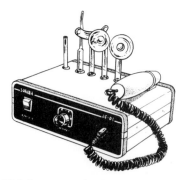

High-frequency unit

General effects and characteristics of HF

Stimulation of surface tissue

HF can penetrate to the subcutaneous tissues and generates heat there which increases the interchange of blood and tissue fluids. Improved circulation and elimination result in enhanced skin texture, colour and oil–moisture balance.

Relaxation (indirect HF)

The generated warmth within the scalp and facial tissues produces a sedative effect, increasing relaxation and relief from tension. The current flows through the surface of the body, but due to the speed of the oscillations, it does not excite muscle fibres.

Germicidal, drying effect (direct HF)

Directly applied, the HF current produces a germicidal, anti-bacterial effect. Ozone is produced as a by-product when an air gap is present between the skin and the glass electrode. This has a disinfecting effect on oily skin, limiting the sebaceous secretion whilst drying and healing pustular infection (with medical approval).

Destructive/fulguration effect (direct HF)

Direct HF can have a destructive effect on skin tissue and is used in scar treatments to speed desquamation. Its use on sebaceous glands within oily skin treatment needs to be applied with caution.

Indications for high-frequency

Indirect method

1 Normal, combination, dry, dehydrated and mature skins for stimulation.
2 For relaxation effects on clients suffering from tiredness, or needing a stress therapy approach in treatment.

Direct method

1 Normal, combination skin – 10 minutes' application for general stimulation.
2 Oily, seborrhoea, blemished skin – 10 minutes of concentrated application on affected areas.
3 Scarred, post-acne skin conditions using five minutes' general and five minutes' 'sparking method' to increase the skin shedding effect.
4 On blemished back and shoulder areas, 10–20 minutes' treatment to dry and heal the skin.

Contra-indications for high-frequency

- Highly strung clients of a nervous disposition.
- Epileptics.

- Asthmatics.
- Extremely vascular skin conditions.
- Skin infection. Adolescent acne may be treated with medical approval.
- An excessive number of fillings in the teeth.
- Clients undergoing treatment for defective circulation; oedema (swelling), high blood pressure, etc.
- Latter stages of pregnancy.
- Sinus blockage.
- Migraine sufferers.

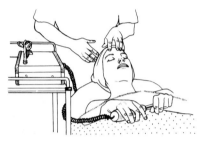

Beginning an indirect HF treatment

Application of indirect high-frequency (Viennese massage)

Equipment preparation

- The equipment is prepared, checked and placed conveniently. The glass saturator electrode or metal rod electrode is attached to the holder to form a firm connection.
- Plugs, switches and leads need checking with the intensity control dial set at zero and the machine switched off for safety.

Client preparation and application

The client should be prepared for general massage and cream or talc applied to permit free movement of the hands over the area. Cream provides a more soothing, relaxing effect, whilst talc gives a superficial and stimulating effect on the circulation.

All jewellery is removed from both the client and the therapist, to prevent induced electricity building up and discharging, causing discomfort or a possible loss of contact. The client is given the saturator rod in its holder to hold and advised to maintain contact throughout the treatment. This completes the electrical circuit and allows an even flow of HF current to pass through the surface of the skin. The client's hand holding the saturator can be kept in sight, outside the blankets, to ensure that contact is maintained. The sensation that will be experienced should be explained to the client to dispel anxiety.

The therapist places one hand in contact with the client's forehead and commences the massage, whilst the second hand turns on the machine and gradually increases the intensity to a comfortable level the client is aware of. (The forehead is a sensitive area so provides good guidance on tolerance.) The client can provide feedback to the therapist, allowing her to increase intensity levels as soon as she has relaxed.

The second hand is now brought into skin contact and the massage applied, with rhythmical movements over the face and neck. Superficial movements give a stimulating effect and deep movements a more relaxing action. At least one hand must be kept in skin contact

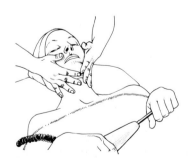

Indirect HF treatment in progress

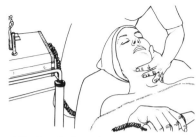

Adjusting the intensity

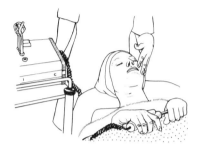

throughout the routine to prevent a break in the current flow, otherwise prickling and discomfort will occur. This discomfort is due to the transient nature of the HF current, accompanying the sudden change in the electrical circuit when the hand loses contact.

Massage can be adjusted to the amount of adipose (fatty) tissue present, with the current evenly spread between both hands or concentrated in one, to provide a regenerating effect. The forehead should be treated lightly to avoid a feeling of pressure or discomfort occurring.

After 8–20 minutes' massage the skin will appear stimulated, with texture improvement and increased local warmth and colour. The face should look relaxed. No area of the face should look overstimulated.

Treatment is concluded by releasing one hand from the face, reducing the current intensity to zero, and switching off the machine. The second hand may then be released, and the saturator removed from the client before continuing treatment.

The HF machines and electrode should be placed safely out of the way and the cream or talc is removed from the skin ready for the next stage of treatment. The metal rod (or glass saturator enclosing a metal spiral) is cleansed and sterilised after use and retained in a sterile container until next required.

Application of direct high-frequency (germicidal and drying effect)

Equipment preparation
In the direct application of HF the client does not form part of the circuit as she does in the indirect application. The equipment is checked as with the indirect method. The chosen glass electrode is placed firmly in the holder and placed safely ready for use. The electrodes can be applied in a number of ways:

- The glass 'mushrooms' are used for general facial, neck and back application.
- The T-shaped electrode is used on the neck and other curved areas.
- The narrow glass electrode provides concentrated HF at its point. This has a destructive effect on skin tissue and has very limited use in beauty therapy. Medically, it is used on scar tissue, warts, etc.

Client preparation and application
The facial area is prepared with talcum powder, to allow the electrodes to move easily over the skin. Application starts at the forehead, using the small mushroom electrode. The equipment is switched on and the intensity increased slowly to a comfortable level for the client, who provides valuable feedback to the operator on tolerance levels.

Circular movements are applied all over the face, in a steady, smooth manner, adjusting the intensity as required. A blue light appears in the glass electrode and the smell of ozone is present. It is often termed 'violet ray' because of its colour, but this can be pink, depending on whether the gas in the tube is neon or argon.

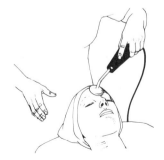

Beginning direct HF-treatment

175

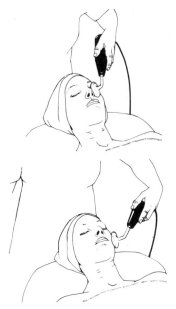

Direct HF treatment in progress

The more superficial movements provide the greatest stimulation as the HF current ionises the air when a slight gap is present between the electrode and the skin. This is seen as a small spark which affects the sensory nerve endings and causes a chemical reaction on the skin's surface.

The technique of sparking can be used to advantage on scar tissue or to activate a sluggish, sallow complexion. The air gap should not exceed a quarter of an inch (6 mm) as its effect becomes destructive to skin tissue beyond this length. Use of sparking should be restricted until skin reaction is known or irritation could result.

When the skin is stimulated (shown by increased colour), treatment may be concluded by reducing the current to zero, switching off the machine and releasing the electrode from facial contact. If the neck is to be treated separately with the curved electrode, the same procedure is used to apply the treatment, moulding the electrode to the contours of the neck, for 4–5 minutes.

The talcum may be removed with damp tissues and the skin left free from tonic products to maintain the drying, refining and germicidal effects of the HF.

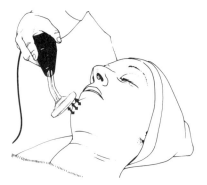

Sparking method

Treatment points

Application time varies according to skin condition, its sensitivity, previous treatment applied and the client's overall tolerance to the application. For a stimulating or tonic effect on the normal or combination skin only a few minutes is required to bring about the circulation improvement. Oily, blemished and scarred skins may need 10–15 minutes of treatment to provide the drying, healing and germicidal actions needed.

The high frequency output terminates in the low pressure gas-filled glass electrode, which offers protection to the client and operator from the risks of electric shock. In normal use, the gas in the electrode becomes ionised and gives a blue–violet glow. Ozone is produced externally as a by-product.

For an even and concentrated effect, the HF can be applied over a dry gauze mask which provides a constant air gap between the skin and the glass electrode. This method is widely used in the popular combined high frequency and galvanic treatments, which will be considered in Chapter 10, Treatment Plans.

Ultraviolet treatment

Ultraviolet rays (UV) are electromagnetic waves with wavelengths between 136 Å and 3900 Å, those within the range 1849 Å to 3900 Å being available for treatment purposes. (Å stands for *angstrom*, a unit of length; 10 Å = 1 nm (*nanometre*).)

Ultraviolet rays are absorbed into the skin, causing local reactions and some more widespread effects which depend on the degree of irradiation (i.e. the ultraviolet output and general time exposure to the rays).

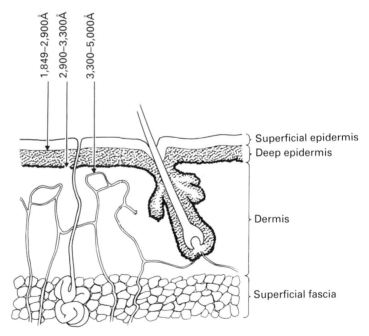

Penetration of UV rays into the skin

Local effects of UV

Erythema reaction

There are four degrees of erythema of which only the first is permitted within beauty therapy. However, awareness of the consequences of overexposure is necessary:

1 A first-degree erythema is a slight reddening of the skin with no irritation or soreness which fades within 24 hours.

2 A second-degree erythema is a more marked reddening of the skin with slight irritation. It fades within two to three days.

3 A third-degree erythema is a marked reaction, which causes the skin to become red, sore, hot and swollen. The reaction lasts about a week and is very painful.

4 A fourth-degree erythema is similar to the third-degree reaction with the addition of blister formation.

Desquamation

Ultraviolet exposure accelerates the skin's normal shedding process. The amount of peeling varies with the strength of the erythema reaction.

Pigmentation

Rays with wavelengths between 2800 Å to 3300 Å (280 nm to 330 nm) are absorbed in the deep epidermis and initiate a chemical reaction which results in the conversion of the amino acid *tyrosine* into the pigment melanin. The degree of pigmentation found depends on the client's natural colouring and the method of application.

Constant duration treatments for germicidal purposes do not bring about a great colour change, whilst progressive applications for cosmetic tanning and tonic purposes effect a considerable colour change over a period of time. The local applications appear to increase the skin's resistance to infection.

General effects of UV

Sufficient UV exposure:

- Increases the body's general resistance to infection.
- Gives a general tonic effect.
- Enables vitamin D to be produced, and if of sufficient intensity and duration, produces pigmentation (a change in skin colour).

It is generally accepted that prolonged exposure to UV rays ages the skin and may even be carcinogenic.

Indications for ultraviolet

1 Sluggish complexion with uneven texture and pH value.

2 Seborrhoea, for improvement of skin texture and to regulate secretions.

3 Acne vulgaris, to promote healing by its anti-bacterial and peeling effects.

4 To provide additional protection in preparation for natural sun exposure in the normal, delicate or sensitive skin, and permit safe and comfortable tanning to be possible.

5 For cosmetic tanning, to produce or maintain a tanned complexion.

Contra-indications for ultraviolet

- A very sensitive skin.
- UV should not be used in combination with treatments that increase skin temperature, e.g. prolonged vapour steaming, or an over-reaction could occur.
- When a client is taking medically prescribed drugs classed as sensitive to UV: gold, the sulphonamides, insulin, thyroid extract and quinine.
- Acute eczema or dermatitis or any unknown skin complaint.
- An unnatural rise in temperature from any source.

Application of ultraviolet treatment

Equipment

Ultraviolet lamps vary in their output according to their type, size and the source of UV rays within the lamp. Bulb-shaped UV lamps contain a hot quartz tube filled with high-pressure mercury vapour (HPMV) and these are still widely used in facial applications. Quartz tubes are also used in single or multiple form (within sun beds and facial tanners) and these are becoming increasingly popular because of ease of use and safety of application. Although much simpler to apply, with less risk of overexposure, modern tanning equipment still operates on the same basic principles of the inverse square law (see below), and some assessment of the client's sensitivity should be made in the initial application.

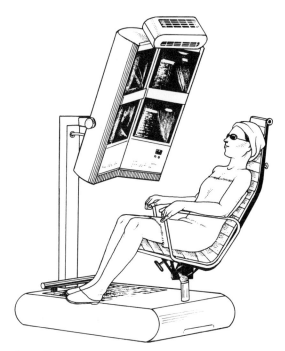

A facial tanning unit

The hot quartz lamp produces a mixture of short and long wavelength rays and provides cosmetic tanning, tonic and germicidal effects. The following factors decide the intensity of the skin reaction:

- The output of the lamp.
- The duration of the exposure.
- The distance between the lamp and the client.
- The sensitivity of the client to treatment.

Equipment should be of sturdy construction, able to be positioned easily, and have sufficient reflector span to treat the face, back and shoulders safely.

Deciding treatment times

To decide on the correct amount of UV exposure to be used initially, the client is exposed to a short duration irradiation and the reaction observed. The timing of subsequent treatment can then be planned using the principle of inverse squares, for the bulb type lamps.

The intensity of rays varies inversely with the square of the distance from the lamp – this is the inverse square law. Thus the intensity of the radiation at 30 cm is four times that at 60 cm and nine times that at 1 m. This law applies to infra-red, visible and ultraviolet rays, so when using a lamp, remember that four minutes at 60 cm and nine minutes at 1 m are required to produce the same effect as one minute at 30 cm.

Both bulb lamps and facial tanning systems need a few minutes to reach maximum output or intensity, so are switched on in preparation for treatment in an enclosed or curtained area. The lamp should be moved as little as possible prior to, during and after treatment, until it has cooled, otherwise its life is reduced. There is also a risk of spontaneous implosion of the bulb, if it is moved whilst hot.

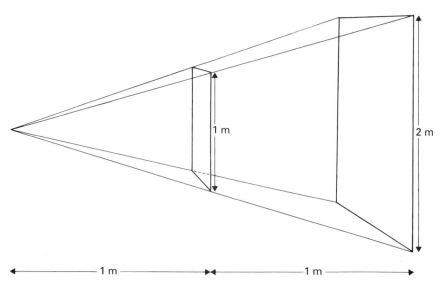

The inverse square law

Preparation of the Client

- The skin is cleansed and all oily preparations removed, leaving the skin clean.
- A facial tanning accelerator product may be applied to speed the effect whilst helping to minimise the drying effects of UV on the skin.
- The eyes of the client should be protected with goggles and the client positioned either upright, facing the lamp or semi-reclining, according to the equipment used. The rays must strike the skin at the correct angle, so that all areas of the face receive equal irradiation.
- Initial treatment should be of short duration, and the client asked to note the effect 24 and 48 hours after treatment.
- Careful records must be kept of treatment, and treatment progressed if a tan is needed, or kept at a constant timing if only the anti-bacterial effects are needed.
- Fair-skinned clients can progress gradually, working from a one-minute exposure and increasing over a series of treatments to reach five minutes, from which point the tan can be maintained by constant exposure times.
- Darker skinned clients may progress more quickly, doubling the exposure time on each treatment to reach a level where their tan can be maintained by constant timing (5–10 minutes according to depth of natural skin tone).
- If the skin appears irritated for any reason, treatment should be suspended otherwise the skin will peel and become sore. When treatment is recommenced, durations should be reduced and distances lengthened from the UV source to prevent a recurrence.
- Areas of scar tissue can become very apparent under the influence of UV, so a moderate exposure programme is the most suitable. A one- or two-minute irradiation repeated at regular intervals on the face or back should control the problem and still allow the skin to benefit.
- Ultraviolet is an excellent treatment for blemished skin, as it is hygienic in its application and avoids the need for hand contact.

Galvanic treatment (desincrustation and iontophoresis)

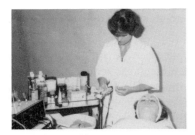

The working position

The use of galvanic current in beauty therapy provides a very useful and effective means for the therapist both to deep cleanse the skin – desincrustation – and introduce active substances into it for specific effect – iontophoresis, also known as ionisation.

Galvanic current is a direct current possessing polarity. It flows in one direction only, from positive to negative, and causes chemical changes. The anode is positive and is acid in reaction, the cathode is negative and alkaline in reaction. The galvanic current should never exceed two milliamps.

Treatment is applied via different poles − negative (−) and positive (+) − and works on the simple principle that:

- Opposite poles attract each other.
- Like poles repel each other.

Effects that the poles have on tissues

Anode (acid)
1 Closes pores.
2 Takes blood supply away from the skin.
3 Soothes the nerves.
4 Firms tissues.

Cathode (alkaline)
1 Opens pores.
2 Increases blood supply to the skin.
3 Irritating to nerves and skin.
4 Softens tissues.

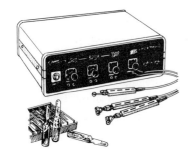

Galvanic treatment unit and ampoules

Desincrustation

Desincrustation is always applied on a negative charge. The active desincrustation product (soap or gel) is placed on the skin, and when negatively charged by the working electrode is attracted to the positive pole (the client's electrode, known as the indifferent electrode). This causes the desincrustation product to be superficially active on surface tissues, creating an alkaline reaction.

Action on the skin

The surface of the skin is acidic. Oily or congested skin has extra sebum and keratinised cells; these extra secretions form a thick layer on the skin, the main ingredient of which is *stearic acid* which plays a principal part in the inflammation of the acne-prone skin. Desincrustation fluid and the negative pole combine to form an alkaline substance which causes *saponification* – a chemical reaction by which fatty substances react with an alkali to form soap. The reaction breaks down the stearic acid (a fatty acid), releasing blocked pores by softening the plug, which can then be refined over a period of time by clinic and home treatments.

Desincrustation treatment points

- Desincrustation is applied with the negative pole on the skin and the positive pole attached to the client (an electrode pad for the arm or back, or hand-held metal bar).
- Desincrustation products are required and are always used on a negative charge. They must always be washed from the skin.
- Desincrustation products are soap-based. They cannot penetrate too deeply into the skin because they have too large a molecular size. The saponification effect is a chemical one on the fatty acid component of sebum trapped within blocked pores. Sebum is softened and released on to the skin's surface where it can be removed by normal cleansing methods, making extraction easier.
- Desincrustation products are very thoroughly removed from the skin after treatment by rinsing until all traces of foam are gone.
- Sponge roller covers used for desincrustation should not be used for ionisation, as it is difficult to remove the soap completely. Use a different colour sponge for the two procedures.

Indications for galvanic desincrustation

1 Deep skin cleansing on the normal and combination skin, as a preventative measure against skin blockage (applied periodically for a short duration).
2 Unblocking of pores on seborrhoea, acne, oily and troubled skin
3 For stimulation on the sluggish or congested skin.

Contra-indications for galvanic desincrustation

- Highly nervous clients.
- Vascular and hypersensitive skin conditions.
- Skin infection, sepsis and skin irritation.
- Excessive fillings in the teeth and metal pins or plates in the face.
- Sinusitis.
- Epileptics.
- Asthmatics.

Application

Equipment preparation
The galvanic equipment may be an independent machine or form part of a combined facial system. The equipment will have the following features:

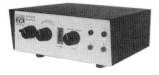

- Polarity controls (negative and positive).
- On/off switch.
- Intensity controls.
- Milliamp read-outs (digital or analogue read-outs which register the skin resistance presented).
- Outlets for the lead connections (marked negative and positive).

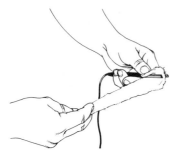

Covering the prong with dampened cotton wool

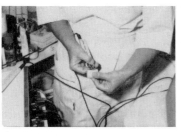

1

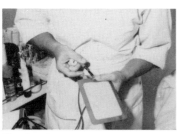

2

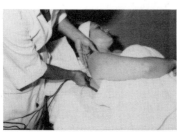

3

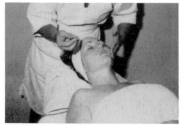

4

Electrodes will include:

- Metal plates/sponge covers or graphite rubber pads/sponge covers.
- Metal prong electrodes (which need to be covered).
- Metal rollers/sponge roller covers.

The equipment is made ready, the indifferent or non-working electrode is fitted with a damp sponge cover and placed ready to be attached to the client's arm by straps or placed behind her back. The chosen working electrode, of the metal prong or roller type, is prepared with moist cotton wool or the special sponge roller cover, both of which are slipped onto the actual roller whilst damp.

The electrodes are connected by leads to the machine and the polarity selected by pushing the negative or positive button as marked. The client acts as the resistance to the galvanic current, which, when treatment starts, shows as a reading on the milliamp meter read-out. The client completes the circuit between the two electrodes; without them both in contact with the client there is no milliamp read-out.

The galvanic application is basically the same for both desincrustation and iontophoresis, but the application, actions and removal of the special products used differ.

Client preparation and application

- The damp sponge-covered electrode is attached firmly to the arm by straps, or placed behind the back so that the client's weight holds it in place.
- The skin is moistened well with water and the special desincrustation product applied and lightly massaged into a foam with the fingers. This helps to identify problem areas under the skin.
- The chosen electrode (normally the cotton wool-covered metal probe) is moistened and applied to the skin of the cheek. The machine is switched on and the intensity increased slowly.
- As the skin resistance is overcome, the client feels a tingling sensation in the skin and may experience a metallic taste in the mouth. It will take a few seconds for the resistance of oily, congested skin to be overcome, so for 30 seconds or so only a low milliamp reading on the meter should be permitted, until the resistance is broken down.
- As galvanic current works by a process of attraction, there is no need for high use of intensity. The galvanic current should be applied at what is termed 'the client's threshold of awareness', that is the level at which they can just discern the current in their skin. A metallic taste indicates that the current is too high. Once the client has experienced the current, the level may be reduced.
- Application is made with firm, smooth movements all over affected areas, ensuring that the skin remains moist. Without lubrication present, the galvanic current cannot work, and skin irritation could result.
- The galvanic current penetrates the skin on a water ladder, in an attempt to reach the opposite pole (the indifferent electrode.) As this happens, the desincrustation product enters the skin surface and achieves its unblocking chemical action on the blocked pores.

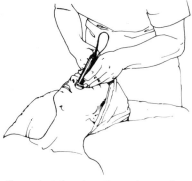

- Keeping to a low milliamp level, four to five minutes of desincrustation is applied (the time should be adjusted to the skin sensitivity or reaction), then the intensity is reduced, the electrode removed from the skin, and the machine switched off.
- The desincrustation product is washed thoroughly from the skin until no soap remains and the skin looks clean and gently stimulated.
- Treatment then proceeds to steaming, extraction, vacuum massage, mask, etc. and may conclude with ionisation of a corrective ampoule.

Concentrated work on the centre panel

Iontophoresis

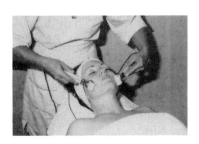

Iontophoresis is the introduction of active water-soluble substances into the skin using ampoules with different ingredients which are charged in different ways. The active ingredients usually flow from negative to positive, so the active electrode will be negative and the positive electrode will be in the client's hand or attached to her arm. The active ingredients used in ampoules are charged in a certain way to allow them to pass easily into the skin, where they are absorbed. The active trace elements pass slowly into the blood circulation and are gradually excreted in the normal way from the body. The polarity of the ampoules will be indicated by the manufacturer, and this indicates the polarity to be chosen on the galvanic machine. Some ampoules may be applied first on the negative pole, followed by the positive pole. Always follow manufacturers' instructions.

Indications for iontophoresis

1 Normal skin needing moisturising.
2 Combination skin needing pH balancing, refining and hydrating.
3 Dry and dehydrated skin needing stimulating and moisturising.
4 Mature skin needing regeneration and firming.
5 Oily and blemished skin needing calming, correction and healing.

Contra-indications to iontophoresis

- Highly nervous clients.
- Vascular and hypersensitive skin conditions.
- Skin infection, sepsis and skin irritation.
- Excessive fillings in the teeth and metal pins or plates in the face.
- Sinusitis.
- Epileptics.
- Asthmatics.

Application

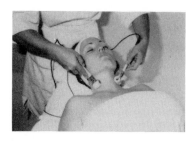

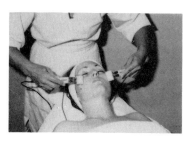

- The equipment is prepared in the same way as for galvanic desincrustation.
- The client is prepared in the same way as for galvanic desincrustation. The covered metal probe or roller electrodes are used and the indifferent electrode is attached as before to the arm or placed behind the back.
- One roller electrode can be used in association with an indifferent electrode, with each electrode attached to the equipment via leads to complete the circuit.
- As an alternative, two roller electrodes can be used, with a double lead attachment. The third lead is separate and acts as the indifferent electrode. Leads must be checked to see that they are correct, as each machine may be slightly different.
- The face is moistened and the ampoule applied according to skin condition. Areas of the face and neck not specifically involved in treatment can be moistened just with water.
- The polarity of the chosen ampoule is noted and the polarity chosen on the machine. If an ampoule is marked for a negative charge, that is the polarity selected on the machine.
- The moist roller is placed on the cheek, the machine switched on and the intensity gradually increased, to reach the client's threshold level of awareness (this may be very close to zero on the milliamp reading). As the current is attracted to the opposite pole – like a magnet – no high intensity is need.
- If water is present and the electrode pads are both in skin contact, the active product is pulled into the skin.
- After a few minutes at a very low level of reading on the milliamp read-out, the treatment concludes by reducing the intensity to zero, taking the electrode from the skin and turning the equipment off.
- The active ampoule remains in the skin to do its work; it is not rinsed off, but excreted gradually from the body over the following few days.
- Ionisation normally concludes the facial sequence so that the ampoule stays in the skin and is not hastened from the surface by active massage, etc. The skin looks calm and matt after ionisation, in an ideal state for makeup. As this is the stage at which ampoules could be used within day skin care, the effects can be pointed out to the client.

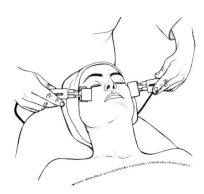

Working with sponge-covered rollers

Treatment points

Some ampoules may need both negative and positive polarity to be used and this will be shown on the manufacturers' guidance. In this case the negative polarity starts the treatment, then at a half-way stage the intensity is brought to zero, the polarity is switched to positive and the treatment recommences, checking that the skin is still moist.

Electrical Treatments

Equipment	Contra-indications	Action/effects	Indicated skin conditions					
			Normal	Oily	Acne	Dry/dehydrated	Mature	Sensitive
Steaming Normal method – or with herbs/essential oils	Skin infection Vascular skin Sinus blockage Sunburn	Relaxing Skin softening/hydrating Cleansing/desquamating Stimulating	✓	✓	✓	✓		
Steaming ozone method	Hypersensitive skin Vascular skin Acne rosacea Sinus blockage Sunburn	Drying Healing Anti-bacterial Stimulating	✓	✓	✓			
Vibratory treatment	Vascular skin Inflammation Skin irritation Skin infection, sepsis Bony facial areas	Gentle stimulation Relaxation Regeneration of skin Prevention and relief of fibrositis in upper back	✓			✓	✓	
Brush massage	Sensitive/vascular skin Skin infection Skin irritation Loose skin conditions Sunburn	Stimulating Regenerating	✓			✓	✓	
Vacuum/suction massage	Sensitive/vascular skin Crepey loose skin Infected acne Areas of capillary damage or skin frailty	Cleansing/desquamating Deep cleansing/unblocking action in combination with galvanic desincrustation Stimulating of skin Improvement in lymphatic circulation/drainage	✓	✓	✓	✓	✓ Modified	
Muscle toning	Hypersensitive skins Vascular skin High blood pressure Nervous clients Skin abrasions Excessive fillings in teeth Sinus blockage Migraine Muscular fatigue and pain	Stimulation of sensory and motor nerves resulting in muscle action	✓				✓	

Electrical Treatments

Equipment	Contra-indications	Action/effects	Normal	Oily	Acne	Dry/dehydrated	Mature	Sensitive
High-frequency	Epileptics Asthmatics Nervous clients Vascular skin conditions Skin infection Excessive fillings in teeth Defective circulation Later stages of pregnancy Sinus blockage							
High-frequency Direct method		Stimulation Destructive Germicidal		✓	✓			
High-frequency Indirect method		Stimulation Relaxation	✓	✓	✓	✓	✓	Modified
Ultraviolet	Very sensitive skin Acute eczema/dermatitis Any unnatural temperature rise Not to be applied with other stimulating routines Not to be applied when UV 'sensitive' drugs are being taken	Erythema ⎤ Desquamation ⎬ Local effects Pigmentation ⎦ Increases resistance to infection ⎤ Tonic effect ⎬ General effects Vit D production ⎦	✓	✓	✓			
Galvanic treatment **Desincrustation/ deep skin cleansing** – with special desincrustation products	Nervous clients Vascular skin conditions Skin infection/sepsis Skin irritation/open skin areas Excessive fillings in teeth Sinusitis	Deep skin cleansing Unblocking of pores Normalisation of skin's oil/hydric balance Improvement in skin colour/ texture/function	Modified	✓	✓			
Iontophoresis/ ionisation – with chosen ampoules to suit skin condition	Nervous clients Skin infection/sepsis Epileptics Asthmatics	Hydrating/moisturising Normalising Regenerating Healing Soothing/calming Improvement of skin elasticity	✓	✓	✓	✓	✓	✓

Indicated skin conditions

The skin must be kept moist at all times. If it needs to be remoistened or more product applied, the intensity is reduced to zero and the electrode removed from the skin. Treatment recommences after the reapplication of water or product and the intensity is gradually increased to the previous working level.

Ampoules are available containing a wide range of active substances for all skin conditions. They should not be opened until required, to retain purity and concentrated action. All skins benefit from natural hydration, so they are applied with water which ensures that the treatment is safely and comfortably applied. In Chapter 10, Treatment Plans, the role of some of the ampoules and their active ingredients will be considered.

Desincrustation products are available as ampoules or in larger containers. As they are special soaps, their activity is not lost through exposure to air. Their action comes from the chemical breakdown of the fatty matter in the skin and pores.The term desincrustation comes from the Latin words *de* – away and *incrustatio* – crustations, surface build up, oily blockage, etc., and explains its action perfectly.

With all galvanic applications the client's individual skin condition and her reaction and tolerance to the galvanic current determine the amount of current applied (the milliamp reading). Through conversation and visual observation of the skin, the correct treatment can be applied, just at the threshold level of awareness, and to cause gentle skin stimulation only. The therapist must trust her own judgement as to duration and intensity of treatment; only she has the client in front of her and can judge reactions.

Self check

1 How does a beauty specialist decide if an electrical treatment is indicated?
2 What effects can electrical treatments have on the skin?
3 List the general contra-indications to electrical treatments.
4 Explain four safety points which must be considered when using electrical equipment.
5 For each piece of equipment described in the chapter, give the following:
   (a) The indications.
   (b) The effects.
   (c) The contra-indications.
   (d) The application procedure.
6 What are the effects on the skin of ultraviolet exposure?
7 Explain the inverse square law and its application in the salon.
8 Define the following:
   (a) Anode.
   (b) Cathode.
   (c) Anion.
   (d) Cation.

CHAPTER TEN

Treatment Plans

Purpose and choice of treatment

The effect of equipment has been studied; now its place within treatment plans in association with products can be seen in relation to specific skin conditions.

Purpose of treatment

Treatment should be enjoyable and a time for indulgence, so do not forget to make your client welcome, giving her your attention and convincing her of the benefits of professional treatment.

Listen to what the client expects from treatment and then devise the best plan to meet this need, matching skin condition against the effects of the equipment. Let the client know that you value her custom and take a personal interest in her progress, altering treatment as necessary to maintain improvement. Taking the trouble to see that all the client's needs are met inspires confidence and is good clinic business.

Professional treatment must be:

- Effective yet safe.
- Able to correct problems as they occur.
- Maintain skin texture or improve it.
- Delay ageing signs and firm the mature skin.
- Prevent problems occurring.

In order for this to be possible, the choice of treatment and the products needed for clinic and home use must be carefully thought out. Their effects must be matched to gain good and safe results. The effects of the treatment and the action of the products must be known and planned together to make a programme suited to the client's particular needs and life style.

The more that is known about active ingredients, the bigger the bank of knowledge to draw from when working out an effective plan of action.

Organising the home plan

The client wants to know how to care for her skin overall and make it look its best and especially needs to know what to use on a daily basis.

She also needs to know what to use when a problem like dehydration occurs; how it can be rectified and the skin returned to normal. In fact, she needs to know how to manage her skin and react to its needs and changes, so a first consideration of treatment is organising the client's home care needs: getting the home care plan established to support professional care should take priority in the early treatments. Unless the correct products are used daily, good results overall will not be forthcoming and the client will be disappointed.

Place emphasis on sales at first and explain why it is so important to the client to gain her co-operation. One of the main reasons clients come for help is to find out what they need to use at home, so do not forget to answer this need. Build the treatment around the products that will be introduced to the client for her use at home. At first, all that is needed is a simple home routine that can be gradually extended to include some specialities when the client has become familiar with the products and trusts them to give her good results.

Treatment plan for normal skin

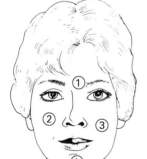

Recognition
1 Few apparent pores.
2 Fine textured, even colour.
3 Well balanced oil–hydric levels.

Normal skin can be prone to dryness if neglected, or through changes in eating patterns, stress or ill health. It is not prone to allergic reactions or sensitivity unless over-stressed by exposure to ultraviolet rays, wind or cold.

Aim of treatment
Maintenance of oil–hydric balance and skin texture. Avoidance of sensitivity and prevention of couperose (sensitive areas of high colour and exposed capillaries). Maintenance of tone in the skin, delaying the effects of ageing. Ultraviolet protection.

Active ingredients in treatment
Herbal ingredients and essential oils: sweet basil, rosemary, lavender, camomile and geranium.
Wheat germ, avocado oil, karite.
Witch hazel.

Professional care
Cleanser (milk or mousse), tonic, eye makeup remover, eye cream, night cream (nourishing), mask (biological or clay type), day protection cream, moisture concentrates, night regenerating cream, ampoules (dehydration, revitalising, collagen and elastin), facial tissue oil, rejuvenating cream.

Home Care

Day care: cleanser, tonic, day protection cream or moisture concentrates, firming eye gel.

Night care: cleanser, eye makeup remover, tonic, night cream or night regenerating cream, eye cream.

Special care: mask, ampoules (dehydration, revitalising, collagen and elastin), facial tissue oil, rejuvenating cream.

1 Essential facial (maintenance of skin performance)

- Cleanse with cleanser (herbal) manually or with brush method.
- Spray tone with a 10% dilution of herbal skin tonic.
- Massage with night cream or regenerating cream or a mixture of both. Use manual movements and indirect high frequency (Viennese massage) for extra effect if needed.
- Apply day protection, moisture cream, moisture concentrate, according to skin need.

2 Firming facial (using the effects of phytotherapy)

- Cleanse with herbal cleanser and brush method, taking special care on the neck and eye areas, using small brushes following natural contours.
- Spray tone the face with a 10% dilution of toning lotion.
- Steam the face gently for 5–7 minutes at a distance of 18 inches.
- Vacuum massage (manual massage, if not available) using facial tissue oil (with essential oils) in a fine film all over the face and neck. Give special attention to neck and jawline. Leave the fine oil on the face and neck.
- Apply night cream to the face and regenerating cream to the neck and upper shoulder areas and massage carefully for 10–15 minutes working manually or with the facial vibrator. Concentrate on muscles in the upper back, shoulders, jawline and eye area especially. Remove cream gently if any remains on the skin after massage.
- Apply a biological mask in a fine film all over the face and neck. The mask disappears into the skin and after 10 minutes the residue left on the skin is gently removed with warm water. Clay masks and biological masks can be alternated in treatment.
- Apply a suitable ampoule – rehydration, revitalising, moisturising or collagen and elastin, depending on the skin's need at the time. Dehydration is a good initial choice, when the ampoules may be alternated for maximum effect. Apply the ampoule manually with gentle tapping movements, or via galvanic current for 3–5 minutes at the client's threshold level (where she can just feel the galvanic sensation in the skin).
- Apply day protection cream or moisture concentrate if more protection is needed by the skin.

3 Rejuvenating facial (if the skin is rather jaded and lacking life)

- Cleanse the skin manually with herbal cleanser, working gently but very thoroughly to avoid over stimulating the skin at this stage.
- Spray tone the skin with a 10% dilution of herbal tonic.
- Steam (no ozone) for five minutes at a distance of 50 cm (18 inches) from the face.
- Vacuum massage using facial tissue oil (with essential oils) in a fine film all over the face and neck. Give special attention to neck and jawline. Leave the fine oil on the face and neck.
- Apply night cream to the face and regenerating cream to the neck and upper shoulder areas and massage carefully for 10–15 minutes working manually on muscles in the upper back, shoulders, jawline and eye area especially. Remove cream gently if any remains on the skin after massage.
- Apply a biological mask (for stimulating effect) in a fine film all over the face and neck. The mask disappears into the skin and after 10 minutes the residue left on the skin is gently removed with warm water.
- Apply muscle toning to the muscles of the face and neck for 10 minutes working from the neck up to the eye area.
- Apply a suitable ampoule – revitalising, ginseng, royal jelly or collagen and elastin, depending on the skin's need at the time. The ampoules may be alternated for maximum effect. Apply the ampoule manually with gentle tapping movements, or via galvanic current for 3–5 minutes at the client's threshold level (where she can just feel the galvanic sensation in the skin).
- Apply day moisture protection or moisture concentrate.

Treatment plan for combination/oily skin

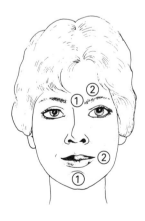

Recognition
1 Centre panel oiliness/blocked pores and heavy, uneven texture.
2 Uneven pH/hydric balance.

The combination skin has an uneven and heavier texture than normal skin and is prone to changes in behaviour due to changes in the skin's pH. The natural acidity of the skin is altered and it becomes prone to irritation, blocked pores, blackheads, blemishes and their resulting scars (especially evident if extraction has been applied). This instability is often caused by over fierce treatment to remove surface oil from the over productive central area of the face.

Aim of treatment
Treatment aims to balance and refine the skin, by controlling oily secretions, refining the pores and hydrating the fluid balance to

improve skin softness and colour. Blemishes which flare up are a major cause of distress and have priority in treatment and home plans. Rehydration of the cheeks is a secondary consideration which is dealt with as skin function improves.

Active ingredients in treatment

Herbal ingredients and essential oils: thyme, rosemary, lavender, camomile.

Seaweed extract, fenugreek.

Witch hazel, menthol, bio-active sulphur, squalene.

Professional care

Cleanser (herbal milk), liquid soap cleanser (seaweed), tonic (herbal or seaweed), natural scrub/exfoliator, eye makeup remover, night treatment (corrective), mask (regulating phyto or clay type), hydro-regulator (hydro-emulsion day protection/correction), desincrustation product (soap/gel), ampoules (seaweed, thyme, rosemary, camomile).

Home care

Day care: cleanser (herbal milk), liquid soap cleanser (seaweed), tonic (herbal or seaweed), hydro-regulator.

Night care: cleanser (herbal milk), eye makeup remover, liquid soap cleanser, natural scrub/exfoliator, night treatment (corrective).

Special care: mask (regulating phyto or clay type), ampoules (seaweed, thyme, rosemary, camomile).

1 Deep cleansing mini-facial (30–45 minutes)

- Brush cleanse with herbal cleanser, or if no makeup is worn, liquid soap cleanser. Cleanse the face carefully but quickly using eye makeup remover pads if needed to remove eye makeup swiftly.
- Steam the face with ozone steam for eight minutes, or until desired erythema is present.
- Apply natural scrub or gentle exfoliator on areas of blockage. Keep paste wet initially and work carefully, concentrating on blocked areas, or scarred, discoloured skin. Wash off and if the skin still appears calm, proceed to the next step.
- Apply galvanic desincrustation on the negative pole for additional deep cleansing in the central area of the face, using a special desincrustation product. Wash off very thoroughly until all soaping disappears.
- Apply corrective ampoule (seaweed or herbal) for the combination skin with galvanic current according to the marked polarity, keeping to the central open-pored skin areas. Work for 3–4 minutes at minimal levels of skin awareness (below the threshold level to avoid galvanic sensitisation from occurring).
- Apply hydro-emulsion (protection/correction) on the central area of the face or the whole face if inclined to oiliness, or use moisture protection on the cheeks and neck if more inclined to dryness or sensitivity.

2 Corrective treatment for combination skin (1 hour)

Ozone

The use of ozone is now believed to create a carcinogenic risk for the therapist and treatments involving its use form no part of any educational course. It is still, however, used in some salons and therapists should check with their local authority as to regulations for their particular area.

- Cleanse with herbal cleanser or liquid soap cleanser, using brush or manual methods.
- Vapour spray with 10% dilution of the tonic (seaweed or herbal). Spray only the central area of the face and simply blot the more sensitive cheek areas with the damp cotton wool pads or sponges so that the action is reduced.
- Work with the gentle natural scrub on any areas of blockage and discolouration, working gently but persistently with petrissage, friction movements on the blockage that can be felt rather than seen. Remove with damp cotton wool pieces or sterile viscose sponges.
- Apply steam (no ozone) and wet the face for a few minutes until a surface film of moisture forms sufficient to allow the vacuum applicators to glide over the skin.
- Apply vacuum suction to lymphatic drainage pattern, working to main facial nodes for stimulation and elimination. Then apply specific strokes on the blocked areas using the small aperture applicators, working with fast, light strokes, tapping where necessary (10 minutes overall is sufficient time).
- Apply steam again, with ozone now, for 4–5 minutes to sterilise the skin and correct the pH balance at a distance of 40–50 cm (15–18 inches).
- Apply the pore treatment massage routine with corrective cream or a light herbal/seaweed gel, avoiding any blemishes or sore areas and working on both the face and upper back and neck areas to improve relaxation and reduce tension. Remove any products that remain from the 10-minute massage.
- Apply mask, regulating, phytotherapy or clay type, according to skin condition. Apply first to the central area, where the action required is more drying and refining, and secondly to the cheeks and neck, where gentle stimulation and hydration is needed. Leave for 10 minutes and remove with warm water.
- Apply corrective ampoule (seaweed or herbal type) for combination skin on the central area only, water on the sides of the face and neck, and penetrate with galvanic current (according to the polarity marked). Work very slowly and carefully well below the client's skin awareness level. Watch for sensory nerve reaction – tracking – on the skin's surface to guide treatment. Work for 3–5 minutes or less, concentrating treatment into the area that most needs the remedial action.
- Protect and correct the skin with hydro-emulsion product (oil free).

3 Refining treatment for combination skin (1 hour)

- Cleanse with herbal cleanser and brush method, taking care not to over stimulate the skin. Work gently but thoroughly. Remove cleanser with damp cotton wool or sterile viscose sponges, taking care not to rinse the sponges and re-use them, but rather use and put aside, to ensure that the skin becomes really clean.
- Steam for 8–10 minutes at a distance of 40–50 cm (15–18 inches) to soften the skin. If cheeks are sensitive, cover them with enlarged eye pads of dry cotton wool.
- Deep cleanse with desincrustation product and galvanic desincrustation process, concentrating on the central area for 3–5 minutes (negative polarity). Rinse off product very well until no foam remains.
- If the skin has become sensitive to galvanic current, there are two alternatives to desincrustation as a means of refining the skin: the first is to work with a gentle exfoliating product under steam for 10–12 minutes, keeping the paste wet throughout. The second is to apply an enzyme peeler (phytotherapy product) on the dry skin after steaming. Allow it to set and cause the enzyme action to take place on the horny surface layer of the skin in a gentle static way, speeding desquamation and refining the skin. This is useful if the skin is a little aggravated or feels sore. The product is rinsed off revealing the deeply clean, yet calm skin.
- On the softened skin the steam is briefly reapplied to wet the skin and vacuum suction is applied under steam. Fast strokes, small aperture applicators and high enough vacuum to provide a 10% lift into the applicators are used to unblock the pores, gradually tightening and refining pore openings and improving skin colour and texture. Work specifically or more generally according the the skin condition, avoiding sensitive or sore areas.
- Add ozone into the steam sequence and apply generally for 5 minutes to improve the skin's pH balance and function. Protect the eyes and cheeks with pads.
- Apply the pore treatment massage with corrective cream, using friction movements on the centre panel to help the refining process. The cheeks, if more sensitive, can have a more suitable cream applied (e.g. for sensitive or normal skin type). Remove the cream thoroughly after 10 minutes' massage.
- Apply a biological non-setting mask (phyto type) or clay mask for the skin condition, applying first to the central area. Leave for 10 minutes and remove gently with warm water.
- Apply 3–4 minutes of direct high frequency to the oily areas of the face only, to aid the refining and healing process.
- Tone with diluted tonic (seaweed or herbal) and blot in well.
- As an alternative to the high frequency and toning, an ampoule for the combination/oily skin can be applied under the galvanic current for 3–4 minutes to the oily areas. Work slowly and carefully to provide a good penetration of the corrective ampoule without too much skin reaction.

- Apply day protection hydro-emulsion on the centre area and day protection/moisture on the cheeks and neck.

Treatment plan for the oily/acneic skin

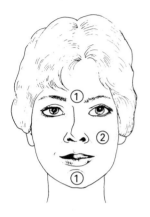

Recognition
1 Blackheads/comedones/seborrhoea/scars.
2 Dull, sallow colour/poor texture.

The skin is horny and keratinised and appears shiny with excessive oil secretion (sebum). Papules, pustules, blocked pores, milia (whiteheads) and scar tissue are all present. Cystic blockages may be felt under the skin, trapped by the comedone formation in the opening of the enlarged pore, aggravated by an overgrowth of epithelial tissue at the skin's surface.

Aim of treatment
Forms of ozone therapy and galvanic treatment are used to clear the infection quickly, healing, refining and balancing skin problems, bringing them under control. Treatment prevents the spread of infection and cleanses, disinfects and gently stimulates the skin to improved functioning. Elimination from within the body and superficially in the skin is important to success. Relief of nervous anxiety and stress is also known to play a part in the successful management and control of acne (especially adult acne), so helping the client to relax is vital.

Active ingredients
Herbal ingredients and essential oils: thyme, rosemary, lavender, camomile, eucalyptus, arnica, fenugreek, ylang ylang.
Seaweed, bio-sulphur, vitamin B complex.

Professional care
Cleanser (seaweed or herbal milk), liquid soap cleanser (seaweed), tonic (herbal or seaweed), scrub (seaweed, herbal), exfoliator (phyto or enzyme type), eye makeup remover, night treatment (corrective), mask (regulating, phyto or clay type), hydro-regulator (hydro-emulsion day protection/correction), desincrustation product (soap/gel), ampoules (seaweed, thyme, rosemary, camomile).

Home care
Day care: cleanser (seaweed or herbal milk), liquid soap cleanser (seaweed), tonic (herbal or seaweed), hydro-regulator.
Night care: cleanser (seaweed or herbal milk), eye makeup remover, liquid soap cleanser (seaweed),
scrub (seaweed or herbal), night treatment (corrective).
Special care: mask (regulating, acne or phyto type), ampoules (seaweed, thyme, rosemary, camomile), exfoliator (phyto or enzyme type).

1 Classic acne treatment (1 hour)

The classic acne treatment is for skins with the classic combination of seborrhoea, enlarged and blocked pores, infected pustules and scars, which is treated with medical approval.

- Cleanse with seaweed or herbal cleanser using brush or manual method according to skin sensitivity. Remove carefully with warm water.
- Inspect skin to determine condition, redness, reaction, etc. If rather sensitive apply phyto exfoliator as an enzyme peel all over the affected area and leave to dry for 10 minutes. If the skin is not sensitive, apply the seaweed or herbal scrub under steam, working the scrub with the fingers into the areas of deepest blockage, watching overall skin colour and how it is responding to treatment. Steam, with no ozone at this point, should be applied at a distance of 40–50 cm (15–18 inches) to soften and add to the scrub's refining effect. Remove the scrub carefully with warm water.
- Inspect the skin again with the surface keratinisation and epidermal overgrowth removed and see how the plugged pores are prominent in readiness for galvanic desincrustation, allowing it to be more effective.
- Apply galvanic desincrustation with special desincrustation gel/soap and negative polarity, working below the skin threshold level and keeping the skin very wet and well covered with product to allow the galvanic current to be effective on the sebaceous plugs. Keeping the current very low prevents galvanic sensitivity developing if the treatment has to be given frequently. It also avoids discomfort over open areas, or patches of scar tissue where skin resistance alters as a result of the change of skin as it healed.
- Work gently for a few minutes, changing cotton wool where necessary to remove the soiled matter from the applicator. Rinse off the product extremely well, leaving the skin clean and settled. As this is the most important stage of the entire treatment, work slowly and persistently to free the blockage and chemically dissolve the trapped matter. This is the stage in treatment that makes extraction methods obsolete in modern therapy practice.
- Apply steam to the face for a few minutes, then apply vacuum massage under steam: generally for lymphatic elimination, then specifically for deep pore cleansing using the special applicators. Continue for 10 minutes.
- Change to ozone steaming and continue to play the steam cloud over the face for a further 3–4 minutes to disinfect the skin, balance the pH and aid rehydration.
- Apply acne mask (phyto, herbal or clay type) in a thin film all over face (and neck if affected). Leave to set for 10 minutes, remove carefully with tepid water.
- Apply acne ampoule with galvanic ionisation for 3–4 minutes, keeping the skin very wet and ensuring that all the herbal or seaweed ampoule is penetrated into the skin gradually. Alterna-

tively, apply direct high frequency current over the face and neck, concentrating on the areas of discoloration and scar tissue. Work with light tapping movements to aid desquamation (skin shedding).

- Vapour spray tone and settle the skin with a 10% dilution of herbal or seaweed tonic, blotting in well with cotton wool or sponges.
- Protect the skin with day protection for oily skin (corrective or protective).

Special note

Ozone therapy using wet and dry forms of ozone is central to the treatment of acne in the clinic and includes ozone steaming, high frequency (direct method) and ultraviolet treatments (short duration applications only). In combination with galvanic treatments, both desincrustation and iontophoresis methods, acne treatment results are dramatically improved.

2 Acne and scar treatment (1 hour)

This is a refining treatment applied where the condition is mainly under control, no longer chronic and the skin needs rehydration, removal of scars and improvement of colour and texture without causing a re-emergence of blemishes. Many scars, discoloured skin areas, poorly textured skin with deeply marked pores, a glassy skin appearance and seborrhoea (excessive oil secretion) are present on the skin's surface.

- Cleanse manually with herbal cleansing milk.
- Deep cleanse briefly with herbal or seaweed scrub.
- Do not steam the face as this makes the *stratum corneum* too soft and could cause subsequent grazing of the skin with the abrasive peel method.
- Apply acne mask (clay setting type or special abrasive peeling mask) and initially keep the mask wet while using the brush head of the running brush unit to work deeply all over the scarred and discoloured areas. Work systematically over the skin, and do not repeat treatment too much over the same areas to avoid sensitivity or broken capillaries being formed by the strong treatment. Allowing the mask to become more dry before removal increases the scar removal effect, but care needs to be taken – especially on dark skins – to avoid over-stimulation and grazing.
- Apply regenerating ampoule manually or under galvanic ionisation if the skin still appears calm and settled. Work with low intensity levels, below threshold sensation level to encourage the skin to take in all the product ingredients (ginseng, royal jelly, geranium, lavender, camomile, etc.).
- Apply day protection for the oily skin or, if the skin seems adequately moisturised from the ampoule, just leave it as it is and simply introduce the home product to the client for her information, explaining why it is not required within treatment.

Treatment for the dry skin

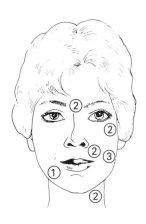

Recognition
1 Softening of firmness.
2 Fine crepey lines.
3 Loss of youthful texture.

Dry skin is thin with no evident pores and a tendency to peel in small patches when exposed to extremes in temperature. It is trouble free if well maintained and stimulated to maintain proper function. If neglected it soon becomes finely lined and crepey losing its natural firmness. Age and sun exposure are its biggest enemies, and correct skin care its greatest asset.

Aim of treatment
With correct treatment and home care this skin can be stimulated to an increased level of sebum secretion and its hydration brought back into balance. Both body and facial skin require constant protection from the elements (especially ultraviolet exposure) so daily use of sunscreen products on the face and body is essential.

Active ingredients
The fast and deep penetrating effect of liposomes carrying the active ingredients into the skin has been able to be used to great advantage within dry/dehydrated and mature skin treatment, bringing immediate visible results for the client. Effective and simple use of liposome products is especially important if the client is contra-indicated to other electrical systems of penetration such as galvanic ionisation.
Herbal ingredients and essential oils: sweet basil, rosemary, lavender, geranium, chamomile, rose.
Avocado oil, arnica and wheat germ oil, karite.
Aloe vera.

Professional care

Liposome cleanser, liposome tonic, eye makeup remover, gentle exfoliator, liposome regenerating cream or nourishing cream, eye cream, liposome moisture cream, facial tissue oil (essential oils), ampoules (dehydration, ginseng, royal jelly, etc.), biological/liposome mask (phyto ingredients).

Home care
Day care: liposome cleanser, liposome tonic, liposome moisture cream.
Night care: liposome cleanser, liposome tonic, eye makeup remover, liposome regenerating cream or nourishing cream, eye cream.
Special care: ampoules (facial tissue oil/essential oils, dehydration, ginseng, royal jelly, etc.), biological/liposome mask (phyto ingredients).

Facial therapy for dry/dehydrated skin (1 hour)

A cosmetically biased routine using liposome products to show how home sales are linked. (Any alternative nourishing product range may be used instead.)

- Cleanse with liposome cleanser, manually or with brush method.
- Work all over the face and neck with a gentle exfoliator in a moist paste for a few minutes to free old surface cells, rinse off well.
- Hydrate with liposome tonic, using a spray (10% dilution) or manual method (using toner undiluted). Blot into the skin very well.
- Apply liposome regenerating cream all over the face, neck and shoulders, and facial tissue oil or eye cream around the eyes. Give a deep, relaxing massage (Continental type) concentrating on the areas of greatest need, for 15–20 minutes. Work to improve relaxation in the person, circulation in the skin. Leave any residual cream on the skin.
- Apply the liposome/biological/geloid mask using active ingredients to match skin need. Apply all over the face, neck and shoulders in a thin film. Leave to work for 10 minutes and any mask remaining (not absorbed into the skin) may be removed gently with tepid water and cotton wool or sponges.
- Vapour spray tone the skin to ensure complete removal of the mask.
- Apply ampoule chosen according to skin need (ginseng, regeneration, dehydration, etc.), ionised on a low level of galvanic current for 4–5 minutes. Keep the skin really moist throughout to improve the skin hydration and function.
- Apply liposome moisture cream as day protection/sun screen.

If the client is contra-indicated to galvanic treatment, the ampoule may be applied manually, tapped gently into the skin to encourage its penetration.

Treatment for the dehydrated skin

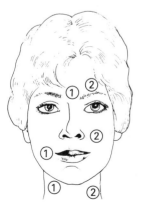

Recognition
1 Fine lines, crepey texture.
2 Skin elasticity and function poor.

The dehydrated skin lacks life and vitality as a result of a deficiency of natural oils and moisture. Skin elasticity is poor, fine lines are evident, especially on the neck and eye area. Skin function is impaired due to ageing, ill health, extremes of weather or stress and anxiety. An incorrect skin care routine, poor diet or neglect (including sun tanning) are other prime causes of dehydration.

Aim of treatment

Treatment concentrates on improving function and increasing biological activity, so aiding the oil and hydric (fluid) balance. Skin elasticity and firmness are improved by use of products such as collagen and elastin, and those containing DNA and RNA. An understanding of the skin's need for protection and stimulation will help prevent capillary damage from occurring, which is always a problem with severe dehydration and dryness.

Active ingredients

Herbal ingredients and essential oils: geranium, camomile, rosemary, lavender.
Avocado, sunflower or jojoba oil.
Oil of evening primrose.
Collagen, elastin, RNA, DNA.
Ginseng – native and extract forms.

Professional care

Ginseng cleanser, ginseng tonic, eye makeup remover, gentle exfoliator, ginseng night cream, eye cream, ginseng moisture cream, facial tissue oil (essential oils), ginseng mask (non-setting type), ampoules (dehydration, ginseng, royal jelly, etc.).

Home care

Day care: ginseng cleanser, ginseng tonic, ginseng moisture cream.
Night care: ginseng cleanser, ginseng tonic, eye makeup remover, ginseng night cream, eye cream.
Special care: ampoules (facial tissue oil/essential oils, dehydration, ginseng, etc.), ginseng mask.

Therapy for dehydration (1 hour)

A routine using ginseng as the theme ingredient for the routine and home care plan. (Any other suitable active product range for dehydration can be substituted.)

- Cleanse eye makeup with eye makeup remover if required.
- Cleanse with ginseng cleansing milk using the brush or manual method.
- Steam the face at a distance of 40–50 cm (15–18 inches) for 6–7 minutes (no ozone) to hydrate the skin and relax the client. Cover any extremely sensitive areas and watch the skin reaction until the skin is pink and warm, but not red.
- Apply facial tissue oil and apply vacuum massage for stimulation purposes, working to the general pattern for lymphatic drainage. Both pulsed and single applicator methods may be used if available. Do not over stimulate the skin, but work towards gentle circulation improvement. Leave the fine oil that remains on the skin.
- Apply the ginseng night cream, and if the skin is severely dehydrated mix the cream with a collagen firming cream (containing RNA/

DNA) to maximise the effect of the professional routine. Apply eye cream around the eyes, very finely to permit good control in massage. Apply a deep and relaxing massage for 15 minutes, paying special attention to the eyes, mouth and neck where lines are most noticeable. Use a lot of light, stimulating movements on the face. Indirect high frequency (Viennese massage) may also be used as an addition to the massage (if not contra-indicated).

- Remove the remaining cream and spray tone the skin with diluted ginseng tonic to settle and refresh the skin.
- Apply the ginseng mask and leave for 10 minutes until dry. Remove with damp sponges or cotton wool.
- Inspect the skin again and choose an ampoule. If the skin is simply dehydrated, ginseng is a good choice. If firming is needed, use collagen and elastin. Regeneration is another alternative. In a home plan the ampoules are often advised to be used in sequence, providing a range of actions, all of which the skin needs. Apply the ampoule with galvanic ionisation, working with minimal levels of intensity on this thin skin, for a few minutes only, below the client's awareness level.
- If the skin is very dehydrated, perhaps from sun exposure, or appears prematurely aged, a 'repair complex' product can be introduced which helps the skin's DNA repair process. It can be used as a night and day protection/repair, and helps to delay or rectify the effects of ageing. It is used under normal moisture protection or night cream.
- Apply ginseng moisture cream (with sun screen)

Treatment for the mature skin

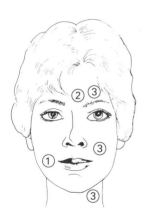

Recognition
1 Fine, permanent lines.
2 Loss of firmness and texture.
3 Loss of elasticity.

Loss of firmness in the mature skin causes the contours to soften and fine lines to appear on the neck, side cheeks and around the eyes. The skin seems loose on its bony attachments, and when pinched gently does not snap back into position, but settles slowly. Menopausal skin thickening around the chin and jaw area may be evident. Although even textured, fine and not over sensitive, the skin feels thin and lacks substance, due to changes in its cellular structure as ageing occurs. Losing its ability to retain fluid, the collagen fibres become cross-linked and rigid, instead of flexible as in a plump youthful skin. This natural consequence of ageing can be delayed with the latest RNA and DNA products (repair complex, night repair, collagen firming creams) which intervene in the skin's bio-engineering, slowing this cross-linking process and helping the skin to rebuild cells lost as a consequence of skin damage, sun exposure, ageing, etc.

Aims of treatment

Stimulation and improvement of biological activity, cellular function and skin replacement rate will help to improve both the elasticity and the skin thickening problems, as both are a result of the skin replacement rate slowing down and allowing the skin to build up in certain areas. A gentle programme of refining is called for in the chin, mouth and nose area, combined into a revitalising and firming plan of treatment for the mature skin.

Active ingredients

Ginseng – native and extract forms.
Essential oils: geranium, camomile, rosemary, lavender.
Avocado oil, sunflower oil, jojoba oil, karite.
Natural moisturising factors (NMFs).
Oil of evening primrose.
Collagen, elastin, RNA and DNA.
Vitamins A and E.

Professional care

Ginseng cleanser, ginseng tonic, eye makeup remover, gentle exfoliator, ginseng night cream, collagen firming cream (RNA, DNA), nourishing cream, eye cream, repair complex, ginseng moisture cream, facial tissue oil (essential oils), ginseng mask (non-setting type), ampoules (collagen and elastin, dehydration, ginseng, revitalising, etc.)

Home care

Day care: ginseng cleanser, ginseng tonic, repair complex, ginseng moisture cream.
Night care: ginseng cleanser, ginseng tonic, eye makeup remover, ginseng night cream, eye cream.
Special care: ampoules (facial tissue oil/essential oils, collagen and elastin, dehydration, ginseng, etc.), ginseng mask, repair complex/collagen firming cream (used when necessary).

Revitalising and firming (1 hour 30 minutes)

This classic facial (Continental style) is the frame for the treatment and into this plan go various elements for firming and stimulating the skin and underlying muscles of facial expression. Ginseng has been used again as an active ingredient, but any gentle regenerating ingredient can be substituted as the underlying theme to the products.

- Remove eye makeup with eye makeup remover if necessary.
- Cleanse with ginseng cleansing milk using the brush method for skin stimulation, using all the specialised small brushes to make the routine a small treatment. Do not allow the brushes to drag at any stage. Use sufficient cleansing product and protect the eyes with a sponge held in the free hand.

- If required, apply a gentle exfoliator as a deep cleansing scrub on skin thickened by menopausal influences. Confine to the areas of need. Rinse off well after a few minutes of friction movements.
- Spray tone lightly with a 10% dilution of ginseng tonic to prepare the skin and introduce the product to the client.
- Apply the ampoule (revitalising or collagen and elastin) directly over the fine lines and worst crepey skin areas, patting it into the skin. It should enter the skin very easily after the brush cleansing routine. Concentrate on the most visible lines, or those of which the client is most aware, such as around the mouth, or from the nose to the corners of the mouth. Discuss this with the client, explaining reasons. Get as much of the ampoule to penetrate as possible. Retain the rest for later in treatment.
- Over the top of the ampoule, apply the facial tissue oil (with essential oils) and use as a medium for vacuum suction, used as both a skin firming and lymphatic drainage measure. Adjust the applicators, lift into the cup and the speed of strokes to suit the skin sensitivity (reaction) and level of firmness. If the skin is very loose, work mainly with the small specialised applicators, over the facial lines, taking care not to cause too much blanching which could result later in bruising. Initially, keep the treatment cautious, but thorough, as done correctly this is an excellent way to aid ampoule penetration and stimulate the skin. Just watch for surface sensitivity, avoid any fragile skin areas, dilated capillaries, naevi or general couperose conditions on the tops of the cheeks. Adapt the routine to suit the skin. Leave any remaining oil on the skin.
- Apply the collagen firming cream (RNA and DNA) and the ginseng night cream (which can also cover the eye area) and give a full 20 minutes' massage of the upper shoulders, neck and face. Incorporate as many firming and stimulating movements as possible to improve the circulation. This is the most important stage of the routine for overall treatment success, as with the client relaxed and strain eased from the back and shoulders the active ingredients and essential oils in the products can be really effective on the circulation. Allow the client time to participate in the aromatic nature of the routine, and gain benefit from it as a form of stress therapy.
- Remove any cream which remains and apply the ginseng mask or a more firming mask (these can be alternated in treatment). Leave the mask on for 10 minutes and remove thoroughly with tepid water.
- Bring the client into a semi-reclining position, and apply the muscle toning routine on a clean skin. Ensure no oil, cream, etc. is still present to block the flow of the faradic current. Cover the electrodes with conductive gel and apply a few contractions on each muscle, working steadily up from the neck to the eye area. The client will be able to notice an immediate difference in skin firmness.
- Apply the rest of the ampoule to the skin, either manually or with galvanic ionisation (if not contra-indicated). Work at an extremely

low intensity, as at this stage of treatment skin resistance should be minimal, and the client will be aware of the current almost on a zero milliamp reading. Apply for 2–3 minutes until all the ampoule has been absorbed by the skin.

- Apply the repair complex product to the skin and explain its special significance to the client (i.e. that it intervenes in the cellular repair process, so delaying effects of ageing).
- Apply ginseng moisture protection (containing sun screen).

Rejuvenation treatment

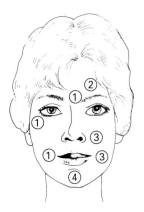

Recognition
1 Fine lines.
2 Softening of texture and lack of firmness.
3 Softening of contours and lack of sensitivity.
4 Menopausal skin thickening.

This treatment is indicated for tired, dehydrated, skins showing ageing signs, because of stress, rapid weight loss, ill health or a post-pregnancy condition. It is effective on sensitive, mature or easily irritated skin. Treatment improves function and stimulates cellular replacement from the basal layer of the skin to create a younger, more vital looking skin from within. Recommended for busy, over-stressed or anxious clients.

Aim of treatment
The overall effect is hydrating, nourishing and gently stimulating: an excellent preventative measure to delay ageing tendencies, fine lines, loss of skin texture, etc. from whatever cause. The rejuvenation treatment (using an ingredient such as royal jelly) is special as it is so effective, but gentle. This makes the treatment ideal for skins prone to allergic and irritant reaction which need more than soothing routines.

It is an ideal treatment to recommend following cosmetic surgery, as the activity comes from the the ingredients rather than from the manual treatment, e.g. massage.

Active ingredients
Royal jelly.
Essential oils: lavender, sweet basil, geranium, camomile.
Wheat germ, sunflower oil, avocado oil, karite.
Vitamins A and E.
Seaweed extract.
Natural moisturising factors (NMFs).

Professional care
Royal jelly cleanser, royal jelly tonic, eye makeup remover, gentle exfoliator, royal jelly night cream, regenerating/rejuvenating cream

(with hyaluronic acid), eye cream, royal jelly moisture cream, facial tissue oil (essential oils), royal jelly mask (non-setting type) or thermal mask, ampoules (royal jelly, revitalising, etc.).

Home care
Day care: royal jelly cleanser, royal jelly tonic, royal jelly moisture cream, firming eye gel.
Night care: royal jelly cleanser, royal jelly tonic, eye makeup remover, royal jelly night cream, eye cream.
Special care: ampoules (royal jelly, facial tissue oil/essential oils, dehydration), royal jelly mask or firming mask, regenerating/ rejuvenating cream (with hyaluronic acid).

Rejuvenation therapy (1 hour)

The routine uses as the theme the royal jelly range which is simple and effective for home use. (Products using alternative active ingredients for regeneration can be substituted.)

- Cleanse manually with royal jelly cleanser, working gently but with deep relaxing movements.
- Spray tone with diluted 10% solution royal jelly tonic, or if toning manually, apply full strength, blotting in well to firm the skin.
- Steam the face at a distance of 50 cm (18 inches) for 4–5 minutes to soften and hydrate the surface, protecting any sensitive areas with cotton wool pads (do not use ozone steam).
- Apply royal jelly ampoule manually (no galvanic ionisation) tapping in well. Encourage as much as possible to enter the warm and softened skin.
- Apply royal jelly treatment cream and rejuvenating cream (with hyaluronic acid) mixed together, applied all over the shoulders, neck and face. Massage thoroughly for 15–20 minutes,working deeply but gently, concentrating on effleurage movements that lift and control the superficial muscles rather than on tapotement movements. The client should feel rejuvenated by the massage. Any cream that remains after the massage may be left on the skin.
- Apply the royal jelly mask (non-setting biological type for firming) and leave to set for 10 minutes. Remove with damp cotton wool or sponges. (A geloid or phyto mask may be used as an alternative, using active ingredients picked for rejuvenation/regeneration effects.)
- Tone the skin with royal jelly tonic. Blot in well.
- Any remaining royal jelly ampoule may be applied at this stage of treatment, and its special properties as an under-makeup treatment should be explained to the client. Busy clients will find daily use of a concentrated ampoule the fastest and finest way to rejuvenate the vitality of their skin when applied on a clean skin prior to day protection.
- Apply royal jelly moisture cream as protection/sun screen.

Treatment for the sensitive skin

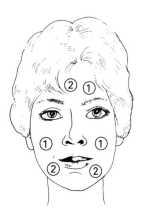

Recognition
1 Thin, delicate areas.
2 Skin prone to allergic reaction.

The skin is delicate and easily exposed to capillary damage or irritation because of a deficiency in its pH balance or acid mantle. Fragile and thin, it lacks natural lipid substances, so its greatest need is for protection and hydration to avoid allergic reactions occurring. The tiny capillaries are visible through the epidermis and this is where the troublesome problem couperose slowly but surely develops if skin is not treated and home care established. The elasticity of the capillary walls is weak and has to be strengthened through gentle stimulation (decongestant effect) and by use of special products at home. It is not properly understood why some people have sensitive skin, but stress seems to play a major part. The skin becomes irritated and develops flaky patches, dermatitis and allergic reactions. Extremes of temperature and stimulants like spicy foods, alcohol and caffeine seem to worsen the problem. A condition of permanent erythema or skin redness often precedes the true couperose condition and indicates a need for special care to avoid permanent damage.

Aim of treatment
Treatment gently encourages the skin to function more efficiently and be able to cope with the changes of everyday life without becoming irritated. Active ingredients known for their calming and anti-inflammatory powers are used in a simple plan which acts daily to settle the skin, balance the pH and improve the circulation, so preventing dilated capillaries forming.

Many of the factors that cause allergic reactions come from within the body, e.g. anxiety, stress, so clients have to be made to recognise this aspect of their skin condition and remain calm. Regular aromatherapy massage of the body with essential oils helps the client to unwind as a form of stress therapy. The most important point is for the client to discover a skin care programme that suits her difficult skin and does not aggravate or cause reactions. Once suited with a product line that works, she will seldom want or be able to change from it.

Active ingredients

Calendula (marigold), azulene, St John's wort.
Essential oils: lavender, camomile.

Professional care
Sensitive skin cleanser, sensitive skin tonic, sensitive skin night cream, nourishing cream, eye cream, facial tissue oil (essential oils),

sensitive skin mask (non-setting type), sensitive skin day protection, ampoules for sensitive skin (azulene, St John's wort, calendula).

Home care
Day care: sensitive skin cleanser, sensitive skin tonic, sensitive skin day protection.
Night care: sensitive skin cleanser, eye makeup remover, sensitive skin tonic, sensitive skin night cream, eye cream.
Special care: sensitive skin mask, ampoules for sensitive skin (azulene, calendula, St John's wort).

Sensitive skin therapy (1 hour)

- Cleanse the skin with sensitive skin cleanser manually or with a very damp soft brush on the brush equipment. Avoid over-stimulating the skin. If in doubt,work manually.
- Spray tone the skin with diluted (10%) sensitive skin tonic or tone manually, just using soft rolling movements. Blot the skin well.
- Apply facial tissue oil and encourage the circulation of the face to work more efficiently by using vacuum suction in an adapted way to draw surface blood away from the most highly coloured areas. Only tiny aperture applicators are used and the minimum amount of vacuum. The skin should scarcely lift into the applicators (less than 5% lift).

   If the vacuum equipment will not provide this degree of control, use the alternative treatment of indirect high frequency, applied as Viennese massage, using the facial tissue oil as the medium for the massage. Keep pressure steady and even, remembering that the lighter the fingers move over the skin,the more effective will be the circulation response in the skin. The same approach of drawing the blood away from the congested areas can be used and a noticeable difference will be evident after only a few treatments.
- The oil remains on the skin and the sensitive skin night cream is applied over the top. A more nourishing cream can be added to the mix to provide more flexibility in the massage, although it is important to introduce the client to the light textured product she will use at night in her home plan. Apply 10–15 minutes of massage, giving equal time to the neck and shoulders as to the face to avoid over-stimulation. The client will gain as much benefit from relaxing tension at the back of the neck as from facial movements, so adapt massage accordingly. Interspace the more active movements with calming movements of the hands, to help the client benefit fully from the massage routine. Vibrations can be added to the sequence to good effect.
- Apply a sensitive skin mask, leave for 10 minutes to dry , and remove residue with damp sponges or cotton wool. Geloid type masks or clay masks may be used as alternatives, with ingredients picked to match the sensitive skin condition.

- Spray tone with diluted sensitive skin tonic, blot in well.
- Apply the ampoule for sensitive skin as a protective and gently stimulating film that will stay on the skin for the next few hours. Ampoules play a very large part in the control and care of the sensitive skin, being a very concentrated form of soothing ingredients – especially azulene, calendula and St John's wort. They are able to settle a difficult skin down quite dramatically, so the client can be trained to use them as an instant calmer if her skin becomes troublesome or irritated.
- Apply sensitive skin day protection as a final step.

Treatment for the couperose skin

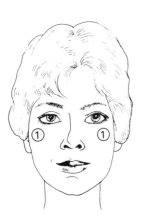

Recognition
Dilated capillaries on the upper cheeks.

The couperose skin is easily recognised by the areas of dilated capillaries, where the blood has seeped into the skin's surface layers in a thread-like formation (hence the common name 'thread veins'). The condition can develop on many skin types but is most common as a progression of the sensitive skin, through age, neglect or incorrect treatment. Over-exposure to sun and wind aggravates the skin condition.

The trapped blood can become a very dark bluish-red in colour, with small varicosities of the blood vessels giving the appearance of capillaries being completely exposed on the skin's surface. This is not the case, but does show how exposed the skin has become and how stagnant the blood.

Aims of treatment
The aim of treatment is to work preventatively, building up the skin's own defence mechanism. Vascular circulation is increased and the capillary walls strengthened, improving vasoconstriction which moves the blood along the tiny capillaries and prevents it becoming stagnant and trapped. The active ingredients in the couperose treatment creams are renowned for their constrictive qualities (especially horse chestnut), but require daily application to be effective. The other elements in the supporting sensitive skin line carry out a programme of soothing and calming to keep the skin in good condition and prevent further damage. As with all skin problems, prevention is better than cure.

Special note: As the couperose condition is most commonly associated with the sensitive and fragile complexion, the treatment plan has been worked out in association with sensitive skin products. However the royal jelly or ginseng treatment lines would work equally well in the clinic and at home, as natural regenerators of the skin. The important thing is that the couperose products must be used night and day in addition to whatever treatment line is being used. They are not substitutes for day protection and night cream but are applied under them, directly on the capillary condition.

As it has to be faced that capillary damage is already present on the skin, all treatment planned has to be gentle in action until the accumulative action of the active ingredients in the couperose creams and ampoules starts to work and show visible evidence of constricting the tiny blood vessels – this may take up to a month. Results can be obtained more quickly by using concentrated ampoules for couperose, a fact which should be explained to the client if she is very anxious to be free from her disfiguring problems. Allow her to decide her priorities.

Active ingredients
Horse chestnut, calendula (marigold), azulene, St John's wort.

Professional care
Sensitive skin cleanser, sensitive skin tonic, couperose day cream, couperose night cream, sensitive skin night cream (or ginseng, royal jelly, etc.), eye cream, facial tissue oil (essential oils).

Sensitive skin/couperose mask (non-setting type), sensitive skin day protection, ampoules for couperose skin (horse chestnut, azulene, St John's wort, calendula).

Home care
Day care: sensitive skin cleanser, sensitive skin tonic, couperose day cream, sensitive skin day protection.
Night care: sensitive skin cleanser, eye makeup remover, sensitive skin tonic, couperose night cream, sensitive skin night cream, eye cream.
Special care: sensitive skin mask, ampoules for couperose skin (horse chestnut, azulene, calendula, St John's wort).

Treatment plan for couperose skin

- Cleanse the skin gently with sensitive skin cleanser, using the manual method.
- Inspect the skin very carefully to determine the extent of the capillary damage and note areas that will require adaptations of the routine, changes in the massage, etc.
- Spray tone the skin to settle it with calming sensitive skin tonic in a 10% dilution, or tone manually using the tonic undiluted. Blot in well, working over the entire face as the calming ingredients in the tonic will help to constrict the capillaries and allow more treatment to be applied.
- Apply the ampoule for couperose manually over the affected areas of the face and just beyond, patting the ampoule in gently, encouraging the skin to accept as much as possible.
- Apply the facial tissue oil in a thin film all over the face and neck

and, depending on the condition of the skin and degree of capillary damage, use the vacuum suction as a means of drawing blood away from the line-like threads in the skin. Use the narrow applicators, low vacuum and fast, light movements. Bring the pattern, though adapted, towards the lymph nodes behind the ears or below the jawline, which ever is the easiest regarding the extent and position of the dilated capillaries. Keep working towards the normal lymphatic drainage pattern, to encourage the trapped blood to disperse via normal elimination means.

Alternatively use indirect high frequency and Viennese massage to act deeply on the circulation. This encourages increased tissue interchange which eliminates the waste products that have become trapped or stagnant. As with bruises, the body will gradually re-absorb the small amounts of blood that have become stuck between the skin layers. Work over the upper shoulders, neck and face. Keep returning to the face just for short periods,then going back to the neck and shoulders for deeper massage movements to speed and free the circulation. Once the muscles in the neck relax, the circulation (and the elimination/lymphatic flow) naturally improve from the head and face.

- Leaving the facial tissue oil on, apply the couperose night cream and royal jelly treatment cream in a mixture all over the neck, shoulders and face and continue massage for a further 10 minutes, working for general relaxation. If the facial skin becomes red, restrict movements to the neck, shoulders and upper arm areas. Remove any cream that remains.
- Apply any remaining ampoule, patting into the skin.
- Apply the sensitive/couperose skin mask (non-setting type) or a geloid or phyto type mask picked for its calming ingredients (e.g. horse chestnut, azulene, calendula, St John's wort). Apply in a thin film all over the face and neck, leave for 10 minutes and remove gently with cool water. The skin will look very calm at this stage, and this effect continues for some hours after treatment.
- Spray tone with diluted sensitive skin tonic. Blot in well.
- Apply the couperose day cream, explaining its importance for constriction and protection of capillaries to the client. This is the stage at which the couperose ampoules could be applied daily instead of the couperose day cream if an accelerated result is desired or the problem is very severe.
- Apply the sensitive skin day protection as a further barrier to the elements and a base for makeup, if worn.

Specialised treatments

As well as all the treatments described in this book there are many more new ones being developed all the time. Products are becoming more and more refined. Machines become more specialised. Included below are some treatments which would possibly be offered by certain beauty salons. Extra post-graduate training is usually required for performing these treatments.

Skin peeling by biological, chemical and abrasive methods

Skin peeling is a treatment that improves the quality and tone of the complexion. The process removes dead cells from the surface of the skin, increasing the skin's natural desquamation, and leaving a fresh clean appearance. It is a cosmetic process, based on biological (vegetable) or chemical products, which only removes dead surface cells and the products of keratinisation in the horny stratum corneum of the epidermis.

Biological peeling
This cosmetic method is achieved by application of a solution which softens the unwanted keratinised dead cells, without affecting the living skin tissue. The sequence is completed by application of a mask-like cream, which progresses the action initiated by the solution and eliminates the dead cells.

The skill in all forms of peeling is in diagnosis and recognition of the existing skin condition, rather than in the actual application of the cosmetic preparations. Observation of sensitivity, skin irregularities or irritation, produced by the first mild skin-peeling application, will give guidance as to future treatment possibilities, and should prevent over-treatment.

Indications for treatment
1 Young problem skins, with blocked pores, blackheads and over-secretion of sebaceous glands.
2 Sallow complexions, which require toning and stimulating.
3 Scarred, post-acne complexions, to refine the skin, and slowly remove the discoloured scar tissue.
4 General cleansing and refining purposes on normal and combination skin conditions.

Contra-indications to treatment
With careful choice and application of biological products, very few skins are completely contra-indicated, but the following conditions might suffer irritation from the sequence.

1 Hyper-sensitive skins.
2 Extremely dry or dehydrated complexions.
3 Mature crepey skin.

The manufacturer's instructions should be followed carefully as variations of application sequence exist. Basic principles, diagnosis, and the need for vigilant awareness of skin reaction, however, stay constant.

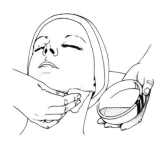
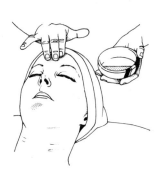
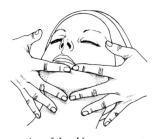
Preparation of the skin

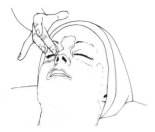

Application of cream

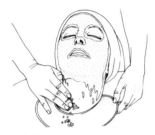

Removal of cream

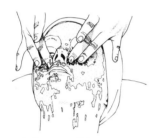

Removal of cream pellets around the nose

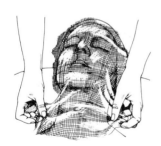

Gauze mask

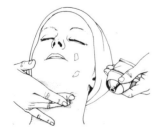

Moisture cream application

Application

1 General cleansing and toning should be completed. The skin should not be steamed as this pre-softens the surface and is disadvantageous.
2 The skin is thoroughly wiped over with the softening lotion, to remove surface dirt, and natural sebum, and prepare it for the peeling.
3 The entire area is moistened with the special lotion, which has a lysing action which helps to dissolve the dead skin cells. The liquid is gently worked into the face and neck until it is all absorbed. Any tingling or itching felt at this stage can be relieved by a few minutes light massage to alleviate the sensation and reassure the client.
4 The solution is left for 3–5 minutes, then the cream is applied in the same manner as a mask avoiding eyes, nostrils, etc. Eye pads are applied and the client rests for 15–20 minutes to enable the peeling process to develop.
5 When the cream is ready for removal, small cracks appear in the surface and the texture becomes dry. The product is removed with light circular movements of the finger tips, commencing at the neck. A cuvette bowl may be placed at the neck to catch the dried mask fragments as they are removed. The dead cells are removed with the dried cream, and on completion the skin will appear fresh and vibrant.
6 When the neck and face are completely clean, nourishing cream and a gauze compress soaked in mildly antiseptic hydrating lotion may be applied. The skin requires protection and rehydration at this stage, so it may be left until it appears calm and has regained its normal temperature.
7 Moisturiser may be applied to complete the treatment, and protect the newly peeled complexion. Only lipstick and eye makeup should be applied after any form of peeling process.

Chemical (progressive) peeling

The chemical method of skin peeling has a progressive effect, becoming increasingly stronger as the treatment extends over a lengthening period. Unlike the biological peeling which has a fairly constant action, the progressive method is capable of causing skin irritation if incorrectly chosen for the skin condition. Previous knowledge of the skin, its reaction to treatment and general sensitivity to chemical substances is vital prior to chemical peeling.

Indications for treatment

1 Post-acne scarring.
2 Discoloured skin areas (mild peeling at spaced intervals only).
3 Sallow, thickened skin conditions.

Contra-indications to treatment

1 Sensitive, dry dehydrated skins.
2 Mature skins.
3 Skin infection, irritation, abrasions etc.

Application

The treatment is composed of an active lotion, which is combined with progressively more active powders to form a mask paste. The paste is applied like a mask, avoiding the eye areas, and left for 5–15 minutes according to the client's reaction. The mask should be removed immediately if, after the initial tingling sensation passes, irritation is felt strongly on any area. The mask powders are used in sequence, always combined with the activating lotion, to produce increasingly evident peeling effects. The mask is removed with tepid water, and nourishing or hydrating preparation applied to soothe the skin.

Progressive peeling forms part of a sequence of skin improvement treatments for the post-acne, scarred, or discoloured complexion. It may be alternated with regenerating treatment for the more mature discoloured skin, or with antiseptic electrical routines for the adolescent skin. No infection should be present at the time of peeling otherwise irritation and soreness will result. The treatment may be applied at moderate intervals, according to skin sensitivity and the effect desired. The skin should never be permitted to become over-exposed, otherwise capillary damage will result.

Abrasive peeling treatment

Abrasive brush treatment is accomplished by application of the brush massage equipment, with special attachments for abrasive effects (see Chapter 2, page 20). Foam pads and an abrasive stone applicator are used to remove the abrasive mask paste from areas of hardened, scarred or pigmented skin tissue. The treatment may be varied to include all but the most sensitive complextions. For indications, contra-indications to treatment and application, see *Abrasive peeling treatment* in Chapter 9, page 161.

Combined galvanic and high-frequency units

Several companies have produced a machine which combines the effective cleansing galvanic current with the equally effective high-frequency current. The products used with this treatment are usually all supplied by the manufacturer, creating a total treatment. The facial routine will last approximately 1½ hours and provides excellent revenue and results.

Air massage units

Often combined with a vacuum suction machine, an air massage unit device has two leads and an intermittent pulse. The strokes are still directed towards the lymph nodes, the difference being the pulsating action. It feels pleasant and relaxing and is effective in lymphatic drainage treatments.

Specific product ranges

There are so many specific product ranges to choose from. Most will offer some sort of specialist facial, for example a prescriptive facial, where a range of additives can be put with a gel or cream base to mix a massage cream and mask. A variety of ampoules and masks for mature, wrinkled skin or acneic problem skins may be available.

Aromatherapy

Aromatherapy is a truly wonderful treatment. It combines the skill of the masseuse and the blending of essential oils to suit the particular requirements of the client. It works on the central nervous system, so essentially it is a body treatment concentrating on the spine, but treatment can be extended very effectively to include the face. Aromatherapy associates wonderfully with reflexology (treatment of the body by application of pressure point massage to the feet). The chosen blended essential oils are massaged by hand only, making this an ideal routine for highly stressed or nervous clients. The increasing popularity of aromatherapy has produced many ranges of associated plant-based products incorporating plant extracts and essential oils into creams, masks, moisture and sun-protection products. Beauty therapists need to keep updated and follow trends which gain media exposure, as this can be an effective boost to business. Reading regular journals, joining professional organisations and attending beauty conferences and trade fairs help to keep in touch with new developments.

It is vital that every client receives a consultation before using any essential oils on the skin, in case there are contra-indications to certain oils, such as some drugs for example or pregnancy.

Self Check

1 Why is it important to give the client home care advice?
2 What is the main aim of the treatment for each of the following skin types?
   (a) Normal.
   (b) Combination.
   (c) Oily.
   (d) Dry.
   (e) Dehydrated.
   (f) Mature.
   (g) Sensitive.
   (h) Couperose.

CHAPTER ELEVEN

Treatment of the Arms and Legs

Anatomy of the hands and forearms

Anatomically the wrist and hand are very complex parts of the body, containing 29 bones and a large number of joints and small muscles which permit an enormous range of movements. A knowledge of the superficial muscles only is required, and the antagonistic nature of the flexor and extensor muscles should be understood.

Bones of the hand

Carpals – bones of the wrist

There are eight bones of irregular size, which fit closely together and are held in position by ligaments. The bones articulate with each other, permitting slight movement, and also give attachment to the small muscles of the hand that move the fingers. The bones of the wrist are:

- Hamate.
- Triquetrum.
- Capitate.
- Pisiform.
- Trapezoid.
- Lunate.
- Trapezium.
- Scaphoid.

Metacarpals

The palm of the hand is made up of five long bones, the proximal ends (those closest to the centre of the body) of which articulate with the wrist bones. The distal ends articulate with the phalanges (finger bones).

Phalanges

The 14 phalanges (finger bones) are also long bones, with three to each finger and two to the thumb.

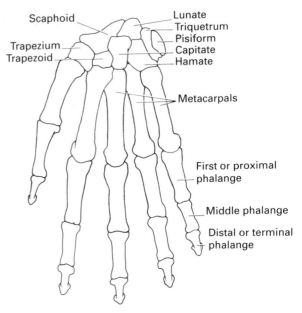

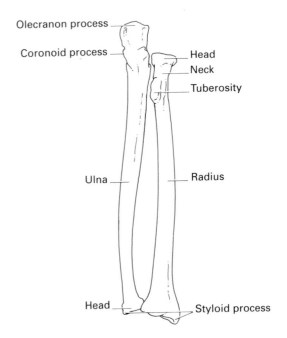

Bones of the hand, wrist and forearm

Bones of the forearm

The bones of the forearm are the radius and the ulna. The ulna bone articulates with the humerus of the upper arm. Only flexion and extension movements are possible in the forearm.

Muscles of the forearm

Many of the muscles of the forearm and wrist are termed according to their action and form two groups – these are the flexor muscles and the extensor muscles (i.e. those that allow flexion and extension actions respectively). Many of the small muscles co-ordinate to form similar actions, so a representative sample of each type of muscle and its action provides sufficient knowledge for the beauty specialist's application of massage in the area.

Table 11.1 Superficial muscles of the forearm and wrist

Muscles	Action
Flexor muscles	
Flexor carpi radialis	
Flexor carpi ulnaris	Flexion of wrist and elbow joint
Flexor digitorum sublimus	Flexion of fingers, wrist and elbow
Flexor pollicis longus	Flexion of the thumb
Extensor muscles	
Extensor carpi radialis brevis	
Extensor carpi ulnaris	Extension of wrist and elbow joint
Extensor digitorum communis	Extension of fingers and elbow joint
Extensor pollicis longus	Extension of the thumb
Rotation and flexion muscles	
Pronator teres	Pronates the forearm (rotation)
Brachioradialis	Flexes the elbow joint

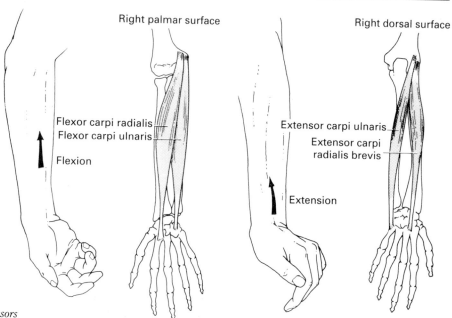

Lower arm flexors and extensors

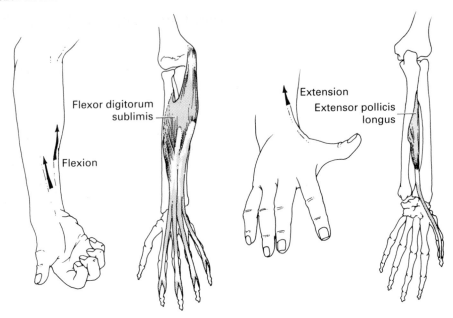

Lower arm digital muscles

It can be clearly seen that the flexor and extensor muscles work in opposition to each other, as antagonistics, and that their names relate both to their bone attachments and the action created.

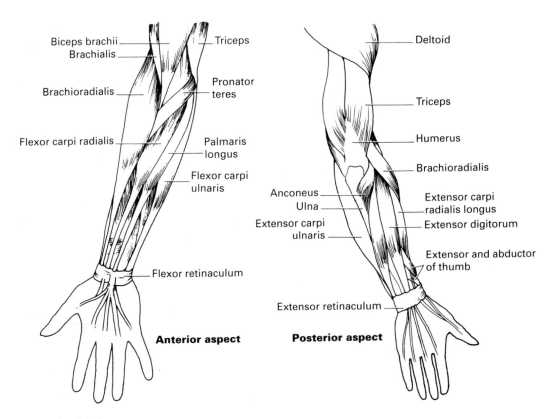

Superficial muscles of the forearm

Structure and function of the nails

The main role of nails is a protective one, safeguarding the sensitive areas of the distal portions of the fingers and toes. Nails are formed from hard keratinous cells, which are termed onychin, and have a very low (7–12%) moisture and fat content. The matrix area of the nail is the most important part and is composed of polygonal cells, similar to the Malpighian layer of the skin. The opaque appearance of the nail is due to the presence of keratohyaline, and the white area (lanula) at the base of the nail is thought to be noticeable due to the change of light refraction at this stage of growth, and acts as a dividing level.

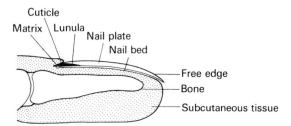

Cross-section of the nail

Sensitivity and growth of nails

The nail rests directly on a layer of prickle cells, overlying an extremely vascular papillary layer containing numerous sensitive nerves. This explains the pain involved if a nail is injured by pressure, or is torn below the flesh line. The nail bed and plate grow outwards together, so any injury to the matrix (cell-forming area) may affect both the nail and bed. The rate of growth in nails appears to be fairly constant, at 2.5 cm (1 inch) in eight months, with no real difference between the sexes. However, the rate of wear, breakage, etc. due to work conditions, health and dirt, vary considerably and will be the area in which the beauty specialist can give the maximum assistance. Eliminating or reducing nail abuse by sensible guidance, plus a programme of professional treatments, will achieve excellent results.

General good health, a balanced diet and exposure to sunlight does appear to improve the condition of nails, but some clients will always have frail nails due to genetic factors. In these cases control of the condition to prevent further deterioration of the nails is the task of the therapist.

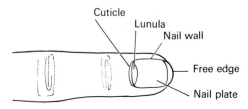

The parts of the nail

Manicure

Purpose of the manicure

Regular and attentive care is necessary if immaculate nails are to be maintained and this point must be stressed to the client. As the nails are so vital to a groomed appearance, the manicure treatment is one of the most popular services that a beauty specialist can offer, often in combination with facial applications. The actual procedure frees the cuticle and nail wall from the nail plate, thus avoiding the risk of hangnail formation which is caused by the stretched skin splitting away from the nail plate. The outline of the nail is kept smooth, infection is prevented, and only gentle treatment is required to maintain an attractive cosmetic appearance. Regular professional attention will also prevent minor nail damage, splits, tears, fragile tips, etc. remaining undetected and becoming more serious in nature.

Repairs and remedial home treatment can be introduced immediately to prevent a worsening of the existing condition. The protective role of the enamel and adherent strengthening preparations should be exploited to the full, reinforced by an extensive programme of nourishing and emollient creams applied nightly. The addition of massage into the manicure routine increases the skin improvement, delays ageing tendencies such as wrinkled or discoloured skin, and controls areas of senile pigmentation in the mature client by the addition of bleaching preparations in the massage medium.

Contra-indications to manicure

A manicure treatment should not be carried out if any of the following conditions are present:

- Bruises on the hand or wrist.
- Swelling of the wrist or finger joints.
- Any skin infection (see Chapter 5, Skin Diseases and Disorders).
- Any nail infection (see later).
- Open cuts or wounds.

Recognition of nail diseases and disorders

Many physical conditions affect the nails, among which are psoriasis, rheumatism, eczema and heart complaints, which show themselves in the nail as transverse ridges, furrows, pitting, etc. Any condition of the nail that appears unusual to the beauty specialist should be directed for medical advice.

Nail disorders

Leuconychia

This is a very common nail disorder in which small white spots appear on the nail plate. They are caused by minor trauma to the nail plate allowing air to be trapped between the nail bed and the nail plate. The white areas grow out, no special treatment is required and a manicure can proceed as normal.

Furrows and ridges

Furrows running across the nail bed indicate a change in the growth rate of the nail. Dermatitis may be the cause of deep furrows. A single transverse furrow or Beau's line across every nail may be the result of pneumonia, thrombosis or other major illness. (An operation on the wrist can cause Beau's lines.) No treatment is required and the furrows simply grow out.

Longitudinal ridges may be associated with rheumatism, but can also occur in good health. A single ridge on one nail may be the result of a major trauma, e.g. a car door accident, or constant picking can also result in a ridge or ridges. Buffing the nail plate can help to smooth out some uneven nail plates.

Pitting

Pitting of the nail plate is usually an indication of an underlying problem, e.g. psoriasis or dermatitis. If the pits are severe medical attention is required.

Hang nail

This condition is usually caused by minor injury or constant irritation through biting, it appears as a small spike of hard nail growing in the nail groove alongside the main nail. Infection can occur if the spike is bitten or pulled off; the manicurist can clip it carefully with sterilised clippers and offer advice on softening the cuticle with massage cream.

Discoloration

Discoloration of the nail plate can be caused by many things: fungal infection, damage to the nail bed or external contact with a substance that can stain it. Ringworm or *Tinea unguium* (see later) can cause the plate to turn yellow-brown or black, this is a contra-indication to manicure.

Hair dyes, nicotine, dark nail enamels and various chemicals can all cause discoloration. Advice can be given about the prevention of staining and the nails buffed regularly to reduce the stains and encourage new growth.

Blue nails indicate a poor circulation in the nail bed, anaemia or maybe a heart problem. Regular use of a cuticle massage cream and finger exercises will help to improve the circulation.

Black nails are usually the result of acute trauma, e.g. a heavy weight being dropped on the nail, or trapping the nail. The darkened area is a bruise to the nail bed; the area grows out, medical attention is not usually necessary and the affected nail can simply be avoided in the manicure treatment.

Brittle nails

This can be a congenital disorder or can be caused by various external or internal factors. Strong detergents can have a degreasing action, leaving the nail plate brittle and with poor circulation. Dietary deficiencies can also lead to thinning of the nail plate. Manicure can help the condition and advice can be given on the prevention of brittle nails.

Self-inflicted problems

Biting or picking at the nail or cuticle can lead to distortion and even permanent damage. The nails appear short, ragged and may show ridges; the cuticles may be untidy, red or open – this can obviously lead to infection. If the nervous habit is prolonged permanent damage may be done. The beauty specialist can offer lots of advice and help in overcoming the problem. Having regular manicures is one step that can help lead to a cure.

Pterygium

This is the overgrowth of the cuticle, which adheres to the nail plate and grows forward with it. Regular massage and oil treatments can gradually free the skin. Advice is necessary to prevent the recurrence.

These are just some of the more common nail disorders; there are many more that affect the nail and surrounding skin in various ways. A nail disorder is not usually a contra-indication to treatment; common sense along with a sound knowledge of nail structure and growth will allow the manicurist to decide if a treatment can take place or not.

Other nail disorders include:

- Eggshell nails.
- Spoon-shaped nails.
- Onycholysis (separation of the nail plate from the nail bed).
- Onychoptosis (shedding of the nail plate).
- Onychorrhexis (slitting of the nail plate).

Nail diseases

Tinea unguium

Ringworm of the nail first shows itself as a yellowish brown discolouration at the free edge. It is caused by the fungus getting under the nail plate at the free edge and attacking the nail plate and bed. If allowed to spread to the entire nail plate the nail becomes thickened and onycholysis may occur. No manicure treatment must be given and medical advice is essential.

Paronychia

This may be caused by a bacterial infection of the skin around the nail. The nail wall and surrounding area become red and swollen, swelling referred to as a whitlow or a felon. The infection can be caused by the introduction of a foreign body such as a splinter or by the use of unsterile manicure tools. No manicure treatment should be given – medical advice is necessary.

Onychia

This is an infection of the nail fold caused by a bacteria or fungus infection. A damaged cuticle can be the site for entry of the micro-organism. The infection can be caused by biting, picking, thumb sucking, frequent use of detergents and continual immersion in water. The area can be very red and inflamed and is often very painful. No manicure treatment should be given; advice about prevention would be helpful and referral to the medical profession is necessary.

The manicure treatment

Small equipment and preparations required

The manicure treatment unit should be mobile, attractive in its presentation and contain all items of small equipment and cosmetic preparations required in the sequence. A small table with an arm rest and bowls for soaking and waste items is the ideal working area and gives the beauty specialist full control over the hands and arms of her client. Manicure trolleys and baskets are also in common use, due to their convenience of size, but as they lack arm supports, separate provision must be made by using a small cushion. The hand should be raised to the right level for fast efficient work, whilst maintaining client comfort.

The manicure unit requires the following items:

- Nail and cuticle clippers and cuticle knife.
- Emery boards and metal files (everlasting diamond type).
- Nail brush, buffer, orange sticks and two small bowls for soaking.
- Covered cotton-wool containers, waste bowls and container for orange sticks. (Ideally all containers should be of stainless steel. They may also be of glass or metal, but not plastic.)
- Manicure and hand massage preparations, and nail repair kit.

Manicure preparations required and their uses

Enamel removers and solvents
These must be capable of fast, efficient removal, without excessive dehydrating and defatting effects on the nail plate and surrounding skin tissue. Acetone or ethyl acetate is the normal base, with the addition of a small quantity of oil. The natural oil and moisture lost should be replaced by application of a nail cream or oil.

Cuticle cream

An emollient product designed to soften and nourish the cuticle, cuticle cream aims to make the nail plate more flexible by replacing the natural fats lost in daily life through exposure to detergents and drying elements. The nail cream or oil should be used within the manicure sequence and as a nightly home care treatment, applied to the cuticle area.

Cuticle remover

The purpose of the cuticle remover is, without discomfort to the client, to loosen and release cuticle skin cells which adhere to the nail plate. The fluid-based alkaline lotion is applied to the previously softened skin with tipped orange sticks. The procedure accomplishes a swift removal of dead and adhering tissue from the nail plate. Potassium hydroxide is the active ingredient in many cuticle removers, and also acts as a nail bleach removing nicotine stains effectively.

Paste polish

Paste polish is used in combination with the buffer application if the nails are ridged, uneven or simply lifeless. If coloured enamel is not required, or if it is a male manicure, paste polish gives a healthy sheen to the nails and does help to minimise evident ridges. Many paste polishes are composed of jeweller's paste formed into a cosmetic preparation for convenience of application. The friction formed during the buffing process increases blood circulation in the nail bed, and the paste polish itself has only a slight abrasive action, with no nourishing elements.

Nail white pencil

Used to whiten the free edge if clear enamel is preferred, and to give a clean light appearance to discoloured nails, the pencil usually requires wetting before application, and is composed of a soap base with the addition of white pigment. The popularity of white pencils has declined as high-gloss enamels have become increasingly popular. They should always be available for clients who like to appear well groomed but, who, due to the nature of their work, they are restricted to colourless enamel or simply a buffed sheen, e.g. medical staff, cooks, etc.

Nail enamels (polish or varnish)

The high-gloss cellulose lacquer or enamel so popular at present must have several qualities if its application is to be successful. It must be easy to apply, with an even consistency and colour, and should be fast-drying. It should not be harmful to the nails or stain them with the pigment resins, and it must be long-lasting and highly protective in action. The cosmetic improvement in appearance is well known, and relies on a high lustre and attractive colour choice.

Base coats

The base coat has a special role in the manicure, prolonging the life of the enamel, preventing pigment from the enamel staining the nails, and minimising irregularities in the nail plate. Its additional effect of increasing the protective element of the enamel application is enhanced by careful choice of the most suitable type of base coat for the existing nail condition.

Nail strengtheners

Plastic-based nail strengtheners help to prevent the nail becoming fragile or over-brittle. The preparation is used prior to the base coat, or may be incorporated into it for convenience by some manufacturers. Care must be taken to prevent the lotion from touching the cuticle skin, or dryness will result.

Hand lotions and creams

The additional exposure to caustic and detergent items that the hands suffer make regular application of hand cream an essential item, if the skin is to remain intact and smooth. Within the manicure routine a water-based emulsion-type hand cream should be used to permit fast absorption and prevent stickiness. For nightly application and hand and arm massage during the treatment, an emollient nourishing cream should be employed to allow free movement over the area of massage, and to increase the benefit gained from improved circulation. The hand lotions are glycerine based, formed into a jelly-like substance by gum tragacanth, and enhanced by colour and perfume. Hand creams have a similar consistency to a general skin cream, and should have similar qualities of nutrient ingredients, fine texture and fast absorption to increase circulation and prevent moisture loss.

Nail repair kit

The repair kit consists of a liquid nail cement which is used in conjunction with fibrous tissues and solvent, to effect repairs of split and torn nails and reinforcement of fragile tips.

The manicure

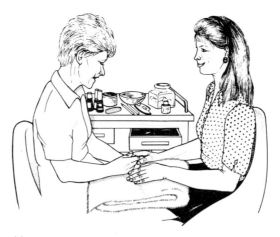

Manicure position

Procedure

The manicure position should be prepared with sterile small equipment, cuticle clippers, knives, commodities required, etc., and clean towels or disposable paper for preference. The enamel should be the correct consistency, with clean bottle necks, and an adequate choice of cream and pearlised colours available. Regular maintenance of tools and preparations, enamels, etc., will avoid cross-infection, and allow fast and efficient work to progress.

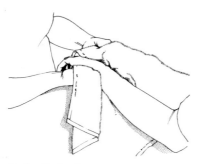

Drying the hand

1 The client's hands should be inspected for nail or skin infections, and then wiped over with a soapy antiseptic solution and dried thoroughly.

2 All the enamel should be removed in a decisive manner with a pad of cotton-wool soaked in remover. Deep shades or thickly applied enamel require the remover pad to soak into the nails for a couple of seconds before it is withdrawn. Final removal should be accomplished with a tipped orange stick soaked in remover, to clean up the cuticle and free edge.

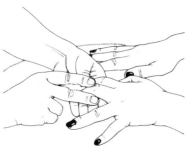

Removing enamel   *Cleaning around the cuticles*

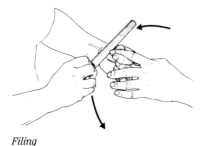

Filing

3 The nails of the right hand are then filed with an emery board from side to centre to form a curve. The sides should not be filed away, but left to give support to the nail. The free edges should then be bevelled to avoid the nail layers splitting apart. Light strokes must be used, with the fine side of the emery board. The free edge should then be checked for smoothness, by running the thumb pad across it to feel for snags, which may need extra attention.

Various corrections can be made at this stage to improve nail appearance or flatter the hand shape. The shape created can be emphasised by the colour and manner in which the nail enamel is applied later in the sequence.

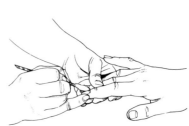

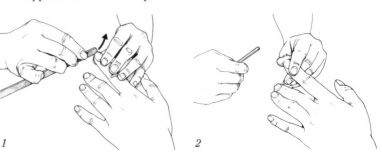

Bevelling   *Checking the edges for smoothness*

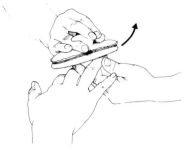

Buffing

4 Paste polish, if required, is applied at this point by spreading a minute quantity onto each nail, and buffing it off with the chamois-covered buffer. The buffer may also be used without the polish for stimulation but, due to the difficulty of sterilising and cleaning the chamois covering the buffer, this step is often omitted from the sequence.

5 Massage cuticle cream into the nail fold and surrounding skin with firm rhythmical pressure, covering the first joints and complete nail area. Place the right hand in sufficient warm soapy water to cover the nails and first joints of the fingers only, to prevent accidents occurring if the client moves her hand unconsciously.

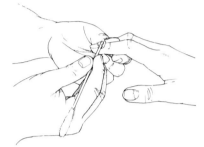

Applying cuticle cream

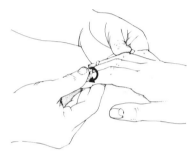

Rhythmical massage on the cuticles

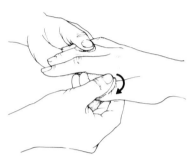

Rhythmical massage on the joints

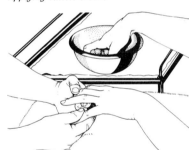

Soaking the finger tips

6 Repeat steps 3–5 on the left hand. If only one bowl is used, the right hand must be removed and dried prior to placing the left hand to soak.

7 The right hand is placed in position on the hand rest in preparation for the cuticle work. The cuticles are flooded with cuticle remover, and a tipped orange stick is used to free the cuticle from its nail plate attachment and push it gently back to form a smooth nail fold. Keeping the area damp, the cuticle knife may be used for stubborn areas or neglected nails. The cuticle should then be smoothed back with the towel, and any dead skin removed with the cuticle clippers. The tipped orange stick can be used to clean the free edge gently by employing a rolling movement. Discoloured or nicotine-stained nails especially require attention.

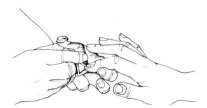

Flooding the cuticles

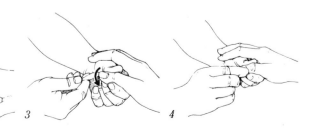

1   *2*   *3*   *4*

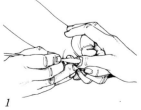

Cuticle work

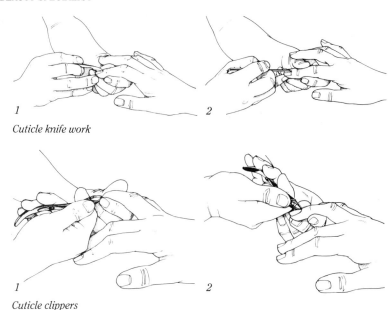

Cuticle knife work

Cuticle clippers

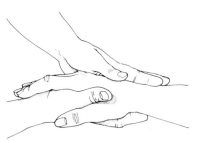

Applying hand lotion

8 Remove and dry the left hand and complete step 7.

9 Apply hand lotion to both hands, smoothing it in with effleurage strokes. The hand massage routine, if required, is applied at this stage of the treatment.

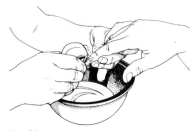

Brushing

10 Both hands should have the nails and free edges gently brushed, to release nail layers, loose skin, etc., and then the final inspection and tidying up can be completed. Separated nail edges should be bevelled, and any excess dead skin carefully clipped away. The hands may then be thoroughly dried.

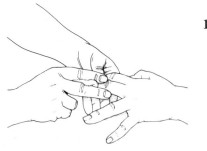

Squeaking

11 Enamel remover is then used to remove all soap, oil, cream, etc. from the nails in preparation for the base coat. Long nails should also have the free edge cleaned with a tipped orange stick.

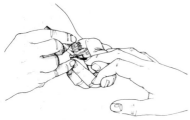

Enamel application

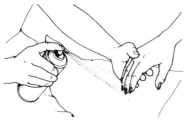

Spray application

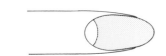

Half-moon application

12 Apply nail strengthener, if required, and base coat to both hands, working from left to right to prevent smudging. Light fast strokes should be used to achieve even coverage. The correct base coat should be used for the nail condition, i.e. strong or fragile, and the enamel chosen previously, i.e. cream or pearlised.

13 Apply the coloured enamel in a similar manner. To achieve sufficient colour density three coats of enamel may be required with pale shades, otherwise two coats of the deeper colours should be sufficient. A top coat may be used on cream enamels, to add lustre, but is not required on pearly enamel. Four coats, including base, colour and top coat, is the maximum that should be applied, or the nails will not dry in a reasonable time. Quick-drying spray may be used to set the surface of the nails, taking care to spray away from the client or furniture.

Some clients prefer to leave the half-moon area of their nails unpainted, and the enamel strokes for this require practice to accomplish an even half-moon area. A slightly different method of application is necessary to prevent flooding of the cuticles. Any enamel which touches the nail wall during the application should be removed before proceeding to the next nail, as once set it is impossible to remove cleanly without leaving a smudgy appearance. Neglected, untidy cuticles also make even enamelling difficult, but excessive clipping should be avoided, and the client encouraged to improve the cuticle appearance gradually by regularly smoothing back the skin, and by nightly application of cuticle cream, to reinforce the regular professional manicure given. Once cuticles have been excessively clipped, they build up an unattractive ridge-like appearance around the nail, and have to continue to be clipped to reduce the hard skin formed. New clients should be encouraged to rely on regular nail attention and professional care to maintain attractive hands, rather than over-zealous treatment applied erratically.

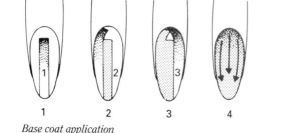

Base coat application

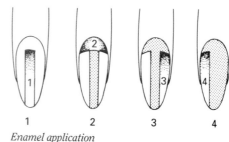

Enamel application

Home care and sales of manicure preparations

As in facial therapy, nail treatments need to be reinforced by regular care and awareness of elements that will aggravate the nail condition.

Fragile nails need the constant protection of strengtheners, base coat, enamel, etc. if a reasonable length and appearance is to be maintained. Rubber gloves should be worn for all jobs involving detergents, etc. Even with all these precautions only a moderate length will be possible. All nails benefit from nightly applications of cuticle cream massaged in, over the enamel, to the nail fold and surrounding skin. Soaking very brittle nails in warm oil is also a very effective treatment, and should prevent the nails being severed at the flesh line.

It is to the manicurist's advantage to see that if her client wishes to change her nail enamel between professional visits, she does so with quality products which will not be detrimental to the nail condition. The client should be encouraged to purchase cuticle cream, strengthener, base coat, enamel and remover from the salon; in this way all her home care needs are fulfilled. However the benefits of a professional manicure should be stressed so as not to undermine the beauty business.

Hand and arm massage

The purpose of the massage is to improve skin texture and appearance by increasing surface circulation and the application or nourishing cosmetic massage preparations, to relax the client and the superficial muscles and to aid joint manipulation. Special bleaching or nourishing and regenerating products may be employed for special effect, or a simple oil or talcum medium may be used. The item chosen must permit massage over an extended area, e.g. 10 minutes per arm, and so should not have a fast absorption rate, unlike the preparations advised for home use, where this is a desirable feature. To gain maximum benefit from the treatment the client's arm should be well supported, either on pillows or arm rests, to prevent muscle tension and permit full relaxation of the entire arm. The client's clothing must be protected and, if the style of the dress makes disrobing necessary, a gown with loose sleeves or a sleeveless gown should be offered to the client. If the treatment is combined with manicure, preparation for both items must be completed prior to commencement to avoid disturbance.

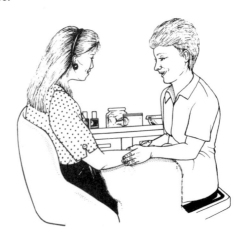

The manicure routine is completed up to the pre-base coat stage of the sequence, with the cuticle work completed on both hands. The pillow or arm rest may then be used to bring the arm into the correct working position.

Sequence of the arm massage

1 The massage preparation is applied with effleurage strokes over the entire arm area. The movement then increases in pressure as a preparation for further petrissage strokes. The elbow, forearm and hand should become relaxed, before progressing to further movements. Repeat 10–15 times approx.

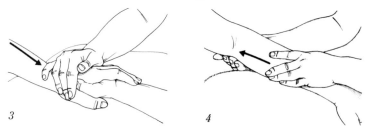

1

2

Effleurage

3

4

2 Friction movements around the wrist, working with the thumbs in firm rotaries, to increase circulation and prevent stiffness in the area.

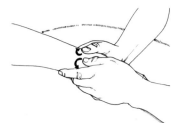

Wrist frictions

3 Petrissage movements on the muscles of the lower arm, flexor carpi ulnaris and radialis, brachioradialis and palmaris longus. The pressure should be upwards, and adjusted to the bulk of the muscles under treatment. Effleurage must be used to link the sequence, by returning the hand to the wrist, prior to repetition of the pressure movement.

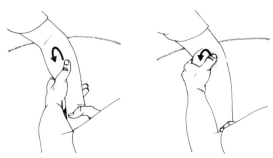

Petrissage on the forearm

4 Link effleurage over entire forearm and hand, to re-establish muscle relaxation; repeat 10–15 times.

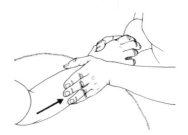

Link effleurage

5 Friction movements around the elbow joint, with the hands either working alternately, one hand supporting the elbow, the other applying massage to the area, or with both hands working together.

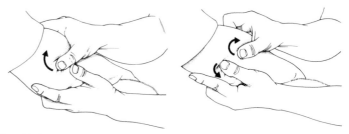

Elbow frictions

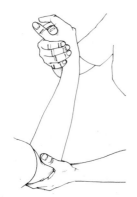

Wrist extension

6 With the elbow retained in a supporting position, the arm is then lifted into an upright position, and the wrist is rotated into its fullest extension, to stretch the ligaments and muscle attachments of the hand and wrist. The hand should be rotated fully to the left and right, with relaxation in between to prevent discomfort. The interchange of blood and tissue fluids created by the pumping effect of the tendons and ligaments on the joints and surrounding area promotes supple and attractive hands, whilst delaying stiffness and enlargement of joints. Apply 3–4 rotations to the left and right.

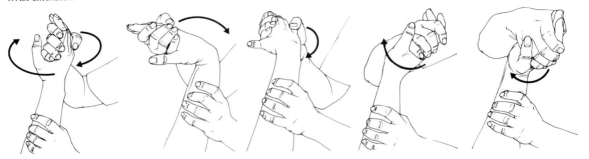

Wrist rotation

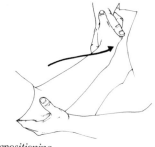

Repositioning

7 Return the arm to the pillow support, palm upwards, and work with firm rotary kneading petrissage movements over the metacarpal area of the palm. Work with the thumbs from the distal to proximal ends of the bones, returning with effleurage strokes. Repeat 6–10 times.

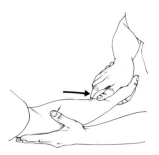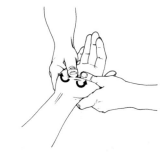

Kneading on the palm

8 Turn the hand over and apply brisk frictions upwards between the tendons of the fingers and thumb, towards the wrist, returning with effleurage strokes. The thumbs work, and the fingers support the hand to prevent discomfort, and provide a base for the pressure movement to be applied correctly. Repeat three times on each set of tendons.

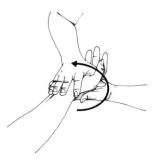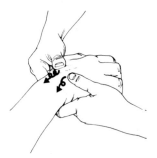

Turning over the hand　　　　*Frictions between the tendons*

9 The movement progresses to scissor-like frictions, performed by the fingers, under the wrist area. The client's wrist is encompassed by the therapist's hands and the movement is applied briskly, to improve circulation in the joint area.

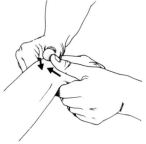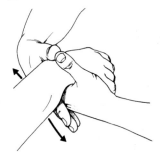

Scissor frictions

235

10 Link effleurage over the entire arm, alternately applied with right and left hands. Support of the client's arm is maintained throughout. Repeat 10–12 times.

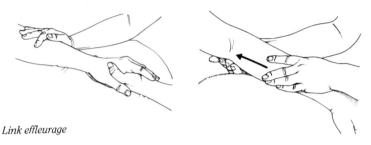

Link effleurage

11 Petrissage movements applied on proximal to distal joints of the phalanges of each finger and thumb, working with even pressure in a rhythmical manner. The hands work alternately, supporting the hand and applying the joint kneading movements.

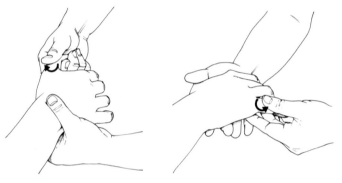

Joint kneading

12 A brisk rolling movement performed with the client's hand held between the therapist's hand, with the thumbs linking through the little finger and thumb, to permit a fast stimulating movement. The circulation stimulation improves skin colour and general functioning, helping to prevent chilblain formation on the fingers in the winter months.

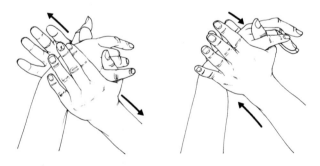

Rolling movement

13 Effleurage stroking movements conclude the massage routine, working slowly and evenly over the elbow, forearm, wrist and hand, finishing at the finger tips.

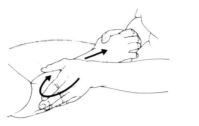

Concluding effleurage

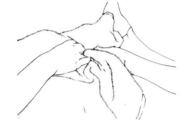

Final cream removal

Any remaining oil, cream, etc., should be removed, first with paper tissues or a towel followed by a tonic application to ensure thorough removal. The sequence may be concluded with a dusting of perfumed talcum if desired, to prevent stickiness, particularly in warm weather. The routine is performed on the other arm, and then the remainder of the manicure is completed, if combined, omitting the hand lotion application. A final check should be made to ensure no greasy areas remain at the end of the complete treatment, especially around the elbow area.

Organisation of the manicure trolley

For the manicurist to be able to accomplish an efficient manicure in the brief time commercially available, it is necessary that her manicure trolley or tray is at all times clean and ready for use. This calls for a neat method of work, replacing items in their correct position, during or at the conclusion of each manicure accomplished. Waste bowls should be emptied after each client, and the tools used, washed, dried thoroughly and sterilised.

Care over sterilisation is very important in the manicure routine, as the skin may be open around the walls of the cuticle, and infection could easily result from careless procedures in the cuticle work.

All the items on the trolley should look clean and attractive to the client, who normally has them in view and would notice tatty and dirty preparations.

Client presentation is important in manicure work, as it is a grooming service and likely to be requested on impulse if the manicurist and her trolley look appealing. The client is tempted to treat herself, and an extra service is gained, which with luck may become a regular part of her grooming routine.

The manicure products should be ready for immediate use, and items such as enamels, base coats, etc., must be of the correct flowing consistency to achieve a fast-setting enamel application. The enamel should flow easily without hesitation back into the bottle from the brush, not form into blobs around the brush. The consistency of new enamels should be noted and if products thicken, they can be brought back to the correct consistency by the addition of a few drops of solvent, applied from an orange stick. Once corrected the enamel needs to be shaken and left, ideally for 24 hours, but even 20 minutes can be helpful in improving the flow of the application. For this reason it is a wise step to consult the client about her choice of enamel colour before the manicure commences, so providing an opportunity to check that the item is a good consistency, and if not, making some last-minute improvement. Enamels thicken through exposure to air, caused either during the actual application, or through air entering the bottle if tops are left messy. Apart from making it even more difficult to achieve a perfect finish in the enamel application, messy bottle tops spoil the consistency of expensive enamels very quickly. With the need to have a good selection of cream and pearlised enamels for the client's choice, any additional expense because of poor product care makes the manicure less able to be operated as a profitable service.

Bottle tops can be cleaned very swiftly with the soiled pads used to remove the client's coloured enamel. The top then forms a good contact with the bottle and air cannot enter, thus keeping the enamel in perfect working consistency.

The temperature in the clinic can alter the flow of the enamel, making it less easy to apply. Cold temperatures thicken the enamel, whilst high temperatures make the products more fluid and less easy to control. Extremes in climate can make products react strangely, so therapists working in hot areas should try to find a cool storage place for their enamels and base coats.

Manicurists should get into a regular habit of cleaning, stocking up and checking their trolleys and the preparations and tools required. When the trolley is not in use it can be protected with a polythene cover to prevent dust, etc. soiling it. If trolleys are always left ready for use in this way in the commercial clinic, it avoids a scramble to prepare or find all the necessary items when a manicure is requested unexpectedly. Even the tipped orange sticks may be prepared beforehand: an air-tight container should be available to store them so that they do not become soiled. This saves time on the actual routine.

Organisation of the manicure routine

The main criticism of manicurists being unable to accomplish a good manicure in the time available (20–30 minutes on average) is mainly due to poor preparation and organisation of the routine. With practice it is perfectly possible to accomplish an excellent manicure in 20 minutes, if the client has regular treatment, as the cuticle work will not be protracted. Really neglected hands and nails should be dealt with on a treatment basis, in conjunction with arm massage, paraffin wax applications, etc. In this way the treatment remains profitable and is of more benefit to the client. A simple explanation to the client regarding the state of the nails can help to decide priorities in treatment and is a more professional way to approach the work.

Really neglected nails may benefit from more work on the cuticles to ease them back gradually, and nail enamel would then not be necessary, making the routine possible within the normal time. Fragile nails may need extra protection in the form of nail patches, for which extra time would be allowed if it could not be included in the normal manicure. Discussion with the client about the time needed, the cost involved, before the manicure commences, avoids client dissatisfaction and places the client in a position where she can decide her priorities.

Paraffin wax treatment

Use of paraffin wax in the hand and arm routine provides a luxurious and enjoyable routine which improves skin texture, colour, and delays ageing signs (such as pigmentation spots). It is also very beneficial for treatment of stiff joints as it provides a steady, high level of heat throughout the tissues, relieving pain.

Equipment

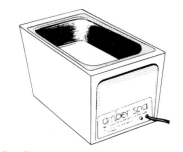

Paraffin wax bath

Small quantities of paraffin wax may be prepared in a simple paraffin wax bath, but for immersion of limbs, a larger bath with a built-in water jacket and thermostatic controls is preferable. The wax is pre-heated, and maintained at the correct temperature of 49 °C (120 °F) automatically, so minimising the risks of overheating or burns. Sufficient time should be allowed for pre-heating the wax; half an hour for smaller baths, and one hour for the larger units.

Application

Equipment preparation
If the waxing is combined with manicure/pedicure and massage, it is placed in the routine in the following sequence. The nails are completed up to the cuticle stage, wax is applied to one limb, which is wrapped and left. The second arm or leg is waxed and wrapped and then the first limb is unwrapped and massage applied. The second limb is then unwrapped, massaged and the manicure completed in the normal way. The working area is protected with heavy grade polythene to protect it from wax drips. Towels used should be covered with paper sheeting to prevent damage. The client should be prepared in a clinic gown to protect clothing.

Paraffin wax may be applied by:

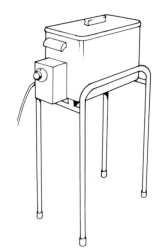

Paraffin wax equipment

- Painting the wax over the area with a large brush.
- Dipping the limb into the wax bath until it is coated.

The wax is pre-heated, and the commodities required for the treatment are prepared. Items required:

- Two sufficiently large foil sheets to enclose the limbs.
- Two medium size towels.
- Nourishing cream and spatula.
- Large brush for application (if used).

Paraffin wax has a low melting temperature. It is a solid with a cloudy white appearance at room temperature. When heated to its melting temperature of 49 °C (120 °F) it becomes a clear liquid which, on exposure to the air, is capable of forming a second skin over the treated area. When sufficient wax encloses the limb, heat is built up under the wax, perspiration is induced and relaxation of the tissues results.

Client preparation/application

The working position should permit safe and efficient wax application, whilst keeping the client comfortable. The wax should be at the correct temperature to minimise drips occurring and speed the application. If the paraffin wax is applied independently the limb should be washed, or wiped over with a soapy, antiseptic solution, and in the case of hand treatment, all jewellery removed if possible.

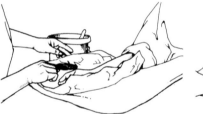
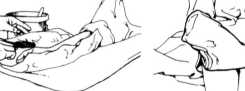

Application on the arm   *The arm wrapped*

- Towels are covered with foil sheets and placed under the limbs in readiness.
- The limbs are covered in a thin film of nourishing cream, then dipped into the warm wax to form a coating. Alternatively wax is applied with a brush
- The process is repeated until a fairly thick layer of wax is formed (5–6 times).
- Once the wax coat has been formed, the limb is wrapped in foil and towels to maintain the heat.
- The second limb is treated in a similar way, and the client allowed a few minutes of rest to permit the maximum benefit from the heat penetration.

Removal

Removal is easily accomplished. Due to the nourishing cream applied at the start of the application, the wax peels off in one piece if it has been evenly applied. The minimum of cleaning up is then required.

The limb will be found to be relaxed, warm, with increased circulation, improved skin colour, and soft texture.

After paraffin waxing, the tissues are in an ideal relaxed state for massage (10 minutes) which eases stiffness and tension in the joints and muscles.

Ageing skin, dehydrated and dry/flaky conditions gain benefit from waxing, as it provides a cosmetic improvement in skin appearance and increases circulation in the area.

Treatment points

- Well made equipment should be chosen which complies with safety standards in the country where it will be used.
- The equipment must be earthed or double insulated, correctly wired and should have enclosed heating elements to prevent over-heating.
- The wax heater should be placed on a metal or wood-topped mobile trolley or work top, protected with rough paper tissues. Glass trolleys must not be used as the risks of glass shattering are too high.
- The wax should not be left to heat and melt close to any flammable material, e.g. curtains. The wax bath should be kept covered with a lid, to reduce the smell and speed the heating.
- Wax should be replaced regularly to maintain a sound working consistency.
- Wax should be strained and cleaned after use to remove waste particles, dead skin, perspiration, etc.
- Paraffin wax is available in its natural form, or with added peach perfume and colour.

Nail repairs and extensions

Badly chipped, torn or fragile nails can be improved by three different methods of nail repair: tissue method, nail builder and artificial nails. None of the methods permit normal heavy daily usage, so the applications are most suitable for clients who do not engage in housework or continuous heavy work. As an instant repair for a special occasion, for career women or professional models, they are all very satisfactory.

Tissue and nail cement repairs

The manicure is completed up to the stage prior to the base coat application. The tear or fragile tip is inspected, and the special tissue torn into a suitable shape to effect the repair. The torn edge permits a stronger repair, and when saturated with nail cement will adhere to the nail plate firmly. The excess tissue protruding over the free edge should be gently smoothed out to fit the nail contour, by pushing it

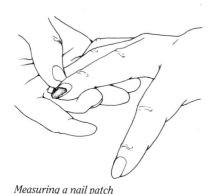

Measuring a nail patch

241

under the free edge with an orange stick. With the client's palm upwards, any rough areas should be smoothed down and extra cement applied if required. When the adhesive has set the manicure can be concluded in the normal way, with a coloured enamel of sufficient depth of tone to allow a good disguise.

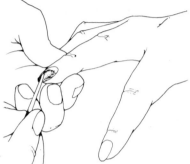

Smoothing out the tissue

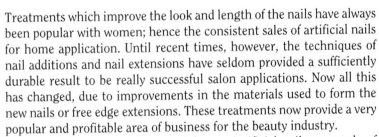

Finishing the free edge

With care, the repair should last for a considerable time while the nail is growing. A well applied repair can be reinforced on subsequent manicures by removing the enamel carefully and reapplying nail cement over the nail plate and free edge areas, without disturbing the actual repair.

Artificial nails and semi-permanent nail extensions

Treatments which improve the look and length of the nails have always been popular with women; hence the consistent sales of artificial nails for home application. Until recent times, however, the techniques of nail additions and nail extensions have seldom provided a sufficiently durable result to be really successful salon applications. Now all this has changed, due to improvements in the materials used to form the new nails or free edge extensions. These treatments now provide a very popular and profitable area of business for the beauty industry.

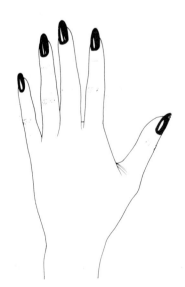

Nail additions come in several forms. Artificial nails are made of plastic materials, which can be shaped to fit varying nail shapes. These are designed to be applied for temporary periods, and can be removed and reapplied. Nail extensions can be used to lengthen the natural nails, either the whole set, or, more normally, used as a repair on a broken nail, to match it back to the rest of the nails. These extensions stay in place until the natural nail has grown sufficiently for the extension to be unnecessary. Durability will depend on the wear and tear the nails receive in daily life. Lastly there are semi-permanent nail additions, where plastic type compounds are applied to cover the client's nails entirely, and extend their natural length. These nails are very tough and durable, and can be shaped with abrasive drills into the desired shape, to suit the client's hand. In-filling is required periodically, around the cuticle area, to keep the nail addition undetectable, making for regular salon attendance and trade in the clinic. The nail additions can be used as a total transformation, or as a nail repair on an individual nail. Like the nail extensions, the nail additions grow out with the natural nail, but because of the toughness of the materials used, and the total coverage of the natural nail, they cannot be removed so readily. So clients need to be advised of the long term nature of their application, and the appearance of the nails needs to be immaculate.

The therapist must advise her client regarding the best nail addition by considering the purpose of the nails. Temporary nails, perhaps for an evening event, may be satisfactorily fulfilled by plastic 'false' nails, allowing the client to return to her normal length nail the next day. Clients who are able, and choose, to keep their nails long, may find the nail extensions best for repairing a broken nail. The fact that they are able to retain long nails gives some guidance to the therapist as to the normal wear they are likely to receive. For the client who is unable to grow her nails long, due to an inherent weakness, but desires this length, nail additions may prove the best solution. A client with weak nails should not, however, be encouraged to look upon nail additions as a remedy to her weak nails, only as an alternative camouflage of the problem. The only things likely to improve poor nails are better health or a better diet and a reduction in wear and tear on the nails from the daily chores.

Artificial nails

Artificial nails are now available in a wide range of shapes and lengths to suit most hands: excessive pre-shaping is unnecessary. The chosen nails should be placed to soak while the manicure proceeds up to the base coat stage. The cuticles must be free, the nails clean and any filing of the false nails completed prior to the adhesive application. Adhesive is then applied to either false or real nails, or both, and the nails placed firmly in position, with the lower edge just beneath the loosened cuticle. The nails can be held in place by small, flat rubber straps or bandages if necessary, but modern adhesives effect such a fast bond that this is really unnecessary, and firm pressure held for a few seconds is sufficient.

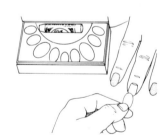

The initial shaping of a set of nails should be carefully undertaken, first by making the choice of nails closest to the client's natural nails, although longer, and then by continual checking to determine that the correct curve and shape of nail is being produced by the filing. Once completed, the attachment of a shaped set of nails is an easy task and can be combined quickly into the manicure procedure, adding additional revenue to the sequence. Clients should be advised to wear artificial nails for short periods only, as continual pressure on the matrix area of the nail can cause transverse nail ridging to appear some time after their use.

Nail extensions

Nail extensions are a new system of false finger nails that rely on a new type of tough fast-acting glue, to bond a plastic shape firmly to the edge

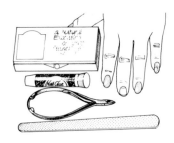

of the natural nail. The result both looks and feels like the natural nail, and it files and grows out just the same as the natural nail. The popularity of nail extensions has expanded the clinic's range of manicure services, and it can be a very profitable treatment. Achieving success relies on skill in shaping the extensions to match closely the shape and curve of the natural nails. This, as with the complete false nails, makes the difference between an undetectable result or an obvious one.

Nail extensions take about 10 minutes for repairing an individual nail, and about one hour for the complete set where the client requires extra length, perhaps due to nail weakness when she is unable to grow the nails to the desired length naturally. Charges for the service should be based on the clinic's normal charge-per-hour basis, depending on the member of staff concerned, and the usual rate at which they are costed. With practice it can become a simple addition to the manicuring skills.

Application of nail extensions

1 The nail to be extended is inspected and the nail enamel removed. It needs lengthening to match the length of the other nails. The nail shapes, glue, clippers and file are assembled.

2 The nail shape is selected for size and tested against the natural nail for the correct fit.

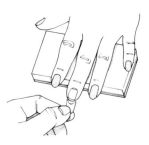

3 Nail clippers are used to shape the inner edge of the false nail shape, to achieve an exact fit with the edge of the broken nail.

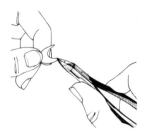

4 The false nail is held in place against the natural nail with edges abutting and adhesives applied at the join. Care should be taken to

ensure that the nail shape is in line with the natural nail, not angled over, as with the instant bond the new glue makes, it is easy to have it wrongly positioned, and fixed in that position very quickly.

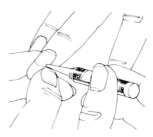

5 The false nail is trimmed to the required length with the nail clippers, and then filed into shape with an emery board.

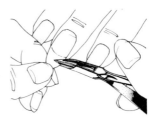

6 More adhesive is applied to fill in any gaps and ensure that the false and natural nails are attached all round the edges.

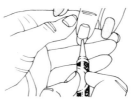

7 The glue dries in a few seconds and is rock hard in half a minute. The join can be filed smooth with the emery board, to make it undetectable.

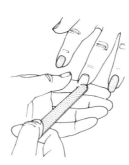

8 The treated nail looks natural and feels like a real nail. Because of the differences in colour between a plastic free edge and natural nail, it is more successful in most cases to enamel the nails, so that the extension blends in with the other nails.

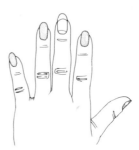

9 The final touch of enamel shows off the nails to advantage and makes it impossible to detect the nail extension.

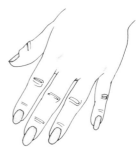

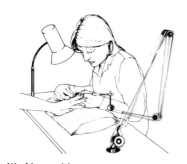

Working position

Semi-permanent nail additions/sculpture

To offer the nail addition service within a clinic requires increased expenditure on equipment and commodities, etc., but the popularity of this grooming and fashion-linked service makes the investment well worthwhile. Very little space is needed to offer the nail addition service: simply a working table position to provide a base for the abrasive drill used to shape the nail compound. The entire nail addition system makes a neat and attractive unit, but because of the noise involved when the drill is in use, it should be sited away from the more restful clinic treatments.

Different systems of nail additions vary in their application methods, and the manufacturer's instructions should be followed exactly to achieve good results. Most nail addition treatments are applied to lengthen and transform the client's complete set of nails or to infill the nails around the cuticles, so this is a grooming rather than a repair service. It has to be a comparatively expensive service because of the time taken in applying the semi-permanent nails (around 1½–2 hours). However, it is proving to be a service that women are willing to pay for to maintain their nail appearance.

Application of semi-permanent nails

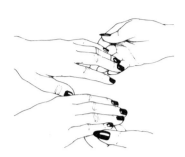

1   Examine the client's nails and discuss the preferred shape and length of semi-permanent nails required. Advise the client about the treatment, its cost, duration, and its need to be maintained by infilling every three to four weeks. Make sure the client understands the long-term nature of the nail additions, and that they cannot be removed if she decides to return to her natural nail length, but must grow out with the natural nails. The nails can be filed down, if they prove to be too long for the client in her daily life. Many clients unused to long nails will find them difficult to get used to, and for that reason it is worth discussing this point with the client in the initial examination. A moderate-length, nicely shaped nail is usually the most successful on clients who have daily chores to cope with. Younger women, with only their appearance to worry about, enjoy really long nails, and have no trouble maintaining them.

2   A drill with an abrasive head is run lightly over the nail to roughen the surface slightly, and provide a 'key' to which the built-on nail will adhere firmly. This may also be achieved by using special abrasive emery boards.

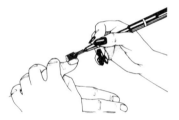

3   A horseshoe shape of adhesive-backed silver foil is fitted around the nail to be treated. This forms a guard on to which the artificial nail will be built over the natural nail's tip.

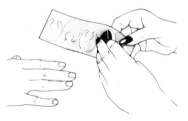

4   Check that the foil is fitting closely under the nail tip and is fixed firmly around the cuticle, without overlapping onto the nail at the sides.

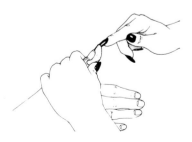

5   The false nail is created with a mixture of powder and liquid, which bonds together to form a clear and strong plastic-type compound. It is painted on with a brush which is alternately dipped in the powder and liquid, and applied onto the nail.

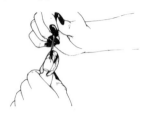

6   The powder and liquid is worked up the nail from the cuticle, over the tip and onto the guard in an approximate nail shape. The other nails are treated in the same way, and the compound is left for a few minutes to set hard. The second hand can be treated in this period, saving time.

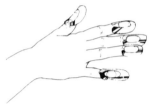

7   When the compound is set, the silver foil is removed from the fingers. The artificial nails will look bulky and uneven because they have been built up considerably to allow for shaping.

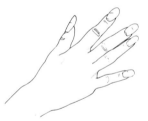

8   Shaping is done with the abrasive headed drill. This is worked lightly over the surface of the artificial nail to flatten and smooth down the compound, to follow the nail's natural contours and around the nail tip to provide the required length and shape. Skill in shaping the nails can make the difference between a really natural looking nail, or a very false one, so this stage is worth taking care over.

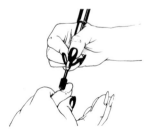

9 Paint the artificial nail with a special vegetable oil before buffing with a smooth-textured head fitted on to the drill. Work all over the artificial nail with the buffer to produce a smooth and natural-looking surface.

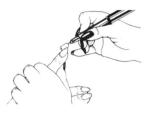

10 Give the finishing touches to each artificial nail with a diamond surface nail file. Emery boards would have no effect on the tough material used to create the nail.

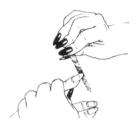

11 Paint the nails in the usual way. The artificial nails respond just like natural ones to nail enamel and remover, though as the nails are so tough, the enamel lasts much longer and does not chip.

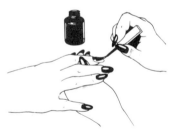

12 The new nails are firmly seated on the natural nails and as they grow, so a gap will be left at the cuticle. This can be easily filled in by the salon, on an average of every three to four weeks.

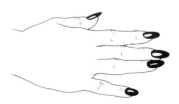

Anatomy of the foot, ankle and lower leg

The foot achieves its function of movement and support by means of a large number of closely articulating small bones formed into arches by their ligament connections to combine strength and flexibility.

Bones of the foot

There are 26 bones of the foot.

Tarsals – ankle bones
These are seven in number:

- Talus and calcaneum, which take the weight of the body, transferred from the tibia bone of the lower leg.
- Navicular.
- Medial, intermediate, lateral cuneiforms and the cuboid, which form a row of bones.

Metatarsals – foot bones
Five in number, forming the greater part of the length of the foot.

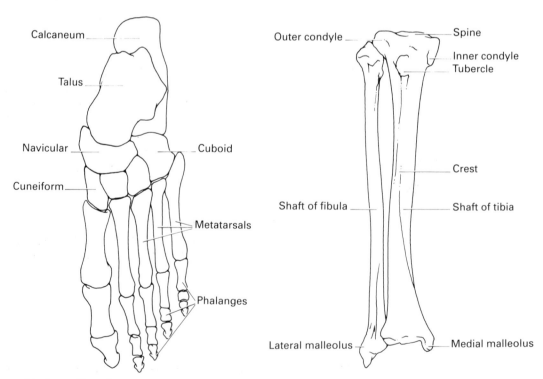

Bones of the foot and lower leg

Phalanges – toe bones

There are 14 phalanges of the toes and they follow the same pattern as the phalanges of the fingers, with three to the small toes, and two to the big toe.

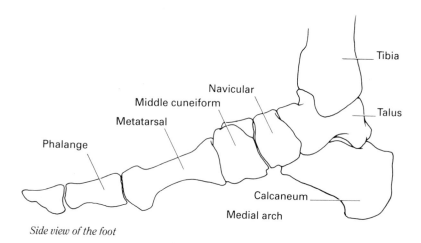

Side view of the foot

Arches of the foot

There are four arches of the foot: two longitudinal, i.e. running down the foot, called the lateral and medial arches, and two transverse arches.

Medial longitudinal arch (long main arch of the foot)

The main arch of the foot, placed on the inner aspect, involves the area from the calcaneum bone to the proximal ends of the three inner metatarsal bones; both these bony areas make contact with the floor like the ends of a bridge. The suspended area of the arch is formed by the talus, the navicular and the three cuneiform bones, the strength and resilience being gained from the small strong muscles and ligaments which surround the joints.

Lateral longitudinal arch (shorter arch)

Situated on the outside (lateral) aspect of the foot, extending from the calcaneum to the cuboid and proximal ends of the outer metatarsal bones.

Transverse arches

The transverse arches of the foot lies under the metatarsal bones, extending from the outer to the inner aspect of the foot.

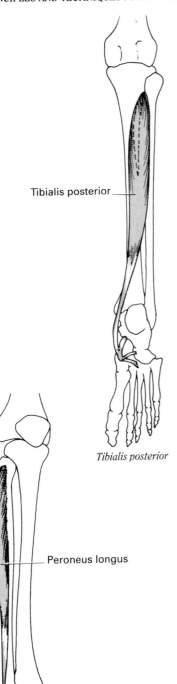

Tibialis posterior

Tibialis posterior

Peroneus longus

Peroneus longus

Bones of the lower leg

The tibia bone bears all the weight and articulates with the femur of the upper leg. The fibula has no connection with the femur. The knee joint permits only limited movement, and is a hinge-type joint. The floating sesamoid-type bone, the patella of the knee joint, is encapsulated within the quadriceps tendon of the thigh muscles and the patellar ligament, and it supports the action of the thigh muscles.

Muscles of the lower leg, ankle and foot

Many of the flexion and extension muscles produce inversion (inward) and eversion (outwards) movements of the foot, through the tendon attachment to the small bones of the foot and ankle. The longitudinal and transverse arches of the feet, which permit a full range of active movements, are supported by the distal ends of the lower leg muscles, particularly the tibialis posterior muscle.

Table 11.2 Muscles of the lower leg and ankle

Muscle	Action
Gastrocnemius (superficial)	Plantar flexion of foot, and flexion of the knee
Soleus (deep) mainly under the gastrocnemius	Plantar flexion of the foot
Peroneus longus (superficial)	Plantar flexion and eversion of the foot
Peroneus brevis (deep)	Plantar flexion and eversion of the foot
Tibialis anterior (superficial) Tibialis posterior	Inversion of the foot and support of the long arch of the foot
Extensor digitorum longus Extensor hallucis longus	Flexion and eversion of the foot and toe extension
Flexor digitorum longus	Plantar flexion and inversion of the foot

Small muscles of the foot

The small muscles of the foot are concerned with maintaining and supporting the longitudinal and transverse arches. The muscles include the interossi and lumbricale groups, and together with fatty and fascia connective tissue form the soft-cushioned nature of the sole of the foot.

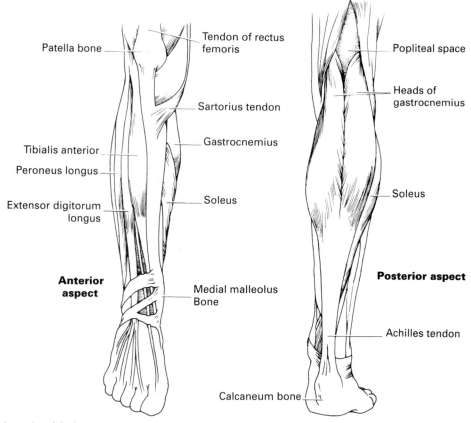

Patella bone

Tendon of rectus femoris

Sartorius tendon

Gastrocnemius

Tibialis anterior

Peroneus longus

Soleus

Extensor digitorum longus

Anterior aspect

Medial malleolus Bone

Calcaneum bone

Popliteal space

Heads of gastrocnemius

Soleus

Posterior aspect

Achilles tendon

Superficial muscles of the lower leg

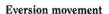

Inversion movement

Tibialis anterior muscle
Tibia bone (long)
Medial cuneiform bone (short)
Metatarsal bone (short)

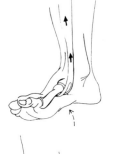

Eversion movement

Peroneus longus muscle
Fibula bone (long)
Metatarsal bone (short)
Ankle joint (hinge)
Medial cuneiform bone (short)

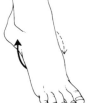

The pedicure treatment

A pedicure is simply a manicure treatment of the feet, with slight difference in the routine.

Purpose of a pedicure

Our feet are vital, often neglected parts of our body. Tired aching feet are a misery to anybody and can lead to postural and other problems. Regular professional pedicures can be a great prevention of minor foot conditions such as corns, callouses and ingrowing nails. (If any of these are already present, medical or chiropody advice may be necessary.)

A pedicure greatly enhances the appearance of the feet and toe nails and has a great psychological effect as well. Professional attention to the toe nails encourages growth, keeps the cuticles soft and pushed back and also helps to prevent the nails from splitting, ingrowing and other minor damage.

The feet must be thoroughly inspected prior to a pedicure, the limitations and scope of treatment explained and medical or chiropody referrals made if necessary.

Contra-indications to a pedicure

- Any nail disease (see pages 224).
- Any skin disease, e.g. *verruca plantaris*, *tinea pedis* (see Chapter 5, page 89).
- Broken bones.
- Swelling of toe, ankle or knee joints.
- Open cuts or wounds.
- Diabetes – due to impaired circulation and poor healing.

Implements and preparation

In addition to the standard manicure preparation and tools, a foot bowl (large enough for both feet), nail clippers, hoof stick, large metal file,

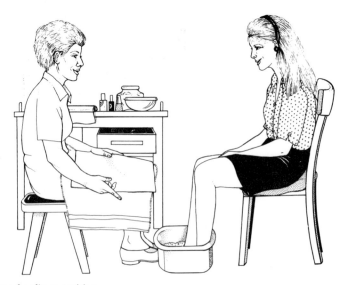

General pedicure position

hard-skin remover, foot powder, soap solution, and antiseptic are required. Disposable paper is the most hygienic method of drying the feet, and protecting working areas. A foot stool and a low seat are also desirable depending on the location of the treatment. Folded paper tissues may be placed in readiness.

The pedicure treatment may be applied in combination with hair-drying and facial therapy, or given independently, and often includes a foot and leg massage for maximum benefit. The routine may have to be adapted, due to the client's position, but the basic routine remains a guide to the elements required and an efficient sequence.

Pedicure procedure

1 Prepare all equipment and commodities. Advise client to remove shoes, tights, etc., and provide a gown and a chair if necessary. Place the client in a comfortable position, and put the feet to soak in the foot bowl, half-filled with warm soapy disinfectant solution. If soaking is not possible, wipe the feet over with a large swab of cotton-wool soaked in antiseptic solution.

2 Remove the right foot from the bowl, dry thoroughly on disposable paper, remove the enamel, and cut the nails straight across with only a gentle curve at the sides to prevent ingrowing toe nails. File the nails with the metal file to remove rough edges.

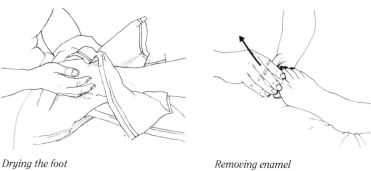

Drying the foot   *Removing enamel*

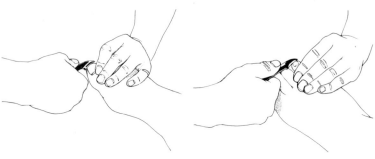

Clipping nails

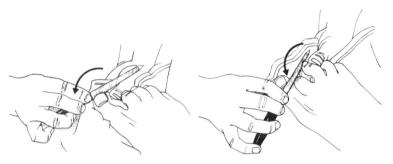

Filing the nails

3 Remove the adhering cuticle skin with a combined use of cuticle remover, a tipped orange stick, cuticle knife and rubber hoof stick. Keep the cuticle area moist with cuticle remover to assist the removal of the skin adhering to the nail plate. Alternate the use of the tools as necessary. Smooth back the nail wall to see progress, and if necessary, remove dead and loose skin with cuticle clippers. Thorough work with the cuticle tools and cuticle remover should minimise the need to clip the cuticle skin, thus reducing the risk of infection developing. Any open area of skin, caused by clipping or over-zealous cuticle work, is a possible site for nail fungus to develop, so care should be taken to keep the skin intact wherever possible.

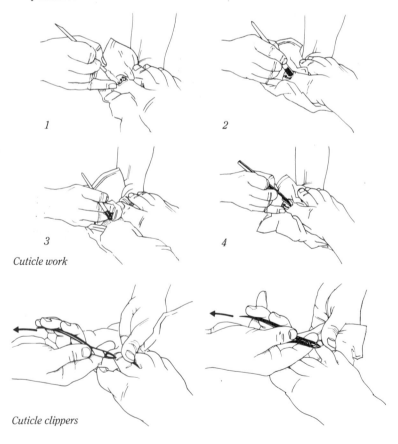

Cuticle work

Cuticle clippers

4 Apply hard skin remover if necessary to the heel and toe pad areas, working vigorously to remove callouses, with massage friction movements over the area. This section of the routine should not be prolonged within a normal pedicure treatment. The foot can then be briefly replaced in the bowl and steps 2–4 completed on the left foot.

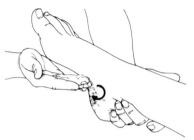
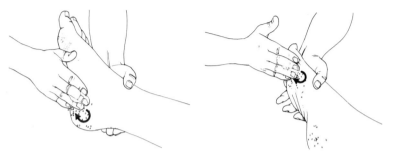

Hard skin remover

5 Remove first the right foot then the left from the bowl, dry them, push the bowl out of the working area to prevent accidents, and place the feet on either a covered foot stool, or one on the floor (on a clean dry piece of paper) and the other on your lap protected with tissue.

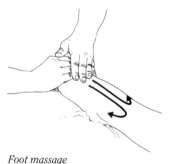

Foot massage

6 Using a suitable foot lotion or powder, massage the feet using effleurage and friction movements. Within the pedicure sequence two minutes is adequate, but if foot and leg massage is to be combined into the routine, it is applied at this stage, using a nourishing cream medium. The leg should be well supported to prevent tension occurring in the muscles. Apply powder generously between the toes to help prevent infection.

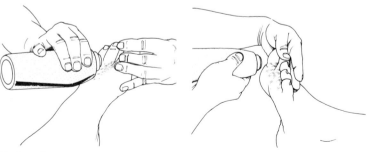

Foot powder

7 Place rolled cotton-wool pieces between the toes of the left foot, clean the nails with remover, and apply base coat, and enamel if desired, in the same manner as in the manicure. Complete steps 6–7 on the right foot.

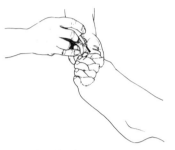

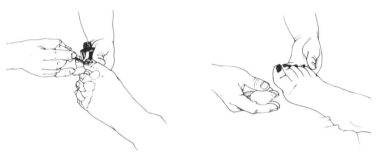

Enamel application

8 When the enamel is completely dry, remove the cotton-wool, check that the feet are dry and comfortable, and allow the client to replace tights and shoes, offering assistance if required.

Complete the treatment by putting equipment and working area in order, sterilise tools, and clean and check all preparations used. Enamels may require attention if they have become too thick and a small quantity of solvent added to improve their consistency. Hand-washing completes the routine, to minimise the risk of infection both to other clients and to the therapist.

A pedicure is a wonderful treatment, extremely beneficial to the feet and very relaxing. Clients almost become addicted to the treatment because they realise they are unable to achieve the same results at home and the feeling of 'walking on air' is marvellous!

Foot and leg massage

Preparation

The massage may be given independently, or combined with the pedicure, where it is applied on completion of the cuticle work, prior to the enamel application. Ensure that the client is comfortable, with relaxed muscles, regardless of the position in which the massage is to be applied, i.e. prone or in a sitting position. The ideal position for the treatment is with the client in a fairly high armchair and the operator on a lower stool, permitting free movement of the arms and enabling the client's lower limbs to be constantly supported. The massage may be accomplished with talcum powder or cream, depending on the time of year, and the condition of the feet and legs. In hot weather and for feet that perspire freely, a dusting of powder is refreshing for the client and more agreeable for the therapist. When the temperature is cold or the feet and legs show a dry and scaly skin, oil or cream will be more beneficial.

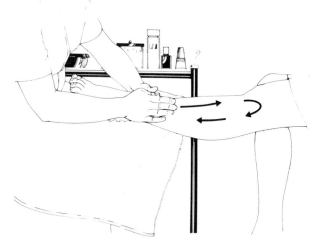

Massage position

Method – sequence of movements

1 Superficial stroking (effleurage) over the entire foot and leg area, repeated until the muscles become relaxed.

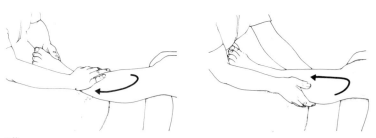

Effleurage

2 Superficial stroking over the upper surface of the foot, one hand supporting, one working, alternately, from the ankle to the toes.

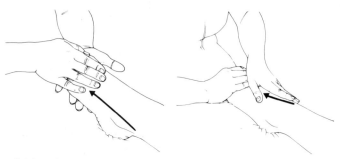

Superficial stroking

259

3   Thumb kneading (petrissage) over the medial arch of the foot, forming firm rotary movements, progressing from the ankle to the phalanges. The movement returns with a superficial stroke, and the fingers rest lightly on the upper surface of the foot. Repeat 3–4 times.

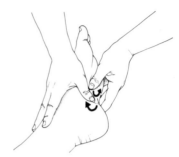

Kneading on the medial arch

4   Petrissage movement over the phalange joints, with the hands enclosing the area, thumbs in firm contact, fingers overlapping. The movement commences under the metatarsals, with the thumbs exerting firm pressure under the ball of the foot; the toes are pressed firmly but smoothly downwards to their fullest extension. Superficial stroking links and returns the movement. Repeat 4 times.

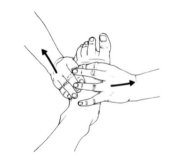

Toe extension

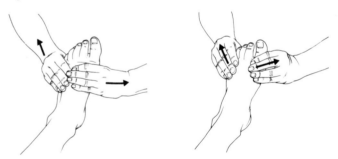

5   Deep kneading over the medial arch of the foot, accomplished with the thumb pad of the therapist's hand, working in firm rotaries, from the heel to the toes. The foot is supported, and so a true petrissage action is achieved.

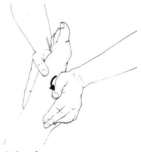

Deep kneading over the medial arch

6   Digital stroking around the malleolus, commencing at the toes, with index fingers together, and thumbs crossed. The movement progresses with firm pressure to the ankle, the hands divide and return with a superficial stroke to the toes, with the outside borders of the hands in contact. Repeat 6 times.

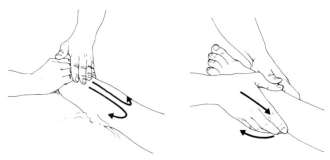

Digital stroking

7   Alternate kneading and stroking on the Achilles tendon of the gastrocnemius muscle, with the foot and leg well supported, and both hands working. Firm rotaries are performed with the thumbs either side of the tendon and the fingers link the movement with relaxing effleurage strokes. Repeat 6 times.

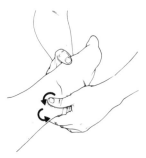

Kneading of the Achilles tendon

8   Superficial stroking over the entire area to re-establish relaxation. Repeat 6–8 times approximately.

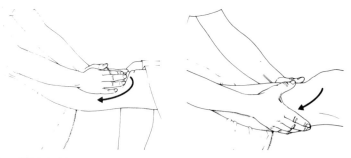

Superficial stroking

9 Thumb kneading over the tibialis anterior muscle, working from the attachment on the foot, upwards towards the knee. Thumbs move alternately working with upward, outward pressure, over the entire muscle, returning with effleurage strokes. Repeat 3–6 times.

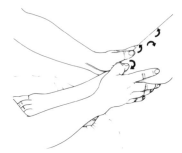

Kneading on the tibialis anterior

10 Palmar kneading to calf muscles, working in an upward direction, with the muscles relaxed, and the leg well supported. One hand supports, the other first lifts and exerts outward pressure on the muscles, then relaxes, and moves to a new position. The petrissage movement is applied to the entire calf area, adjusting the pressure according to the bulk of the muscles. Superficial stroking links the movement, which is repeated with the other hand in a medial direction. Repeat 3 times each side.

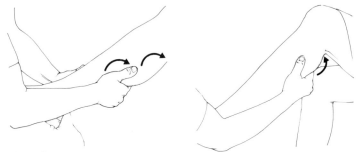

Calf kneading

11 Alternate palmar kneading, with both hands working from the knee to the ankle, rolling the muscle in a rhythmical manner. Superficial stroking links the movement, and should be repeated 4–6 times.

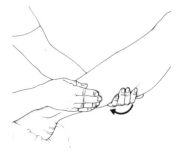

Leg rolling

12 Clapping movement to the calves, performed briskly, with the palmar areas of both hands formed into a cupped posture. Apply for 20–30 seconds.

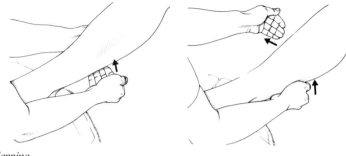

Clapping

13 Snatching movement, performed over the toes, with the fingers and thumbs in a light tapotement stroke, rapidly repeated.

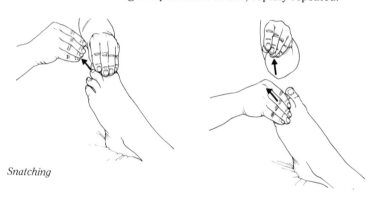

Snatching

14 Whipping movement, applied in the same fashion, exerting rapid stimulating strokes over the toes, to increase local circulation and improve colour. Both snatching and whipping are applied lightly and quickly for 10–20 seconds, and at no time should discomfort be experienced.

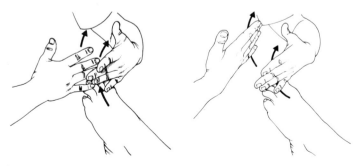

Whipping

15 Relaxing superficial stroking over the entire foot and leg completes the routine. Repeat 6–8 times slowly, finishing at the toes.

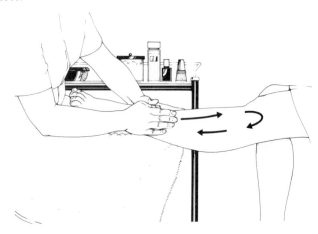

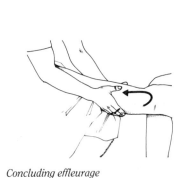

Concluding effleurage

Conclusion

Excess cream or oil may be removed, and the legs toned with mild tonic, and dusted with unperfumed talcum if desired. If applied in combination with pedicure, the routine may then be concluded.

Self check

1 Name the bones of the hand and wrist.
2 What is an antagonistic muscle? Give an example in the forearm.
3 Why do we have finger nails?
4 Describe the growth of the nail.
5 What are the advantages of having a manicure?
6 Draw a diagram to show the structure of the nail.
7 Name four contra-indications to a manicure.
8 Name four common nail disorders, and describe the appearance of two contagious nail diseases.
9 List the products used in a manicure; state the active ingredient and the function of each one.
10 Describe how to shape nails. What influences the choice of shape?
11 Why are nails soaked during a manicure?
12 What are the advantages of a hand and arm massage?
13 What are the storage considerations for nail enamel?
14 At what temperature is paraffin wax applied?
15 Name four contra-indications to paraffin waxing.
16 List the effects of paraffin wax.
17 Name the methods available for nail repair. Give the advantages and disadvantages of each one.
18 Name the bones of the foot and ankle.
19 Describe the arches of the foot.
20 What are the indications for a pedicure?
21 Name four contra-indications to a pedicure.

CHAPTER TWELVE # Depilatory Treatments

Consultation

The hair removal method should be discussed briefly with the client prior to treatment to avoid confusion or disappointment over results. The advantages of each system can be given, with guidance as to which is most suitable for the client's own needs. The amount of superfluous hair, its location and the rate of growth decide the best means of removal. Conversation and inspection of the hair may point out the need for a more permanent solution (i.e. epilation, electrolysis) being required to resolve the problem, especially on the face.

Depilatory methods available (temporary)

- Plucking.
- Waxing – hot and warm wax methods.
- Shaving, cutting, abrasive gloves and depilatory creams.

Plucking and waxing remove the hair completely from the follicle, leaving an active area of cells which in time produce a new tapered hair, which appears on the skin's surface after a period of 4–6 weeks depending on the strength of the hair growth. If rapid regrowth occurs a more permanent method of hair removal could be indicated.

Shaving, cutting, abrasive gloves and depilatory creams remove the hair only from the surface of the skin, and blunt regrowth is apparent after only a few days. Although these methods are not used professionally, they should be discussed in consultation, to give the client a comparison of the advantages of professional depilatory treatment over these home methods.

The skin may also have become rather fragile and easily irritated if abrasive gloves and depilatory creams have been used previously, as these remove some of the skin's surface, mechanically or chemically.

Advantages and disadvantages of temporary methods (waxing)

Advantages

- Large areas of unwanted hair can be removed quickly in one session, providing instant results.
- Relative low cost and high client satisfaction makes waxing a regular grooming service.
- Only slight discomfort is experienced with correct application technique.
- The client is free from unwanted hair for long periods, and regular treatment thins the regrowth considerably.
- Regrowth is fine ended, and feels soft and natural in texture.

Disadvantages

- Has to be repeated at regular intervals to maintain a groomed appearance.
- Waxing can occasionally cause regrowth hair to be ingrowing, causing discomfort. Waxing should not be repeated until the condition rectifies itself. Use of friction gloves and special creams which speed the skin desquamation (containing AHAs – alpha hydroxy-acids) have largely eliminated the problems of skin over-growth trapping the emerging hairs.

Permanent hair removal methods available (destruction of the active follicle)

Epilation

Epilation is removal of the hair and destruction of the follicle using a short wave diathermy current (heat). This causes coagulation of the hair root and surrounding cells, restricting and eventually destroying the follicle's ability to produce a new hair.

Electrolysis

Electrolysis is removal by galvanic (chemical) means where chemical substances formed at the tip of the needles destroy the hair root and surrounding cells.

Both methods of permanent removal are applied via extremely fine needles which enter the hair follicles individually.

Advantages and disadvantages of permanent methods

Advantages

- The only real solution to excessive hair growth. For deeply rooted lip or chin hair, under hormonal influence, and with very rapid regrowth, permanent treatment is the professional answer.
- Each regrowth that occurs produces a finer growth. Fine hairs may only require one removal to achieve destruction.
- Once completed the task never needs repeating – a strong point for really hirsute clients.

Disadvantages

- Skin reaction may occur in some cases.
- Discomfort may be experienced by some clients.
- High cost if a large area of superfluous hair growth requires treatment.
- While rather lengthy treatment is being undertaken the client may not look as well groomed as normal.

Depilatory waxing – hot wax (hard type)

Traditional hot wax consists of beeswax and resins, plus soothing ingredients. These minimise the reaction to the heat of the wax,and prevent irritation after hair removal.

The wax is solid when cold, and has a high melting point, with a working temperature of approximately 68 °C (154°F). Available in natural yellow/reddish brown, or as an azulene (green) wax, all hard wax removes hairs very efficiently – even very short hairs. Hot wax can be re-used, strained, etc., and its high cost makes this necessary for leg waxing. If well maintained, hot wax is very economical in use, but it does require proper care to work at its best.

Cross-infection risks now make it more normal to dispose of wax used within facial, underarm and bikini wax treatments

In countries where wax may not be re-used, hot wax either has to be disposed of and its cost built into the treatment charges, or disposable cool wax must be chosen.

As waxing treatment is offered at such a wide range of venues, salons, health studios, etc., where meticulous care of the wax is more difficult to ensure, disposable wax should be chosen to ensure the necessary standard of hygiene.

Depilatory waxing – warm wax

Warm wax is disposable, which limits cross-infection risks,and is an attractive alternative to hot wax methods, being easy to prepare and maintain. Improvements in the wax's ability to remove hairs efficiently have resulted in warm wax being the most widely used method.

Warm wax is a combination of wax, oils and resin, and has a low melting point of 43 °C (110 °F), so the wax reaches its working consistency very quickly. This also reduces the fire risk in the clinic.

Warm wax is used very sparingly, in conjunction with thin fabric strips, with both the wax and strips being thrown away after use. With practice warm waxing can be a much quicker procedure for hair removal than the hot wax system. It has special techniques of its own, which must be followed to achieve efficient hair removal without discomfort. Skin reaction to waxing is considerably reduced, due to the lower working temperatures needed to accomplish the hair removal.

Wax choice

It is useful to have both systems of wax available in the clinic to cope with a range of hair growth problems. With care, warm wax can now remove even short hairs as efficiently as hot wax, but there will be instances when hot wax is still the most effective means of removing deep rooted hairs without skin trauma, as it has the greatest adhering power to the hair and skin. Hot wax is still preferred by many operators for lip and chin, underarm and bikini and inside thigh hair removal. In this case new wax should be used and simply be thrown away after use, making cross-infection impossible.

Contra-indications to waxing

The area to be waxed should be inspected prior to treatment, for problems that prohibit or limit the application; for example:

- Varicose veins.
- Defective circulation, i.e. diabetic condition, ulcers on the legs, etc.
- Skin diseases.
- Cuts and abrasions.
- Warts, hairy moles.
- Stings or sepsis present.
- Hypersensitive skin, from sunburn, windburn, over exposure to sunbeds, etc.
- Any areas of the body where extreme discomfort would be involved, i.e. breasts, pubic area, and in certain instances of known sensitivity, the underarm area.

Safety precautions

- The equipment must be of a certain standard of safety, and should have a sturdy construction as it will have fairly constant use, and it must be reliable.
- It should be earthed, correctly wired and should have enclosed heating units to prevent overheating of the outer casing.
- The wax containers should have both bottom and side heating elements (heating band) for fast and safe wax heating.

- The heater should be sited on a metal or formica-topped mobile trolley protected with paper roll and should not be placed on a glass-topped trolley.
- The wax should not be left to heat and melt close to any flammable materials such as plastic goods, curtains, etc.
- Covered containers reduce both the pungent odour of the melting wax, speed the melting and reduce fire risk.
- Wax pans must be kept free from wax on the rims and bottoms, or the wax can ignite and cause a fire.
- The attractive equipment now available allows it to be placed close to the working position, where its progress can be supervised in view of the client.
- Thermostatically controlled waxers prepare and maintain the wax, making it always available at the right temperature, but it still needs final checking to avoid burns.

Fast, safe results in waxing come by getting to know the wax, choosing the best wax for the job and then applying it with attention to technique. This includes controlling the preparation, testing, maintenance and application of the wax, avoiding areas of danger.

The following faults reduce the efficiency of waxing so must be avoided at all times:

- Overheating the wax.
- Inadequate protection of the client and working area.
- Incorrect working consistency of wax, i.e. too hot or cool.
- Neglect in testing the wax in relation to the client's tolerance.
- Poor skin preparation which prevents the wax from adhering.
- Careless application, producing untidy removal and unsatisfactory results.
- Moving the wax whilst hot.

Hot wax hygiene and maintenance

To maintain efficient performance, prevent cross-infection and ensure wax economy and maximum usage:

- Pots and spatulas should be kept clean by wiping with equipment cleaner (surgical spirit) whilst still warm after use.
- The thermostatic control should keep the wax at a moderate working temperature of 68 °C (154°F). This prevents a prolonged period of heating which has a detrimental effect on the adhering properties of the wax and results in unsatisfactory removal.
- Avoid heating the wax above its correct working temperature, as it will darken and give off a pungent odour. It also becomes brittle and hard to remove.
- New wax is used in bikini, underarm and facial waxing and is thrown away after use. Increasingly this is becoming the trend with all hot waxing, to lessen cross-infection risks. The wax costs then have to be built into treatment charges, like any other clinic commodity.

Depilatory hot waxing

Equipment choice and preparation

Modern waxing equipment has large-capacity containers, with thermostatically controlled heating elements which heat the wax to its correct pre-set temperature. This is then maintained throughout the application, preventing over-heating and ensuring adequate wax is available to complete the treatment. Dual pan units allow a choice of wax to be available, i.e. natural or azulene, or allow for straining of the wax to remove hairs and clean it (in those countries where re-use is permitted).

- Sufficient depilatory wax should be pre-heated to a moderate temperature. Hard wax normally comes in solid one-kilogram blocks, which can be broken into lumps to add to the wax in the pans.
- When the wax attains the consistency of syrup and is easy to control, it can be tested on the operator's wrist.
- The wax must be liquid enough to adhere to the hairs, particularly if they are short, but not too hot for discomfort or subsequent grazing of the skin.
- The items required for waxing are made ready: surgical spirit, talcum powder, cotton-wool, wooden spatulas, tweezers, a small brush, soothing lotion or cream.
- The working area should be protected and the wax equipment brought close to the working position for efficient waxing.

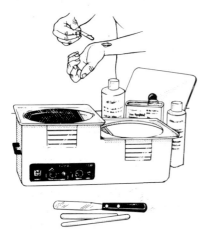

Testing the wax temperature

Client preparation

- The client is helped into position, and the area to be waxed is inspected for contra-indications under the illuminated magnifier. The patterns of hair growth are determined in order to guide the application.
- The areas to be waxed are checked, whether full-leg, half-leg etc., as this changes the application routine slightly and needs to be known prior to starting treatment.
- The skin is cleaned with spirit to free it from oils and lift flat-lying hairs away from the skin.
- A light dusting of talcum in the pattern of removal is then applied against the growth to make the hairs erect. Very flat hairs can be brushed to lift them from the skin.
- The wax is tested just prior to use and then rapidly applied in strips about 5 cm (2 inches) wide, against the hair growth. Initially strips can be quite short until proficiency is reached, then they can lengthen, so that the length of the leg is treated in one strip (if the hairs all grow in the same direction).

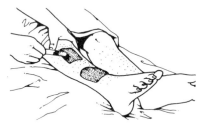

Application of strips

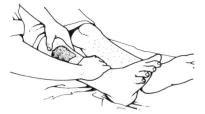

Pressing down the wax

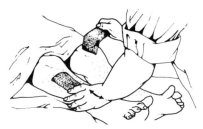

Taking off and rubbing

- Equal distance should be left between the strips to allow for the following application, and ensure even coverage, with no overlap if possible.
- As many strips as can be managed should be applied at each stage of the treatment, with the ends of the strips covering bare skin wherever possible to reduce discomfort for the client on removal.
- Strips should be rapidly applied, with firm edges, against the hair growth to a thickness of quarter of an inch. Wax build up should be avoided, as it slows the removal, and could cause skin grazing.
- When the wax is no longer sticky to the touch, it can be firmly moulded to the area to increase its adhering properties.
- Wax strips are removed when they reach a flexible but still semi-set state, by quickly flipping up one end, ripping the strip off with a decisive movement (with the hair growth), and following up swiftly with a rubbing movement to stop the smarting.
- Removal should follow the contour of the area, staying parallel to the skin, to avoid wax breakage or stretching of the strip.
- Wax strips should not be permitted to become over-set and brittle, or they will shatter on removal and the client will experience discomfort, and annoyance. Treatment time will also be extended.
- Areas in which the hairs have not been removed satisfactorily may be rewaxed only if the skin does not feel or appear sensitive. Working with straight-sided strips to a neat pattern avoids the need for rewaxing to a large extent.
- The front of the legs should be completed and the client requested to turn over (if a full leg wax is planned the front of the thighs are completed before the client turns).The headrest is dropped and the client made comfortable, and her clothing protected again with tissues. The back of the leg normally requires a different direction of wax application, still against the growth, but around the leg, following its contours. The strips should not be made too wide, otherwise hair removal will be poor,with hairs remaining after treatment.
- On completion of the wax, the legs should be inspected with the client sitting up and her legs in a pulled-up position, free from the couch.
- Loose wax fragments should be removed with the rough paper from the couch, to make the client clean and comfortable, and stop wax escaping to surrounding areas.
- Any remaining wax, loose hairs, etc. remaining on the legs may be removed with surgical spirit.The illuminated magnifier can be used to check the final result and to look for stray hairs, which can be removed with tweezers.
- A soothing cream or lotion can be applied with massage to disperse the heat reaction present, using firm stroking, effleurage movements. This will help to reduce redness and blotches. Regular massage helps prevent the formation of ingrowing hairs as the hairs reappear, so the client should be encouraged to follow this routine at home.
- The client is helped from the bed, finally checked for wax and assisted with clothing.

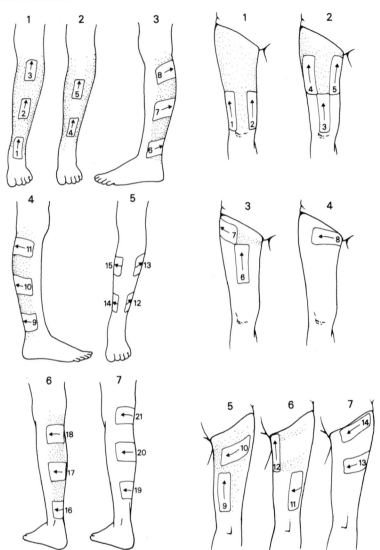

Depilatory sequence on the legs   *Depilatory sequence on the thighs*

Leg wax organisation and after-care

- A half leg wax (up to the knees) should take half an hour, depending on the hair growth.
- With practice the lower leg strips (1, 2, 3, 4, 5) can be combined into one, saving a lot of time. Whenever the growth pattern alters, however, the wax application has to alter to match it or the hairs will not be removed correctly. The diagram of strips provides a guide to application which must be altered to follow the actual hair patterns seen.
- A full leg wax, including inside thigh, should be possible to complete in 45 minutes to one hour, depending on density and growth pattern of hair.

- In consultation, inspection of the growth can provide a guide to the time required and the charge to be made, so the client is informed and the correct appointment booking can be allowed.
- Clients should be advised to take only a warm, not a hot bath, on the same day as waxing is applied.
- Hairs regrow over a period of 4–6 weeks, and regular removal should be encouraged.
- If the client suffers from ingrowing hairs, she should be advised to use a friction mitt gently on her legs in the bath or shower, and also to use the special creams which thin the epidermis, containing alpha hydroxy-acids (AHAs).
- A minimum of 0.6 cm (0.25 inch) of hair is necessary to ensure a satisfactory waxing result. Shorter hair than this will result in hairs coming through a day or two after the waxing.
- If blunt hairs are evident very shortly after waxing, it is an indication that the hairs have been broken off, rather than removed cleanly from the follicles. This points to poor technique, mainly of removal, with the wax being lifted away from the skin, rather than contoured to it.

Underarm waxing (hot wax method)

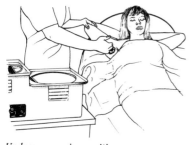

Underarm waxing position

- The wax is prepared and checked for temperature in the normal way. New wax is melted, and on removal will be discarded, so is not placed back into the container.
- The client is placed in a semi-reclining or flat position, and made comfortable with her arm raised.
- The clothing and couch are protected with disposable materials.
- The skin is cleaned with a damp cotton wool pad, and dried with tissue. Talc is applied in the application direction, against the growth.
- The wax is applied against the hair growth, either in one piece (in the case of sparse growth) or two pieces, normally towards the centre. The upper pieces of both underarms may be applied and removed, followed by completion of the lower areas, to produce a complete removal with the minimum of discomfort. Alternatively, one underarm may be completed followed by the other.
- The underarm area may be soothed with antiseptic calming lotion or emulsion to reduce discomfort. Blood spots (in the case of strong growth) require a soothing compress to be held to the skin for a few minutes after completion.

Organisation and after-care

- No deodorant or anti-perspirant products should be used for 12 hours after waxing to prevent irritation.

- Results normally last 2–6 weeks, depending on the degree of growth present. The regrowth period is gradually extended with regular removal, as less hairs are available for waxing every time, due to the resting and growing cycle of hairs.
- If, after waxing, regrowth hairs are evident within a few days, the hairs have broken off and technique is at fault.
- Regular waxing, with its apparent reduction in hair, reduces the discomfort of waxing considerably, so it should be encouraged especially for clients with a heavy underarm growth.

Bikini wax (hot wax method)

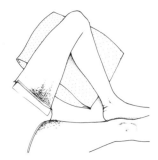

- The client is positioned so that her back is supported, and her leg is bent at the knee and rests on a covered pillow or cushion so the muscles of the inside thigh can be relaxed.
- Underwear is protected by paper tissues and the area of removal is inspected and discussed.
- The area is cleansed and talc applied to lift the hairs, against the hair growth.
- The wax is applied in small patches, against the growth, firmly applying the wax with the tip of the spatula.
- The wax strips are firmly moulded to the skin, and when semi-set but still flexible, ripped off decisively (normally in the direction of the hair growth). The skin is held firmly to minimise discomfort.
- Heavy hair growth can be treated with small, but logically placed strips or patches to ensure that all the hairs are removed. The first inside thigh is completed and checked and soothing lotion applied.
- The client is repositioned and the second thigh completed and soothed.
- If the lower abdominal area is to be waxed, the client is repositioned, placed flat with a pillow behind her head, and the waxing is completed in the same way. Small wax strips or patches are applied against the growth, and removed with the hair growth.

Clients should be consulted about the area of skin they want to be free of hairs, and if necessary encouraged to wear the swim suit or underwear they want to wear. Hot wax can also be applied on the abdominal area.

New clients should be advised of the sensitivity of waxing in this area, and treatment approached from the point of view of a good result, without undue discomfort.

Warm waxing

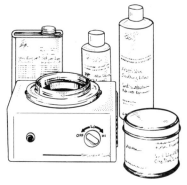

Warm wax unit

Warm wax has become a popular system of depilatory treatment for the following reasons:

- Low equipment cost – a wax heater of 25 g (8 oz.) capacity is adequate for most treatments.
- Convenience of application, low working temperatures, short preparation times.
- It is easy to apply and remove, improving application times and treatment profits.
- It is disposable and has a low maintenance and a high hygiene profile
- It is very economical in use when applied correctly.
- It is very easy to control, making it ideal for facial hair removal, i.e. lip, chin, sideburns, eyebrow hair.

Equipment

Warm wax is heated in a thermostatically controlled small heater, until it becomes clear and warm 43 °C (110 °F) and will spread over the skin and hairs easily in a very thin film. The thermal unit takes only 10–15 minutes to warm the wax to a working consistency, which is a useful point for unexpected wax clients. The wax may stay at this temperature all day, without causing odours, making it possible to offer waxing treatment at very short notice.

The wax system consists of:

- The heater.
- Wax in 25 g (8 oz.) metal containers, which normally fit directly in the heater, as the wax is not really fluid until warmed.
- Waxing strips of fine, but strong material, either pre-cut or in a roll ready for cutting, to suit the area of treatment (long strips for legs, tiny narrow strips for lips, eyebrows, etc.).
- Wooden spatulas.
- Pre-wax lotions for skin cleansing.
- After-wax soothing lotions.
- Equipment cleaner (surgical spirit) for keeping the heater neat and wax-free on the rims.

Warm wax application method (legs)

Warm wax is applied with the hair growth, and removed against the growth, and provides very natural regrowth.

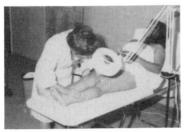

Skin inspection

Warm wax is applied in a quite a different way from hot wax and can remove hair extremely quickly, once the technique is mastered. As the wax does not set, its timing of removal is not so critical as hot wax. However the warmer it is when the removal strip is placed over it, the better the result will be. Hair must be at least a quarter of an inch long to be satisfactorily removed with the warm wax method; ideally it should be longer.

- The hairs are inspected to determine hair direction and density.
- The skin is cleaned with pre-wax lotion, which removes all oil, etc. from the skin, ensures a good attachment of wax to the hairs and lessens the skin-shedding effect.

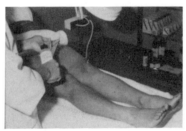
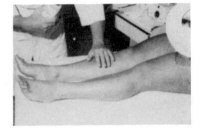

Skin preparation

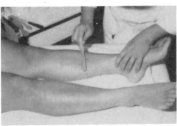

1

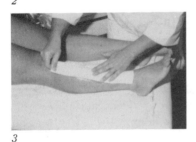

2

- A small quantity of wax is applied to the area of treatment, using the edge of the spatula, at an angle of 90 degrees to the skin. The wax is pushed along the skin with the direction of hair growth, to form a thin film.
- A muslin strip is then placed over the wax so that the edges are free, and pressed down firmly to make a good bond.
- The strip is then removed with a quick action of the wrist, against the hair growth direction, contouring to the shape of the treated area. The strip is removed almost parallel to the skin, and must not be lifted upwards or a poor removal will result.
- The fabric strips may be used again on the next area until they become loaded with wax and cease to remove the hairs and wax efficiently. Depending on the density of the hair growth, only 2–4 strips may be needed for a half leg wax.
- When the wax is completed, the client draws her legs up and the skin is inspected for loose hairs, etc. An after-wax product is applied with a few minutes' pleasant massage to conclude the routine.

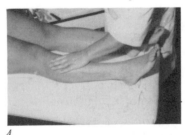
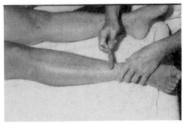

3

4

5

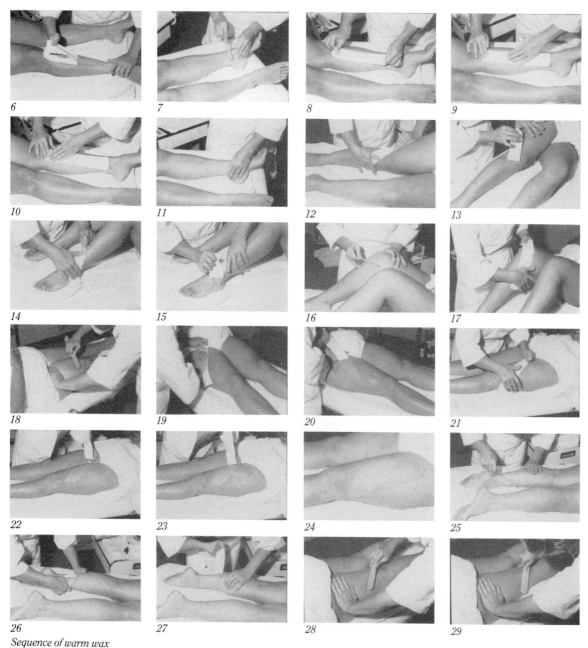

6 7 8 9
10 11 12 13
14 15 16 17
18 19 20 21
22 23 24 25
26 27 28 29

Sequence of warm wax application on the legs

Organisation and after-care

An organised approach to the application is used, though not as rigid as with hot wax, as an area can be re-waxed if really necessary.

- If the hair growth is scanty, the warm wax can be applied over a larger area – still with the growth – and the strip used to remove the hairs with repeated application and removal, in a fast pattern of bonding, and removal, picking up more hairs with each stroke. This allows a half leg wax to be completed in 10–15 minutes, with practice.

277

- The less overlapping that occurs, the better will be the skin reaction, and the faster the treatment time.
- The hair growth direction is followed closely: hair may grow inwards around the ankle, and inwards or downwards on the calf. Special positioning may be necessary around the ankles if hair is present.
- It is often possible to wax the entire lower legs from the front by re-positioning the client, if the growth patterns are simple and the client is of a slim build. For larger clients, or those with a difficult hair growth pattern, the front and backs of the lower legs should be treated separately, like the thighs.
- Less time is taken up with managing the wax so a full leg wax can often be completed in half an hour, depending on the amount and pattern of hair growth present.
- If the thighs are included in the waxing sequence, the fronts are waxed after the front of the lower leg, then the client turns over and the backs of the legs are completed.

Bikini wax (warm wax method)

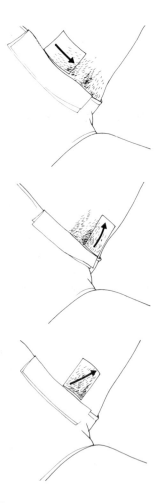

- Smaller, narrower removal strips are prepared, and the wax made ready and checked in the normal way
- The client is positioned in a semi-reclining position, with the leg supported on a pillow and the knee flexed.
- The area of treatment is protected with paper tissues, and the hair growth inspected. Pre-wax lotion is used to clean the area and make the hairs adhere to the wax.
- As the hair growth in the area is dense and deep rooted, small areas should be waxed at a time to minimise the discomfort for the client.
- An organised approach is needed to avoid re-waxing in this sensitive area.
- The normal hair growth is followed, and application made in three main sections, altering the application to match the hair direction exactly.
- Wax is applied with the growth, and using specially cut small strips, pressed down well and removed against the growth, contouring to the area.
- The skin is held taut with one hand whilst the other hand is used to quickly rip off the strips. The free hand is then immediately pressed firmly on the waxed area to stop the skin smarting.
- One inside thigh at a time is completed to avoid re-positioning the client unnecessarily. Soothing after-care lotion is applied to settle and protect the skin.
- With both inside thigh areas complete, the skin is soothed again with after-care lotion. (If the abdominal hair is to be waxed, small damp compresses can be placed on the inside thigh areas, whilst this is completed)
- The protective tissues are removed, and if the abdominal area does not require waxing, treatment is complete.

Organisation and after-care

On an initial wax on a heavy growth, minute blood spots may appear where deep hairs have been removed. This normally only occurs on exceptionally strong growth and will not continue to occur if the client gets into a regular pattern of waxing (fewer hairs being present due to the disruption in the natural hair growth cycle). If blood spotting does occur it indicates a need for extra after-care attention, and advice to the client to avoid irritation or infection.

- Smaller sections of wax can be applied to reduce skin trauma and spotting.
- Tight underclothes should be avoided initially, which would tend to rub on the area, adding to skin irritation.
- Very hot baths, or use of vaginal sprays, should be avoided for the first 6–12 hours after the wax, as these could irritate the skin whilst it is still sensitive.

Certain treatments should not be applied together, i.e. sauna and waxing, as the skin should be at a normal temperature when the wax is applied, or a more severe skin reaction will result.

If the client always suffers a severe reaction to warm waxing, the alternative of hot waxing can be suggested, with the wax being used in the normal hard wax method, and thrown away after use.

Abdominal waxing (warm wax method)

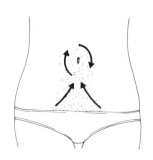

- If the abdominal area is to be waxed, it is normally applied in combination with waxing of the inside thigh, but it can be applied independently.
- The skin is carefully cleansed and prepared with pre-wax lotion, keeping the hair in its natural direction pattern.
- Waxing is applied in the normal warm wax method, but very careful attention to the hair direction is necessary to achieve good results.
- Small areas should be treated, following the hair growth direction meticulously, whether it grows upwards from the groin, or in a circular pattern on the abdominal area. The softness of the skin in this area presents a problem in some cases, such as in post-pregnancy skin softening, or in the overweight or older client.
- Position the client so that the abdominal area is as taut as possible, perfectly flat on the couch rather than semi-reclining which tends to bunch the soft tissues.
- Apply the wax and remove the hairs with the strips, one area at a time. Do not apply the wax generally, or it will become too cool for a good result.
- When the strips are removed, the skin should be held firmly to reduce skin trauma and discomfort, and the waxed area immediately covered with the free hand to reduce the smarting.

- The hairs can be removed in a logical sequence. Any hairs which are not removed successfully on the initial wax application, because their direction is different from the bulk of the hairs in the area, can be re-waxed. This re-waxing should be kept to the minimum possible, as it increases the risk of skin trauma and irritation, and could result in blood blisters forming.
- On completion the area is soothed and protected with after-wax lotion and the normal after-care advised.

Underarm waxing (warm wax method)

Underarm waxing is a very popular treatment and gives excellent results, especially for dark-haired clients where underarm 'shadow' is always present with other depilatory methods (as they only remove the hairs from the surface of the skin). Depilatory waxing frees the client from underarm hairs for 2–4 weeks, according to the growth rate.

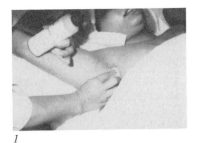

3

- The client is placed in a semi-reclining position, with one hand placed behind the head, the elbow bent and the arm resting on a covered pillow.
- The underarm skin must be flat, and the client is re-positioned until this is achieved.
- The area is protected with tissues, as are the client's underclothes, etc.
- One underarm is treated at a time, making it more comfortable for the client.
- The underarm hair is cleaned with pre-wax lotion and the direction of the hairs observed. The area is dried and the hair brushed into sections ready for wax application.
- Wax is applied in the hair direction in small areas, pushing the wax firmly over the hairs in a thin film. The small strip is quickly applied and removed swiftly, holding the skin firmly to reduce discomfort.
- The process is repeated until the entire area is clear. If the hair growth is in a spiral pattern, divide up the application and follow the direction closely. This avoids unnecessary re-waxing, which can make the skin sore.
- Very short hairs need the wax to be really warm, to help the pores to open and make the hairs more easily removable.
- On completion of one underarm, it is checked and soothing after-wax lotion applied. The client is repositioned, and the second underarm treated in the same way.

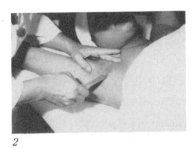

1

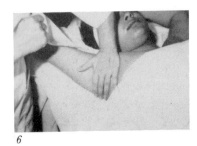

2

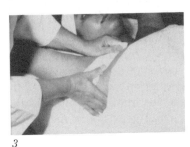

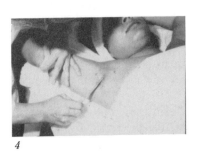

4

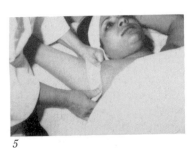

5

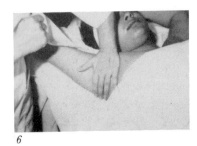

6

Organisation and after-care

As the under arm area has deep-rooted hairs like the inside thigh area, blood spotting can occur until the hairs are thinned out by regular waxing. After-care to the client would include:

- Avoiding the use of anti-perspirants, deodorants or scented talcums or perfumes in the underarm area for a few hours after waxing.
- Avoid friction in the underarm from tight clothes rubbing the skin.

Clients who are new to underarm waxing can be advised when booking the wax not to have the treatment on the same day as some special event, but to book it a day or two in advance to allow the skin to settle. Taking care with new clients can gain them as regulars to the service, which is a very effective but not comfortable treatment.

Arm wax (warm wax method)

The arms are very easy to treat, as the skin is firm and the hairs grow in the same general direction around the arm.

- The area is cleansed with pre-wax lotion, and the hair direction left natural.
- The wax is applied and removed sytematically in the normal way, until the area is cleared.
- The wax may be applied over a larger area if the growth is light, and the strip applied, removed, and re-applied until it becomes loaded with hairs and wax and is unable to remove the growth satisfactorily. It is then discarded and a new strip applied.
- Depending on the density and length of the hairs to be removed, one or two fabric strips per arm should be sufficient.
- The skin is soothed with after-wax lotion and inspected for loose hairs, wax, etc.

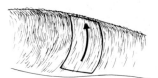 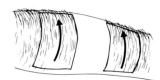 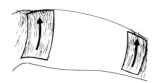

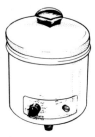

Warm wax facial unit

Lip and chin waxing (warm wax method)

Contra-indications

- Hypersensitive skin.
- Herpes (cold sores).
- Cuts, pustules or skin irritation.

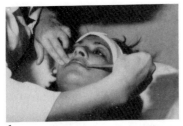

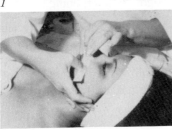

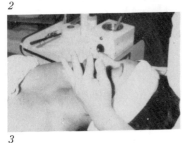

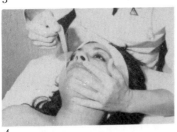

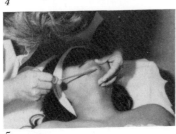

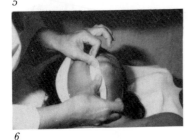

Application

- Special small fabric strips are cut ready for the lip/chin wax.
- The lip area is cleansed gently and any makeup removed thoroughly with cleansing milk.
- The skin is cleaned and prepared with pre-wax lotion, keeping the hairs in a natural pattern.
- The wax is applied with the growth, one area at a time if the growth is heavy. (It may be applied over the whole lip area – keeping to hair direction – if hair is scanty.)
- The hair is cleared one section at a time, using the specially cut strips, first the side lip and then the under nose area.
- The strips are pressed firmly to the wax, and removed by holding their free ends, and swiftly removing them against the growth direction, taking care not to knock the client's face. The area can be briefly held with the free hand to stop the smarting sensation.
- The chin area can be waxed in a similar way, preparing the skin, inspecting the hairs and applying and removing the wax neatly, until all hairs are gone. Re-waxing should be avoided if at all possible with facial waxing.
- The waxed area should be inspected for stray hairs and remaining wax, and these tidied with tweezers.
- The skin can then be soothed and protected with after-wax lotion, and the client advised not to apply makeup for a few hours. If the skin is highly coloured, the reaction can be disguised with medicated makeup or flesh-tinted medicated powder.

Care should be taken not to wax a larger skin area than necessary, otherwise fine vellus facial hairs will be removed, giving the face an unnatural appearance.

The wax should be applied right down to the lip line, to include these fine hairs, and out to the corners of the mouth where fine, long silky hairs can be present. A smaller applicator/spatula can be useful to place the wax only where it is wanted, and not beyond.

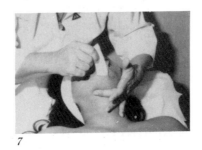

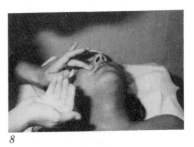

Eyebrow waxing (warm wax method)

Warm wax is very effective for shaping the brows, and is especially useful in the dark-skinned client, where the hair growth may be extensive and need clearing up to the hair line at the sides of the brows.

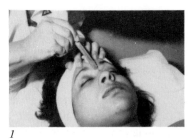

1

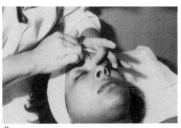

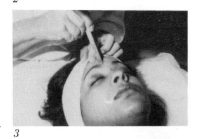

2

3

Being very controllable, and cooler, the wax provides a quick, convenient and safe way of shaping the brows.

- Makeup is removed from the brow, and the shape of the proposed brow discussed with the client, using a mirror if necessary.
- A tiny amount of wax is applied using a small spatula or orange stick, and the unwanted hairs are parted from the main brow shape.
- The hairs are removed following the natural direction of the hair growth, not the direction the hairs may have been placed by the wax.
- Using a narrow strip, the strip is pressed down on to the wax and then removed with a fast movement, against the natural hair growth.
- Small areas may be cleared at a time, first between the brows, and then above (if necessary) and below, to form an attractive shape.
- Avoid removing too much of the actual eyebrow hair until the approximate shape has been approved by the client. Waxing is so fast and effective, more hair can be removed than is desired by the client, so check periodically with her.
- When the brows are completely shaped to the client's satisfaction, they can be wiped over with soothing after-wax lotion, and the client advised not to apply makeup for a few hours following treatment.

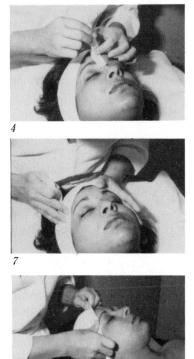

4

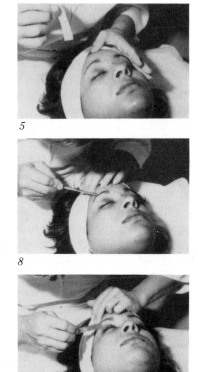

5

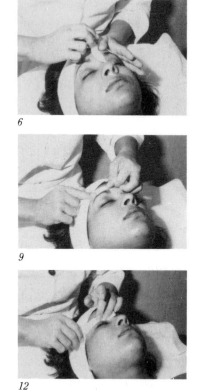

6

7

8

9

10

11

12

Lip and chin waxing (hot wax method)

Hot wax may also be used for removal of facial hair, using the special small heater, which prepares a small amount of hard wax for the service. New wax is used for the lip and chin wax, and is thrown away after treatment. Wax is applied against the growth, and removed with the growth. It is used on its own, not in association with strips, etc.

Contra-indications

- Hypersensitive skin.
- Herpes (cold sores).
- Cuts, pustules or skin irritation.

Equipment

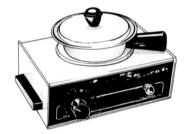

Hot wax facial unit

- A waxing unit able to contain and heat a small quantity of wax for the small treatment.
- Talcum powder.
- Tweezers.
- Spatulas.
- Brush (to make the hairs stand free from the skin).
- Soothing after-wax lotion.

The wax heater is switched on and some lumps of new hard wax placed in the container and allowed to reach a working consistency. It must be checked to prevent overheating. The temperature is then tested by the therapist so that it is liquid enough to adhere to the hairs yet is not uncomfortable for the client.

Application

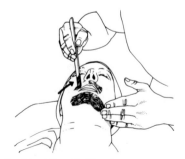

Combined lip and chin wax

- The skin is cleansed with cleanser and inspected for the hair direction.
- The clean skin is then brushed lightly with talc, against the hair growth, which lifts the hairs and eases the wax removal.
- The wax is tested for temperature, and if correct, applied to the hairs.
- Small manageable amounts of wax are applied against the growth from the outer corner of the mouth, over the lip, to the central area under the nose. The second side is covered so that the central part overlaps to form a solid, moustache-shaped piece of wax, extending from the lip line, over the area of unwanted hairs, but not beyond it. Care should be taken to avoid getting wax into the mouth or nostrils.

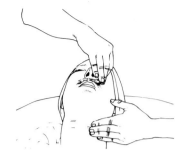

Flicking up lip wax

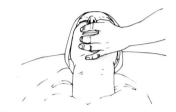

Lip wax removal

- The wax is pressed firmly but gently on to the skin and allowed to set for a few seconds, until touching one corner moves the entire piece. A good removal relies on the wax being flexible, set enough to hold together, but not over-hard or brittle.
- Removal is accomplished by first flicking up the outer corners with one firm stroke, whilst supporting the face with the other hand, then removing the wax in one piece with a firm swift movement contoured to the shape of the face. The second hand gives immediate relief to the area by firmly placing the index finger on the waxed area until the smarting passes.
- The skin can be inspected, loose hairs removed with the tweezers and soothing lotion applied.
- Re-waxing is not really advisable with hot waxing, due to the increased skin reaction with this method. If small patches of hairs have been missed, they can be specifically re-waxed only after the skin has had a small rest with soothing lotion applied, or they can be waxed on another occasion.

Chin wax

If the chin is to be waxed, treatment is applied in a similar manner to the lip, preparing the skin, inspecting, brushing the hairs with talcum, and applying small patches or strips of wax according to the amount of hair present The hair direction is normally towards the lip, so application is against this growth direction. Contoured areas around the jaw should be removed carefully to avoid breaking the wax pieces.

The same after-care of the skin is necessary, with soothing products applied immediately and skin colour disguised if necessary with flesh-tinted medicated powder to avoid the risk of transient bacteria causing infection in the skin.

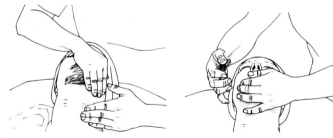

Flicking up chin wax   *Chin wax removal*

Self Check

1 For each of the following areas state the procedure, specific contra-indications and after care for hot waxing and cool waxing:
   (a) Leg.   (b) Bikini line.
   (c) Chin.   (d) Lip.
   (e) Underarm.
2 What precautions should be observed when waxing?
3 At what temperature is (a) hot wax (b) cool wax applied?
4 In table form compare the benefits of the two types of waxing.

Health, Hygiene and Safety

CHAPTER THIRTEEN

Image projection

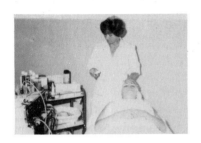

There has never been a time when it was more necessary to project a healthy, clinically sound image to enhance the value of professional beauty services and allay public anxiety. The serious problem of AIDS, (Acquired Immune Deficiency Syndrome) has made people very aware of the need for rigorous hygiene standards in public facilities. These include health clubs, exercise and treatment centres, hair and beauty salons, in fact anywhere the public is treated in large numbers, and where hygiene could be suspect.

The high standard of hygiene the beauty industry has always maintained to guard against cross-infection must now become more visible to the casual observer. To reassure the public, it is necessary to make hygiene more evident through the use of disposable materials, sealed containers for products and obvious use of sterilisers, etc. This ultra-clean image has to be projected to illustrate the care that is being taken in the clinic to safeguard the client's welfare.

Cleanliness is a vital consideration for the beauty specialist when planning the layout and design, organising the routines and maintenance, and indeed in the practical day-to-day working of a salon.

Micro-organisms breed in an unhygienic atmosphere and it is totally undesirable to allow this to happen in the beauty salon environment. For her own protection, the protection of her clients and the reputation of her business the beauty therapist must strive to maintain the highest possible standards of cleanliness. It is necessary to take every precaution to ensure that micro-organisms do not thrive in the salon; this can only be achieved by the therapist having a knowledge of the possible problems and a thorough understanding of the steps she must take to deal with them.

Public hygiene

The safety, health and welfare of the general public is enforced by law through government and health acts, to which anyone offering a business service has to comply. Business premises have to conform to a set of standards relating to the purpose for which the space is registered, e.g. office use, clinic, exercise club, etc. Factors such as access, fire risk, ventilation, hygiene, adequate toilet and washing facilities, etc., which protect the client's well-being, will determine the use that may be made of the floor area.

Both the standard of facilities and the qualifications of the staff are checked on a regular basis in most parts of the world, either through licensing or local authority registration. Permission to operate is gained only by complying with the standards laid down. This ensures adequate facilities for clients and staff. It also helps to ensure employment protection for trained beauty specialists, and guards the public from unqualified operators.

It is important that the beauty therapist has some background knowledge of the micro-organisms that can easily infect the beauty salon if strict hygiene measures are not followed. The micro-organisms that can be involved are split into three main groups: bacteria, viruses and fungi. These are defined, along with other terms, in the glossary which follows.

Glossary of terms

Antiseptic: this word means against (*anti*), putrefaction (*septic*). An antiseptic is a chemical agent which destroys or inhibits micro-organisms on living tissues. It is generally believed that an antiseptic will inhibit the growth of micro-organisms rather than actually destroy them (*Bacteriostat* rather than a *Bacteriocide*, see below). Manufacturers' instructions must be followed for the use of an antiseptic. (An antiseptic is usually regarded as a weaker solution than a disinfectant, and antiseptics can often be used on the skin.)

Aseptic methods: taking care to avoid infection by clean and orderly working habits, rather than allowing infection to appear and then applying disinfectants, etc. Using aseptic methods should create the ideal working conditions for the beauty therapist: she should avoid infection, not have to remove it.

Bacteria: these are single-celled organisms, microscopic in size, that reproduce by splitting very rapidly when in the correct conditions. Some bacteria can produce spores, which are a dormant form of the bacteria that can survive through unfavourable conditions and then reproduce when the conditions become favourable. The spore is considerably more resistant than the bacteria to heat, drying and chemicals and therefore raises an important point when considering hygiene measures. Bacteria reproduce readily when conditions are favourable, different organisms requiring different conditions; pH, balance, moisture, various gases and temperature are the main considerations. Common types of bacteria include *staphylococcus aureus* which causes skin infections, boils, pustules and impetigo, *streptococcus pyogens* which causes throat problems and salmonella which causes food poisoning. Whooping cough, gonorrhoea, diphtheria and typhoid are also among the diseases caused by bacteria.

Bactericide: a chemical agent which under defined conditions is capable of killing bacteria, but not necessarily their spores.

Bacteriostat: a chemical agent which under defined conditions is capable of inhibiting the growth of bacteria.

Cross-infection: an infection which passes from one person to another, or from one part of the body to another.

Disinfectant: this is a term applied to a chemical agent which destroys micro-organisms but not necessarily spores. It does not necessarily kill all micro-organisms but reduces them to a level which is not harmful. Different strengths are available and manufacturers' instructions must be followed.

Fungi: fungi are micro-organisms of the vegetable kingdom. There are many types but only a few which affect humans. The main fungal infections that concern the beauty therapist are tinea (ringworm) and candida albicans (thrush). These can be transmitted by direct contact or use of a towel or other shared object.

Fungicide: a chemical agent which under defined conditions is capable of killing fungi, but not necessarily their spores.

Fungistat: a chemical agent which under defined conditions is capable of inhibiting the multiplication of fungi.

Germicide: a chemical agent that destroys all micro-organisms, but not necessarily their spores.

Non-pathogenic: bacteria that are harmless to the human body and may even be beneficial.

Pathogenic: bacteria capable of producing disease in humans. The temperature most favourable for their development is our body temperature of 37 °C (98.4°F).

Sterilisation: 'the total removal or destruction of all living micro-organisms'. There is no such condition as partial sterility: an item is either sterile or it is not. The state of sterilisation cannot be achieved in a beauty salon, apart from the pre-sterilised items in sealed packets.

Viruses: viruses are even smaller than bacteria and are inactive outside the living cell that they infect. They require a host cell for metabolism and reproduction and so it is more difficult to diagnose and treat a viral infection. Common viruses include herpes simplex (cold sore), herpes zoster (chicken pox and shingles), verruca vulgaris (wart), Hepatitis A and B and HIV infection.

Methods of transmitting micro-organisms

Infection is defined as 'the introduction of pathogenic organisms into or onto the body as a host'.

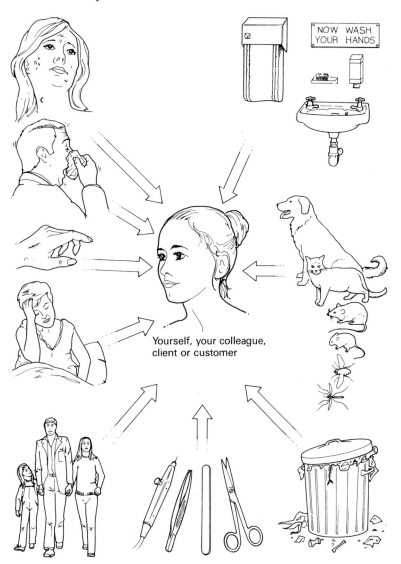

Yourself, your colleague, client or customer

Potential sources of infection

In a beauty salon human beings are the most likely source of infection. It is essential to avoid cross-infection from client to client or client to therapist. All people are potential carriers of infections that are unwelcome in the salon and it is often very difficult to screen out those who are contra-indicated. People may be without symptoms, having acquired the micro-organism and not yet realising it; they may simply be a carrier; or they may still be carrying spores if they have just recovered from an infection. Visual and verbal consultations are vital in order to rule out a wide range of problems, and with strict hygiene measures the beauty specialist can prevent the reproduction of micro-organisms.

There are three main routes which the infection takes to get into the body:

- Via the respiratory tract (breathing in the germs) e.g. cold and influenza viruses.
- Via the alimentary tract (eating or drinking the germs) e.g. food poisoning.
- Through the surface of the skin e.g. boils, warts, herpes simplex and impetigo; or when the skin is pierced, hepatitis B and HIV.

The micro-organisms can be transmitted to these routes in two main ways, by direct or by indirect contact. Direct contact occurs when an infected person touches another person, or the airborne droplets are spread via a sneeze or a cough. Obviously very close contact is taking place in a salon all the time. Indirect contact occurs when an infected person uses an article, e.g. a towel, telephone, cosmetic cream or hair brush and then the same article is used by another person. The two people involved in the transmission of the infection may never actually meet – a very important consideration for a beauty salon where lots of people will be coming into contact with many items.

A beauty specialist cannot be too careful when dealing with the matter of cleanliness and hygiene. There are many ways in which she can protect herself and clients from the risk of cross-infection.

Personal hygiene

As the client's first impression of the clinic is gained from the beauty operator, her appearance should be of attractive freshness and vitality. Her pride in being in the profession should shine forth, giving the client confidence. A healthy, well-groomed appearance sets the tone of the following treatments, and shows what can be achieved with skilled help.

Personal hygiene and good grooming rely to a large extent on good health, being the correct weight for height, having the correct posture, etc. A balanced diet, adequate sleep and exercise, etc. all play a part in healthy living. Having an interest in life and being well motivated in your chosen career is of great importance, as this helps to make the daily chores of personal cleanliness, oral hygiene, grooming routines, etc. less tedious.

Training as a beauty specialist is physically strenuous, and if overall health and posture are not good the work will be very tiring and back pain and fatigue could result.

The beauty specialist should be a credit to her profession, whether in or out of clinical uniform. The clean, white beauty uniform gives the client a good feeling of security, and tells her that she is in professional hands. Being well groomed is essential, and works well on the personal and professional fronts as a confidence builder.

All beauty therapists owe it to themselves, their clients and their profession to project a professional image at all times. This involves very strict personal hygiene. A lot of this is common sense and should be an automatic procedure for beauty therapists:

- Always wear a clean, pressed overall.
- Bath or shower regularly.
- Use deodorants and anti-perspirants.
- Change underwear daily.
- Keep nails short, clean and manicured (no nail enamel).
- Keep hair tidy, clean and well-groomed, not falling on the face or collar.
- Do not wear jewellery.
- Wash hands before and after every client, and during treatments as appropriate.

Client hygiene

As mentioned previously, clients are the greatest possible source of infection in the salon. Careful consultations should eliminate the majority of problems, and visual inspections are a vital procedure. However, once a client is accepted in the salon there are still certain steps that must be taken to ensure that no cross-infection occurs:

- Encourage clients to shower before treatments.
- Encourage clients to wash their hands before treatments.
- Avoid breathing directly over a client.

Salon hygiene

This area of hygiene needs very careful consideration: owing to the wide variety of treatments offered in salons and the vast range of equipment and instruments used, it is necessary to apply a wide range of hygiene measures. The main areas for consideration are as follows:

- Waste disposal (see below).
- Towels, bed linen, gowns and headbands – they should be changed between each client. (An alternative to creating a large amount of laundry is to use disposable paper bed roll and towels. However, this raises an important environmental issue and it is up to the individual to consider all the options available and make up her own mind, but always keeping the hygiene issue as the priority.)

- Wet areas.
- Showers.
- Wash basins.
- Work tops.
- Instruments, tools.
- Floors.
- Equipment.

All should be cleaned regularly in the appropriate way.

- Always use spatulas in jars and pots.
- Always replace lids on jars and bottles immediately.
- Never apply any product such as makeup directly onto the skin.

Methods of sterilisation

There are three main methods of sterilisation that can be applied in a beauty salon. They are radiation, heat, and the use of chemicals.

Due to the wide range of items and surfaces that we need to clean, the varied materials they are made of and the advantages and disadvantages of the sterilisation methods available, no one method is ideal. It is up to the beauty specialist to consider the range of treatments she has on offer and the items she wishes to sterilise, and choose the appropriate method for each task.

Radiation

Ultraviolet is a radiation method of sterilisation that has been widely used in beauty salons. The ultraviolet cabinets do, however, have some disadvantages and it has been proved recently that they are not very effective. They only destroy a limited range of organisms, penetration is limited, the rays only travel in straight lines and any dust, oil or other debris on the surface of the item prevents the ultraviolet being effective. This method is certainly not suitable for makeup brushes or sponges, due to the lack of penetration. The ultraviolet cabinets could be used to store items that have been sterilised by another method.

Gamma irradiation is used on a commercial scale – it is not practical for a beauty salon, although the disposable needles that are used by most electrologists are sterilised in this way. The packet displays a colour-change indicator showing that sterilising conditions have been reached. Each needle is pre-packed and sealed and remains sterile until the packet is opened. Once opened in the salon the needle is no longer sterile.

Heat

Sterilisation by heat, especially on a small scale, is the most effective and economical method. Both dry and moist heat can be used.

Dry heat

Temperatures in excess of 150 °C (300 °F) are needed to destroy bacterial spores. The exact temperature required depends on the apparatus being used and the items being sterilised. Generally the higher the temperature the shorter the exposure time.

Hot-air ovens

All items placed in these ovens must be washed thoroughly and able to withstand the high temperatures involved. Plastic, ordinary glass, fabric, sponge and brushes are not suitable for sterilisation by this method.

Glass bead steriliser

This is another method of dry heat, suitable for small objects.

The tiny glass beads contained in a protective insulated case are heated to a temperature between 190–300 °C (375–570°F), depending on the manufacture, and the sterilising time is between 1 and 10 minutes. Again, this method is not suitable for plastic, sponge, brushes or ordinary glass. The units are specifically designed for the beauty trade and are in keeping with salon equipment. They are small and easy to use.

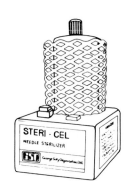

Glass bead steriliser

Moist heat

Moist heat kills micro-organisms by coagulating the protoplasm of the organism, (as the white coagulates in the process of boiling an egg).

Boiling

Although most forms of bacteria are destroyed by five minutes in boiling water, bacterial spores and some viruses may be resistant to this exposure. Boiling is therefore considered only as a disinfectant procedure and has limited use in a beauty salon.

Autoclave

An autoclave is a closed unit that increases the atmospheric pressure and raises the temperature of the boiling water within to between 110–135 °C (230–275°C). These higher temperatures are capable (pro-

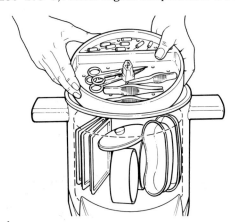

Packing an autoclave

viding that the timing is correct) of destroying all micro-organisms and spores. A pressure cooker works in the same way and could easily be used in a beauty salon.

Care must be taken when using an autoclave that the equipment can withstand the temperatures, and everything is clean and stacked according to the manufacturer's instructions. The user must adhere to the rules for preparation, holding and cooling times.

Chemicals

There is a vast range of chemicals on the market that are designed to promote salon and home hygiene. The directions produced on the containers are often unintentionally ambiguous making it difficult to decide exactly what the chemical can be used for and even what it does with regard to disinfection and sterilisation in the home or salon. Very careful consideration is necessary when choosing any chemical methods to promote hygienic conditions. Careful thought must go into planning a salon with regard to the upkeep of the surfaces, trolleys, floors, worktops, seats, etc., and a careful choice made when purchasing the chemicals intended to maintain hygienic conditions. Reference should be made to the glossary at the beginning of this chapter in order to determine exactly what the chemical is supposed to be doing and to ensure that it is meeting these requirements.

Immersion

The sterilising fluid is composed of chemical compounds called *aldehydes*; it is placed in a plastic container which usually has a perforated tray at the base. Immersion is a very useful method for a beauty salon, as most materials used there can be treated in this way. However, all items must be clean and dry before going into the solution (any water on the articles will dilute the sterilising fluid). The sterilisation time depends on the manufacturer's instructions – usually between 10 and 30 minutes. The chemical requires changing after a given time, maybe 14 to 28 days – again, refer to the instructions.

All items must be thoroughly rinsed upon removal from the chemical and it is advisable to avoid skin contact with the sterilising liquid.

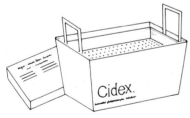

Liquid chemical steriliser

Waste disposal

Disposal of waste material in a salon needs very careful consideration. This procedure should be determined during the planning stages and then carried through into the working environment.

Cotton wool, tissues and paper roll must be placed in a covered container, ideally lined with a removable plastic bag. This should be removed at least once a day and placed inside another bag. The bin should then be washed and disinfected. Electrolysis needles and other sharp disposable items must be placed in a 'sharps' container and then sent away for incineration. Dirty laundry should also be placed in a covered receptacle and removed for laundering daily.

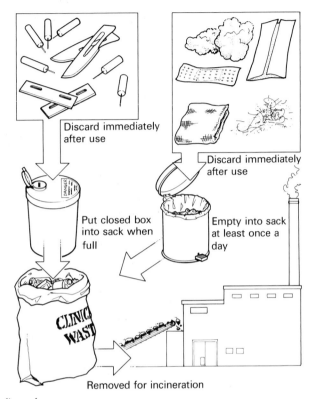

Discard immediately after use

Discard immediately after use

Put closed box into sack when full

Empty into sack at least once a day

Removed for incineration

Waste disposal

Self check

1 List the factors of personal hygiene that a beauty specialist should consider.

2 What is cross-infection? How can it be prevented in a salon?

3 Describe a suitable method of sterilisation for each of the following:
   a) Cosmetic sponges.   b) Cuticle implements.
   c) Mask brushes.   d) Vacuum suction cups.
   e) Epilation needles.   f) Tweezers.

4 List the methods of sterilisation available for a salon and give the advantages and disadvantages of each one.

CHAPTER FOURTEEN # Business Organisation, Salon Procedure and Equipment Choice

Methods of work

There is a wide range of work opportunities for the qualified and competent beauty specialist or therapist and she may decide to concentrate more on treatment, or on sales, or combine them. Initial work experience is usually gained from general therapy in the clinic, to build up client handling, social and sales skills whilst improving practical techniques.

With experience, the therapist can move into many new areas of work, owning her own business, progressing upwards into sales or management, technical demonstrating, teaching, etc. – careers that are rewarding and can fit alongside family life, in a way few other professions can.

General salon work, beauty clinic

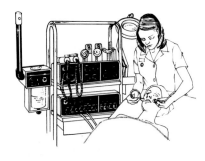

All aspects of facial and body treatments are normally available to the client, from cosmetics and remedial facial therapy, through the full range of figure improvement services, and including grooming aspects such as depilatory and epilation applications. In a large clinic a facial specialist is able to apply all aspects of her training and, if she holds additional body therapy and epilation qualifications, all areas of treatment may be undertaken, giving a varied and interesting work range.

In-store salon

A beauty unit within a store situation is an increasingly popular position for a facial specialist. The work is normally confined, by space and facilities, to cosmetic facial treatments, and may be offered in combination with electrology. A growing method of work is for the facial cubicles to be operated on a franchise basis, with the therapist working for a large company, and having the advantage of national advertising and bulk supplies of cosmetics. A trend towards increasing the electrical facial treatments improves the specialist's work range, and produces more satisfactory results. Skin care advice, cosmetic sales and artistic makeup applications make this an ideal field of work for the facial specialist or therapist most interested in facial therapy and cosmetic applications. Epilation qualification increases the range of work, and is highly desirable both for client satisfaction and convenience, and as a means of additional revenue.

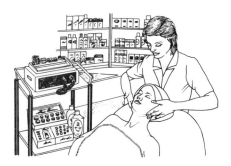

Home visiting practice

The flexible hours of a mobile practice make it a suitable business for any therapist restricted by family commitments to certain hours of work. It can be successfully offered in both rural and suburban locations. Housebound wives, tied by family responsibilities, in either community would welcome the service.

Facial, body, depilatory and epilation applications may be offered on a visiting basis.

Good organisation and planning are needed, to avoid time wastage in travel and preparation on arrival. Booking of treatments to co-ordinate areas of work for certain days or periods of the week is essential, and of course a reliable means of transport is a necessity.

The variable income of a visiting practice makes it more suitable for a highly experienced therapist used to promoting treatments, who is only limited by circumstance from fulfilling normal salon hours. A newly qualified woman might find it difficult to be self-employed and suitably adaptable and organised to secure a regular income from the business. Clients may prefer evening appointments on occasions, or weekend treatments, and a visiting therapist must be prepared to sacrifice part of her normal leisure time in obtaining and completing treatments if she is to fill her working week.

However, the rewards for a skilled operator, both in freedom and income, can be extremely good, as long as the necessary time required

297

is spent on organisation of the business. An account must be kept of income and outgoings, car expenses, special insurance, stock requirements, and provision made for tax deductions, as these will be demanded on a half-yearly, not weekly basis as with PAYE (Pay As You Earn) contributions.

The health hydro

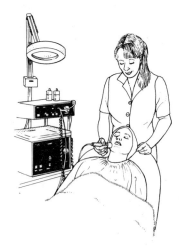

The health hydro, having many residents to care for, normally divides the work between facial therapy and body treatments. Beauty therapists with full therapy qualifications may be able to use all their skills, or may have to concentrate on one area. As the work of the nutritional and complementary health experts becomes more closely linked, the therapist will find her work boundaries becoming less defined, and she will have larger areas of responsibility for holistic health.

Because of the total supervision and controlled diets of the hydro guests, a more corrective programme of holistic (whole body) improvement is possible, encouraging guests to change life style and eating habits for the good of their overall health. This total approach will appeal to therapists interested in body treatments based on diet, exercise, manual and aromatherapy massage, and electrical routines, including muscle toning.

Facial specialists will find themselves using all their skills: facial and stress therapy massage, depilatory treatments, hand and arm treatments, pedicure and paraffin wax routines. Treatment and makeup sales are also strongly featured, making up an important part of the operator's income through sales commission.

Staff are normally resident whilst working within a hydro, as hours of work are linked to the guests' arrival and treatment sessions, which may be very varied. Some hydros are in very beautiful locations, or may be rather isolated, making residence necessary.

Television makeup artist

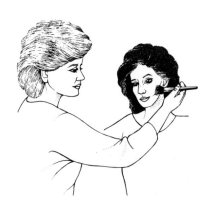

Entry into the field of television work is gradually becoming less restricted, though the field is over-subscribed as it is interesting and exciting and makes a good career. Competition to gain places on the full-time training course is very fierce, and applicants need to have a hairdressing and beauty background, and must have an academic standard of education including Art and History at A level. Age of entry is seldom lower than 21 as makeup artists have to be mature and adaptable workers, able to work on demand.

Throughout the paid training period, experience is gained in all aspect of television and film makeup. The varied work hours, and involvement in the programme production require that the job is a major interest in the trainee's life. It has little in common with normal clinical work, though it uses basic skills and develops them on an artistic basis. If the facial specialist has a strong interest in makeup and costume, training as a television makeup artist can be a fascinating and rewarding field to enter.

A career in sales

Deciding to concentrate on selling as a career can lead the way to a very interesting and financially rewarding life style. Having the ability to make sales is important in general therapy. Promoting treatments and cosmetic products, answering the client's needs in full, making useful profits for the clinic and personal commission on sales are all part of the job.

Developing this talent into a career is easy for a trained therapist since selling is revealing an unconscious need to an individual, and these skills and knowledge have been acquired in beauty training. The

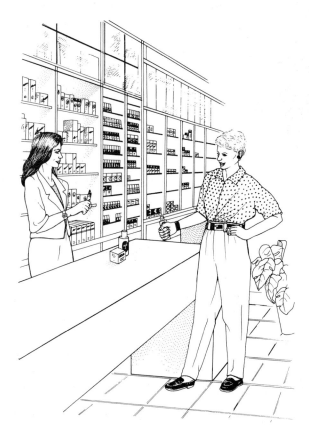

ability to handle a sale naturally comes from having a genuine interest in the client as a person and a wish to share with her latest product information, new techniques, treatment, etc. to keep her abreast of the times and fully informed about the latest and best available.

High pressure selling is unnecessary: most sales can be made through enthusiasm, using technical knowledge to suggest treatments and products that are beneficial to the customer. The therapist can be at ease with this form of technical selling and will use sales aids such as skin charts, brochures, product promotions and demonstrations to make successful sales.

Clients have a need to believe in the products and gain enjoyment from them, so that they obtain good results from their regular use. Gaining sales experience and finding it fulfilling could lead to a career specialising in sales, either as a sales representative, area sales manager or technical sales demonstrator (equipment, products or services).

Sales demonstrator

A demonstrator is a sales person with special ability to communicate with an audience, holding their attention whilst the value and effectiveness of the product is revealed. Practical demonstrating skills can be gained in training and can lead to varied career opportunities, e.g. in the cosmetic field, as a makeup artist, with equipment companies, or in a freelance capacity demonstrating and teaching internationally.

Skills needed for success as a demonstrator include having a confident, well organised manner and a good knowledge of the product

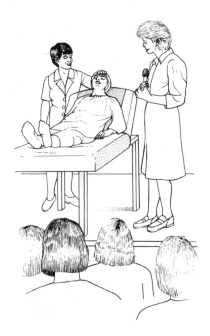

to be sold. The purpose of the demonstration would have to be known as well as the potential target market to be reached (the size of the audience, average age, etc.).

The demonstrator has to able to work to, and keep within, a time plan, getting across her sales message effectively and quickly, and holding the audience's interest in a lively and relaxed way. It is also necessary to have a good memory so that facts and figures about the product can be brought readily to mind to answer questions from the audience, at the same time as continuing with the practical demonstration and describing what is happening.

A successful sales demonstrator is a fairly experienced operator, but sales is one area of work in which, if you do have a special sales talent, nothing is beyond your reach, and no opportunity closed simply because of youth. A sales career relies on results, and if these are obtained, success can come very quickly.

Leisure centre

The leisure industry is a definite growth area, with health and fitness awareness increasing all the time. Most leisure and sports complexes have a beauty salon located on the premises often run on a leasehold basis. This presents a useful opening for beauty therapists who want to run their own businesses. Reception facilities can be shared and the overhead costs are reduced considerably. Leisure centres attract large numbers of people and the two industries complement each another.

Teaching

With the increasing number of training establishments and beauty qualifications available there is an obvious demand for beauty therapy teachers. An academic background is desirable and some sound industrial experience essential. Teaching qualifications can be gained prior to, or during a career in education; the actual entry qualifications will depend on the individual establishment.

Beauty therapist on board ship

Most large cruise ships have a beauty salon on board. The salons are usually run on a concessionary basis often in conjunction with a hairdressing salon. Cruising is an expensive way of having a holiday, so luxury and total passenger comfort and relaxation is a high priority. The work on board is demanding – there are long days at sea when the salon is open, passengers cannot go ashore and spend their days being pampered in the salon. The accommodation for beauty therapists is usually shared with other crew members. Conditions can be confining, time off limited, and the work very demanding, but life aboard ship can be very enjoyable and the chance to travel presents a very favourable job opportunity for beauty therapists. To gain work in this area there is usually a lower age limit of 20–21 and a minimum requirement of work experience.

Treatment planning and promotion

The treatments offered will be based on the following factors:

- The type of work situation, whether an independent clinic, linked with hair dressing or health facilities, or a home visiting practice.
- The area in which it is intended to trade. A highly populated urban area requires a different approach from a mainly residential location, but may support similar levels of turnover by simply promoting a slightly different range of treatments and products suited to the residents in that area.

The age range and life style of potential clients can provide a guide as to the amount of time and money that they are likely to spend on clinic services. This helps to decide the range of treatments that may be offered and the type of product line. It also helps to determine charges.

A professional clientele will require fast, efficient grooming treatments to maintain appearance, but may have little time to spare for relaxation sequences, however much they might benefit from them. They should be encouraged to consider stress therapy routines for instance, as a preventative measure to maintain health.

Retired or wealthy clients with less demands on their time will enjoy soothing routines and will appreciate the manual aspects of therapy and the personal attention given to them. Luckily these clients are always with us.

Younger clients desire results and so expect highly efficient treatment sequences, requiring the salon to be equipped with electrical equipment of a more specialised nature, e.g. ozone steamer, galvanic unit, etc. This is an exciting new area of business, and can be charged at a high rate, as long as results are achieved. It is a large new area of product sales – especially with the latest phytotherapy products.

Presenting new treatments

Most therapy practices have a mixture of elements, and it is wise when setting up the business initially to allow a fair measure of flexibility, until a clear pattern of client need emerges. Skilful promotion can sell almost any beneficial treatment to a client, if it is presented with confidence and its advantages are discussed knowledgeably. If a good sense of trust has been developed between the therapist and her clients, they will look to her for information and guidance.

Promotional ideas

Advertising promotions linked with the time of year, or promotions presenting new treatments or new equipment which the salon has acquired, are normally very successful. They keep the client interested, and show her that her custom is valued. Any enquiries resulting from advertising, promotional mail, etc. must be dealt with positively by a receptionist and converted into treatment bookings. Any anxiety the client might have has to be dealt with sympathetically, in order to gain a new customer.

Stressing qualification

As the beauty therapy business appears fairly complicated to the lay person, the qualified nature of the staff should be shown in advertising. Consultations can be given where necessary, so that the client gets to meet and know her therapist, and she can confirm the treatment needed. Diplomas showing membership of professional organisations should be displayed in the clinic as this denotes that the clinic staff have a high level of skill. Displaying qualifications also illustrates to the client the value placed on her receiving a safe and successful treatment, and makes her feel in good hands.

Factors which influence treatment charges

The location of the salon and the overall cost of its overheads, business loans, rent, rates, equipment and staff costs must be considered when deciding the scale of charges that will operate. The highest costs of the salon will be the salaries of the skilled staff involved.

Where personal attention is required throughout the treatment, cost per hour will be high. More general supervision, or less specialised work such as manicure, makeup applications, etc., can be costed on a lower basis. Facial therapy using advanced techniques and equipment will be the most profitable and high-rated treatment, with charges to match. If results are forthcoming, costs of treatment plans and the associated home products will be willingly accepted by clients.

Working out charges

Many salons operate on a charge-per-hour basis, with all treatment carried out by a qualified therapist. The charge is worked out to return a certain percentage of profit, related to the overall costs (salaries, rent, product costs, etc.) and the capital investment involved.

The level of this price per hour must be set according to the location of the salon, its competitors' prices, and the type of clientele it attracts. This method demands good facilities, a wide equipment choice and skilled staff experienced in treatment and product promotion to achieve success.

Treatment courses

Bookings of treatment courses are beneficial for both client and business. Forward planning enables the appointments to be placed at convenient times in the week – at the best times to suit the client – and forms a solid base for other bookings. Booked plans normally ensure that the client attends regularly, which improves results. Discounts can be given to the client, usually a bonus treatment, on advance course payment of the 8–12 treatment booking.

Advanced and specialised treatments

Specialised treatments such as epilation, vein treatment, facial muscle toning, thermal mask routine, etc., will naturally be costed at a higher rate due to the additional skill and special products involved. Specialist qualifications, training and experience are required in order to offer these treatments. This can be be reflected in advertising to attract new clients for these advanced routines, perhaps drawn from a wider area, particularly if similar facilities are not available nearby. Offering a wide range of treatment enlarges the reputation and status of the business and keeps it ahead of its competition.

Setting up the facial cubicle

The choice of equipment for the cubicle will depend on the range of services planned and the finances available. Certain pieces of equipment, such as a flexible couch are an investment for the future and should not be economised on, as all treatment stems from the client and operator being comfortable. Modern therapy practice now demands that anyone offering a facial service is basically well equipped, so the initial investment is quite large – but so are the returns that can be expected.

Cosmetic sales make up an increasingly important part of therapy, bringing with them excellent profits, but requiring an initial capital

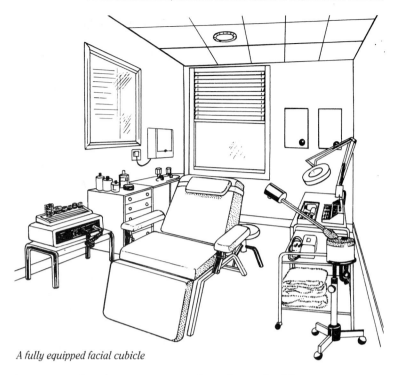

A fully equipped facial cubicle

investment for the treatment and resale stock. Clients expect professional products to be available to them for their home use. Profits from the resales quickly help to make future equipment purchases to keep the clinic up to date with the latest trends.

Equipment choice

Setting up a facial cubicle to offer a sensible range of services would include:

1 A flexible treatment couch/lounge and stool, ideally capable of multi-position action, to permit a full range of facial treatment, plus arm and leg applications, depilatory treatments and electrology. As it is a major item of expenditure, consideration should be given to the different treatments which will be offered. A couch which provides client and operator comfort makes for relaxation and efficient application of techniques, whilst preventing operator strain.
2 Trolleys large enough to support a range of equipment as well as cosmetic preparations, towels, bowls, etc.
3 Small steriliser for small implements such as brushes, sponges, delicate items, manicure and pedicure tools, etc.
4 A magnifier, trolley or wall-mounted, or a mobile type on a stand, for skin inspection. A cool light is essential for client comfort and avoiding eye strain – particularly for epilation.
5 Storage cupboards incorporating a wash basin or a vanity unit, to provide hand washing facilities and storage for towels, bulk

cosmetic containers, equipment, etc. The storage space should be close to hand to prevent unnecessary noise and movement during the treatment.

6 Facial steamer with ozone steam facility, for skin cleansing, balancing and antiseptic effects (ozone therapy).

7 Vibratory massage unit for facial stimulation, relaxation of tense muscle fibres in the shoulder area, etc.

8 Facial vacuum unit for deep skin cleansing, toning and treatment of fine lines. Also for clearing blocked pores in conjunction with steaming and galvanic desincrustation.

9 Spray toning for pressure toning.

10 Brush massage unit for thorough cleansing and stimulating massage, as an alternative to manual methods.

11 Galvanic equipment for desincrustion and iontophoresis.

12 High-frequency equipment – direct and indirect methods.

13 Muscle toning with faradic type currents.

Equipment is available to incorporate systems 9–13 in combined treatment units which are space saving, convenient and attractive in the clinic. The disadvantage is that combined units may only be used by one operator; they cannot be shared between working therapists like the separate systems. Also combined units have to be purchased all at once, with a high initial cost, but of course they will increase earnings significantly.

14 Facial waxing heater for depilatory waxing, hot or warm method.

15 Dual pan wax heater for general depilatory waxing of the legs and body, using hot and warm wax systems.

16 Small equipment and basic commodities: bowls, waste bins, cotton wool containers (with lids), soft viscose sponges (ideally 30–40), gauze, paper tissues, paper sheets, fine oils, talcum, small tools for manicure and pedicure, tweezers, spatulas, lash and brow tinting equipment, orange sticks, soothing lotion, eye lotion (Optrex, etc.), mask ingredients (for clay masks if used).

17 Towels, clinic gowns, headbands, small pillow and washable blanket.

18 Professional and resale treatment products and makeup.

Professional treatment products may be kept on a separate trolley with a wide range of lines to suit different skin conditions. The resale products can be attractively displayed nearby, on a glass wall unit or work surface, where they can be seen by the client.

Professional and related resale products should include:

● Normal skin: cleanser, tonic, night cream, massage cream, mask, ampoules and day protection.

● Dry, dehydrated and mature skin: cleanser, firming tonic, nourishing night cream, massage cream, non-setting or firming mask, ampoules and special care (repair complex, etc.), day moisture cream.

● Sensitive and couperose skin: cleansers, light massage cream, night cream, mask, special care (couperose day and night products), ampoules and day protection.

- Oily/combination skin and acne problems: herbal cleansing milk, deep cleansing scrub, gentle exfoliator, soap-based cleanser or desincrustation gel, enzyme peel, treatment cream, corrective mask or clay mask, corrective ampoules, hydro-emulsion day protection.

Additional equipment to extend the treatment range could include:

19 Paraffin waxing bath, to offer the increasingly popular arm and leg treatment in association with manicure, pedicure and massage.

20 Ultraviolet ray treatment for tanning and skin improvement on acne and oily skin problems.

21 Infra-red heat lamp for warm oil mask treatment and treatment of stiffness in the upper back.

22 Pulsed air massage for lymphatic drainage massage.

23 Epilation equipment for permanent removal of superfluous hair (if qualified).

Home visiting practice equipment

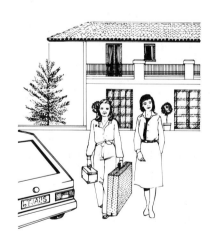

Equipment for a mobile visiting practice must be neat in design, sturdy in construction and should ideally be a combined multipurpose unit, designed for the task. If purely manual and cosmetic routines are to be offered, these present no real problem, apart from finding a suitable position for treatment in the client's own home. Electrical applications require more forethought and planning to avoid time wasting. Electrical connections should be checked to ensure the correct fittings are available.

Multipurpose facial units enclosed in a carrying case present the maximum convenience, time and space saving, and are efficient in use. A cosmetic treatment case, either purpose built, or adapted from another use, i.e. a baby box, can carry small sizes of the required creams and lotions needed for treatment and resale purposes. The latest products, being more likely to be based on natural ingredients, will be packed in smaller sizes, and are very economic in use, ideal for a mobile practice.

Carrying electrical apparatus in a mobile practice presents particular problems, due to the delicate nature of the equipment, and damage which could result in transit. Special containers built to contain the small equipment reduce the likelihood of intermittent performance, but a heavier toll on maintenance is unavoidable and should be allowed for in overall costings. Foam-lined containers lessen the effects of transporting the apparatus, but the choice of equipment should reflect the role it has to fulfil. A combination portable unit providing vacuum, vapour spray, galvanic and high-frequency current permits a wide range of treatment and is ideal for the mobile practice or a small facial unit where space is limited.

Depilatory and epilation treatments are also popular areas of treatment, due to the privacy ensured for the client, and can be applied with ease if attention is given to the working position. A mobile couch may be desirable for leg waxing, and does extend the range of possible treatment as it provides the necessary support for more extensive therapy.

Beauty therapy qualifications and methods of training available

Beauty therapy qualifications may be obtained in a variety of ways, either within an educational situation (further education, technical college or adult education centre) or by commercial means through a training school or private college.

Internationally recognised qualifications are offered by the International Health and Beauty Council (IHBC), Le Comité Internationale D'Esthetiques et de Cosmetologie (CIDESCO), the International Therapy Examination Council, the City and Guilds of London Institute, the British Association of Beauty Therapy and Cosmetology (whose exam board is the Confederation of International Beauty Therapy and Cosmetology), Business and Technology Education Council (BTEC) and International Aestheticians (IA).

The difficulty of obtaining truly world-wide recognised qualifications is slowly being overcome, as the work of these examination boards in setting an international level of competence is being increasingly accepted. This will mean that eventually a minimum period of training and skill will entitle a qualified therapist to work anywhere in the world without restriction. It is because of the differences that exist on the minimum age of training, duration of the course and its content, and educational entry requirements, that until now qualified therapists have found employment restricted outside their country of training. So it is to the profession's advantage to have international organisations which promote its standards and have the strength to obtain world-wide recognition of the therapist's professional status. Therapists should support these organisations by joining the national associations which are affiliated to the international organisation. In the United Kingdom, CIDESCO has chosen the British Association of Beauty Therapy and Cosmetology to represent them, and provide an international qualification to students who first pass the confederation examination at the required level, and undertake a longer period of training.

So when considering training, look at the opportunities provided by the major associations, and realise that the standard that they have set world-wide has had to be earned. Do, if the possibility of an internationally recognised qualification is desirable, expect to be required to meet entry requirements on age, academic achievements, etc., and to train for a specified period according to the level of course chosen. The therapist's work is to a professional level to protect the client's safety, training must reflect this.

Course content

Depending on the level of the training undertaken, the facial specialist will be required to have a sound knowledge of physical science, nutrition, cosmetic chemistry and anatomy to support the practical skills obtained. The information will all relate to the application of the practical techniques and is necessary to apply treatment safely. As the equipment and the cosmetic applications become more sophisticated, the facial specialist has to extend her knowledge of the systems of treatment available. So the training is a blend of technical expertise, manual skills and artistic ability, and it should be of sufficient duration to allow confidence to develop in client handling and sales skills.

Very often facial therapy is studied in conjunction with body therapy and electrology to provide the therapist with a wide range of employment opportunities and to give variety to the work itself. Full therapy training is normally of one year's duration in a private training school, and two years in an educational establishment (a longer time due to the educational vacations). In the longer educational courses, more time is also spent on related topics to round out the students' experience and build confidence and social skills. Art, drama, social studies, etc. all play their part in developing individual confidence and personality, which is so vital in the therapist's professional work.

Professional bodies and awards

City and Guilds of London Institute

City and Guilds Beauty Therapists' Certificate 304 (2-year full time further education course, United Kingdom)

This course covers all aspects of facial and body treatments, and is provided on a two-year basis at selected colleges throughout the UK. Students must be at least 16 years old and have a minimum academic qualification of three GCSE passes. Due to the competition for places, colleges can be very selective in their choice of applicant and may demand a higher level of GCSE passes than the minimum. Tuition is divided between theoretical and practical aspects of therapy, permitting confidence to develop in client handling and practical techniques. The longer period of training makes this an ideal course for the younger woman, and allows skills to become established under the guidance of experienced lecturers. A 3-year course combining beauty therapy with hairdressing is also offered at many colleges.

City and Guilds Electrical Epilation Certificate 305

Run in conjunction with the Beauty Therapists' Certificate, the training covers both theoretical and practical aspects of permanent hair removal by electrical methods. Students have the opportunity of clinical practice, and can build up knowledge of individual case histories of clients during the training period. A minimum of 200 hours of practical epilation application is the requirement specified by the examination board before students may enter for the final examination. The qualification denotes a very high standard of electrology skill and knowledge.

International Health and Beauty Council

International Beauty Therapists' Diploma

This course is widely available on a one- or two-year basis at further education colleges, private schools and training establishments. The course covers all aspects of salon work, facial and body treatments, figure improvement and cosmetic applications, plus background theory relating to the practical aspects. Students are encouraged to undertake training in related subjects such as electrology and cosmetic camouflage during the training period to enhance their career prospects. Practical skills are established through clinic sessions. The course has a very commercial bias. Academic requirements for entry are four GCSE passes (one of which should be English) and a minimum age of 18 years. The course attracts a proportion of mature students, who have previous experience in another field of work, such as nursing, commerce, etc. The International Beauty Therapists' Diploma is a respected therapy qualification available around the world.

The Beauty Specialist's Diploma

The Beauty Specialist's Diploma covers all aspects of facial therapy, grooming treatments and arm and leg applications. It is often a forerunner to full therapy training (or combined with it) as the demand is increasingly to offer a full service requiring all-round qualifications. The Beauty Specialist course is available on a one-year basis in the college situation, often followed by a further period of body-work training. It is available in commercial schools, private training establishments, etc., on a full or part time basis and provides full facial qualification which is nationally recognised. The course covers practical and theoretical aspects of facial therapy, cosmetic and physical science. and business organisation. Entry to the course is three GCSE passes or previous commercial experience .

Diploma in Electrology

Normally taught in conjunction with full-time therapy courses, to provide competence in permanent hair removal by electrical epilation. Training is to a very high standard of practical skill and sound theoretical knowledge is also required for successful completion of the course. Qualification is by examination only, covering practical technique, hygiene requirements, theoretical background knowledge, anatomy, functions of the endocrine system and electro-physics.

Remedial Camouflage Diploma

This qualification covers all the techniques used to camouflage by cosmetic means severe skin blemishes, scars, birthmarks and pigmentation abnormalities. Also included is the cosmetic post-operative treatment of cosmetic surgery patients. Entry to training is restricted to those who already possess a basic beauty qualification in facial therapy or who are currently training.

The Confederation of International Beauty Therapy and Cosmetology

British Association of Beauty Therapy and Cosmetology

Aestheticienne's Diploma

The diploma course covers facial and body therapy and electrology. On successful completion of the course (having gained a pass of 70% or more in all sections of the examination) students can take the CIDESCO examinations through their national exam board. The course is normally one year full-time or 1200 hours of study.

Beautician's Diploma

The course covers all subjects relevant to a beauty operator: facial therapy, makeup, electrical treatments, arm and leg and depilatory treatments, plus the necessary background theory to understand those subjects. In addition, business organisation, cosmetic science, salon procedures, hygiene and first aid are covered theoretically. Course length is 300 hours.

Body Therapist's Diploma

The course covers body massage, electrical treatments, figure analysis, exercise, heat treatments, plus the necessary background theory to understand these subjects. In addition, business organisation, ethics, salon procedures, hygiene and first aid are covered.

Electrolysis Diploma

The course covers practical electrology and theoretical studies of anatomy and electrical science. The course requirement is 200 hours if studied in association with a beauty training, 300 hours if studied independently.

Le Comité Internationale D'Esthétiques et de Cosmetologie (CIDESCO): International CIDESCO Diploma

The International CIDESCO Diploma has been recognised for over 30 years and held in esteem in more than 27 countries around the world. The CIDESCO training is uniform in all countries, being of at least one year's duration, plus a probationary period of six months, before the full diploma is granted. Training must be at least 1200 hours' duration for practical and theoretical work and covers facial and body therapy, cosmetic applications, treatment of the hands and feet and waxing therapy. Study options are also offered, to extend the student's range of experience, and these can be tailored to the student's natural interest and area of chosen work. The study options include electrical epilation, care of the breasts, scalp treatments, specialised massage, etc.

Students must be a minimum of 18 years old before they sit their final examinations, though many CIDESCO students are older than this minimum as maturity of outlook is a very desirable asset for a therapist. Students are also expected to have a sound educational background so that they may benefit from the training undertaken. With the courses offered in the United Kingdom and examined by the Confederation of International Beauty Therapy and Cosmetology, the entry requirements are a minimum of three GCSE passes. Good oral and written ability in the language of the country, plus a sound background to the science studies are necessary. Anatomy, cosmetic science and physics are all taught as related theory on the course to support the understanding of the practical work.

Exacting conditions for recognition at a CIDESCO training school, as regards facilities, qualifications and experience of teaching staff, etc., ensure that a high standard of tuition is received which will meet the international standard. After successful completion of the course, students must work in a first class beauty centre for a further six months, after which they can apply for the full CIDESCO diploma. This does ensure that only serious therapists are recognised by the organisation.

International Therapy Examination Council (ITEC)

The International Therapy Examination Council was founded in 1973 and has expanded to cover a very comprehensive range of professional skills to meet the requirements of the beauty, body and leisure industries. ITEC now examines so many students world-wide that it can rightly claim to be one of the leading authorities. Thousands of candidates each year obtain ITEC qualifications which are highly respected by prospective employers who know that it stands for excellence in training standards and practical achievement. ITEC courses are offered mainly in private schools and in some further education colleges, usually taken over one year.

Aestheticienne Course
This course covers all aspects, both theoretical and practical, of facial anatomy and physiology: skin, dermatology, massage, electrical therapy, small treatments, makeup, manicure and pedicure.

Physiatrics Course
This course covers all aspects, both theoretical and practical of body anatomy and physiology: massage, electrical therapy, exercise, diet and nutrition, and also covers figure analysis.

Electrology Course
Covering practical and theoretical electrolysis; a minimum of 200 hours' study.

ITEC Honours Diploma
As well as a variety of short courses offered such as Beauty Specialist, Beauty Consultant, Manicure, Facial Makeup, Anatomy, Physiology and Massage there is the much coveted ITEC Honours Diploma. This is open only to students or qualified therapists who already hold Aestheticienne and Physiatrics Diplomas. It is a practical examination with oral questions included.

Institute of Electrolysis

Diploma in Remedial Epilation
The institute offers associate or full membership to its potential students depending on their age and general background. The associate member will normally attempt full membership when age and circumstances are acceptable to the institute's council. The main qualification, the Diploma in Remedial Epilation (DRE), is normally taught on a personal basis by a registered tutor in a clinic situation. The diploma course covers all aspects of skin and hair histology and demands an extremely high standard of operating technique in practical epilation. Theory subjects also cover clinical pathology, practice organisation, sterilisation procedures and first aid. Training is normally full-time, available on a private basis through tutors, and entry to the institute's membership is through examination only.

National Diploma in Beauty Therapy
BTEC is an awarding body in the UK that provides a wide range of full-time and part-time vocational courses. Courses leading to the BTEC National Diploma in Beauty Therapy aim to provide a broad educational foundation and equip students for a range of beauty therapy careers. Courses are intellectually challenging and are designed to help students cope with all aspects of the work environment. Close co-operation between the industry and teaching staff ensures that the training is commercially biased, with emphasis on client handling, marketing and sales skills to promote the practical techniques necessary for success.

Course duration. The National Diploma is a full-time course of two-years' duration which is run by several colleges of further education. (Students already employed in the industry as trainees can take the National Certificate level course over two years on a part-time basis and this can be upgraded to the Diploma level qualification by further studies.)

Entry and exemptions. Courses leading to the National Diploma are primarily designed for people who are about to start training for a career in the industry. Students must be at least 16 years of age and have completed a UK compulsory secondary school education or its equivalent and be able to satisfy the centre providing the course that their competence in English language and numeracy is sufficient to enable them to understand and progress satisfactorily on the course. They will need to have obtained either:

- a BTEC First Certificate, or First Diploma level qualification
- four passes at GCSE level (General Certificate of Secondary Education) at grade C or above, including science subjects and English
- full CPVE certification (Certificate of Prevocational Education) with a level of attainment equal to that required of students entering with either of the above
- a Certificate of Achievement from a BTEC 14–16 preparatory programme with a profile of attainment designated for such progression.

Students may be able to enter the course without the above entry requirements at the discretion of the college, if they are able to show previous experience or studies that demonstrate that they will be able to cope with and benefit from the training and will use it effectively in building a career.

International Aestheticiennes (IA)

IA is an independent examining board which combines to form a professional membership association, offering examinations in all areas of beauty therapy.

National Vocational Qualifications (NVQs)

Due to the changing climate in vocational training and education a national standard is being established in all vocational training areas. The beauty therapy industry is currently devising a programme to comply with NVQs. This will involve standards being set at various levels. This programme is still in its infancy and at the time of writing the levels and standards have not been published. You will need to contact the examination boards for the most up-to-date information.

Benefits of professional membership

Belonging to the professional organisations in beauty therapy and electrology has many advantages for the busy operator. It provides a means of keeping up to date with new techniques, equipment and information through periodic meetings, news bulletins and social gatherings of members. It maintains a professional status for the members and serves to promote a high standard of practical and theoretical knowledge to the public. It builds a good relationship with the medical profession and other well known organisations, which creates a good working atmosphere based on mutual trust and respect.

Self check

1 List the career opportunities open to the beauty specialist.
2 What are the skills required to be a sales demonstrator?
3 How are treatment costs worked out?
4 What are the advantages of belonging to a professional organisation?

Useful addresses

Professional organisations and examination boards

Further information on courses will be available from the following examination boards and professional organisations:

Aestheticians' International
Association Inc.
5206 McKinney
Dallas
Texas
USA

National Cosmetology
Association
Esthetic Division
3510 Olive St
St Louis
Mo 63103
USA

Skin Care Association of
America
1009 West Chester Pike
West Chester
Pa 19382
USA

Advanced Association of Beauty
Therapists
Suite 807
45 Market St
2000 Sydney
Australia

South African Institute of
Beauty Therapists
PO Box 56318
Pinegowrie 2123
South Africa

British Association of Beauty
Therapy and Cosmetology
Second Floor
34 Imperial Square
Cheltenham
Glos
GL50 1QZ

City & Guilds of London
Institute
76 Portland Place
London
W1N 4AA

Australian Federation of
Aestheticians and Beauty
Therapists
Box 2078
GPO
Brisbane 4001
Australia

Association of Professional
Aestheticians of Ontario
PO Box 6384 Postal Section
Toronto
MSW 1X3 Ontario
Canada

Cidesco Sektie Nederland
Gentsestraat 137
NL 2587 HNS
Gravenhage
Netherlands

Cidesco Section
291 St Heliers
Bay Road
St Heliers
Auckland
New Zealand

Business and Technology
Education Council
BTEC
Berkshire House
168–173 High Holborn
London
WC1V 7AG

International Therapy
Examination Council
ITEC
James House
Oakelbrook Mill
Newent
Glos
GL18 1HD

International Aestheticians (IA)
Bache Hall
Bache Hall Estate
Chester
CH2 1BR

Magazines and trade publications

Health & Beauty Salon
Magazine

Hair & Beauty Magazine

Hairdressers Journal

Trade publications for the Hair
and Beauty industry: details
from Reed Business Publishing,
Quadrant House, The Quadrant,
Sutton, Surrey
SM2 5AS

Les Nouvelles Esthetiques (by
subscription only)
Mapperly Plc
55 Lucknow Ave
Nottingham

The National Journal of
Esthetics (Skin care magazine)
140 Main Street,
El Segund
California 90245
USA

International Beauty & Hair
Route: (specialist magazine for
electrologists, skin care and
aesthetics, beauty therapists)
PO Box 313
Port Credit Postal Station
Mississauga
Ontario
Canada

Equipment and product suppliers

Beauty wholesalers to the industry

Many of the larger wholesalers will act as agents for the equipment and products previously mentioned. They offer a comprehensive and convenient service to the beauty professional and offer most of the best names in the equipment and product business. Some also manufacture their own equipment and products or make it under licence to the international standard of the parent equipment or product company. Most wholesalers offer both cash and carry facilities (where good cash savings are made) and mail order services to help the busy professional. Technical help is usually available in the form of expert guidance about the equipment and products from an experienced therapist/sales person, and in the form of information sheets, catalogues, treatment guidance notes or a mailing list offering the best buys currently available to help the therapist. The range of services now offered by the wholesalers is very comprehensive, and full clinic planning services are normally available if planning a new clinic or redesigning one. Most wholesalers can supply a full range of body and skin care equipment, related treatment products, exercise equipment; saunas, sun beds, and spas, supplying the industry's every need on a national and international basis. The following are some firms which the therapist may find useful:

- E. A. Ellisons and Co Ltd, Crondall Rd, Exhall, Coventry (Tel: 0203 361619): a full range of equipment and products for the beauty industry, information and technical advice to the industry – clinic planning, training, design and product development; technical advice from a trained therapist, training and demonstration clinic for full range of equipment, including Sterex, Duelli waxing systems, Sterex disposable epilation needles, plus full range of basic product lines for the hair and beauty industries; a most comprehensive and efficient service to the beauty professional offered with cash and carry, mail order, technical advice, planning assistance; supplies everything needed for the therapist to achieve success in her business: equipment, products, knowledge, and friendly support.

- Esthetics and Beauty Supply, 180 Bentley Street, Markham, Ontario L3R 3L2, Canada: an extensive range of equipment, supplies and services to the beauty therapist and esthetician; able to supply a total service – from a complete package for a new business, to basic supplies for the beauty professional; offers technical advice on clinic planning, training, a wide choice of equipment, installation and service of equipment, plus a selection of products, makeup and nail lines for business success; a skilled and supportive service from trained therapists, with training and demonstration clinics, and in association with 'Ann Gallant' post-graduate training and access to the latest international advances.

- Hairdressing and Beauty Equipment Centre, 262 Holloway Road, London, N7; a comprehensive range of hairdressing and beauty

317

equipment, agents for the Italian 'Dale' beauty equipment, for the aroma mist steamer, and for most leading makes of equipment, sun beds, spas, sauna, exercise and health related equipment; not a manufacturer, but a stockist of a very comprehensive range of equipment; not a supplier of products. Technical advice available from a trained therapist on the use of the equipment; small training clinic.

- House of Famuir, Beeston Grange, Sandy, Bedfordshire, SG19 1PG; an equipment and product supplier (Slendertone, G5® Massagers, Ballet Electrolysis Needles, GM Collins Products); and manufacturer of own range, comprehensive range of salon supplies, wax, basic and specialised products for professional therapy; small training clinic and technical therapy advice available to aid the therapist; a large training centre now in Sheffield.

- Oritree Ltd, 3 Moxon Street, London, W1; a full range of equipment and products, makeup, wax supplies, nail products and many small resale items to increase retail sales in the salon; training clinic and technical advice available.

- Aston and Fincher Ltd, 8 Holyhead Road, Birmingham, B21 0LY: a large group of wholesale cash and carry suppliers for the hairdressing and beauty industry, with bulk supplies, wax, towels, small range of beauty equipment; an efficient and friendly service to therapists.

- Carlton Professional, Carlton House, Commerce Way, Lancing, West Sussex, BN15 8TA: a comprehensive range of equipment, including that of their own manufacture, plus bulk preparations for salon use; agents for GTE Italian equipment; suppliers of the Epitherm 'Hot bead steriliser'; able to give advice on clinic layout; trained therapist; able and willing to help with choice of equipment.

- George Solly Organization, 111 Watlington Street, Reading, Berkshire, RG1 4RQ: a full range of equipment and product supplies; suppliers of their own 'Popular' range of good value equipment; agents for prestigious German-made Nemectron equipment; technical guidance and friendly service.

Further addresses

Product supplies

(American skin care range)
Dermalogica
Dermal Products (UK) Ltd
Weir House
Hurst Road
East Molesey
Surrey
KT8 9AQ

(Sin care range)
Renaissance
Loukia Nicola Skin Care
138a Park Lane
Manchester
M2 5PX

(Skin care range)
Dr Renaud Skin Care Range
2 Roman Road
Storeton Village
Wirral
L63 6HS

(Skin care and makeup)
Susan Molyneux
9 King St
Cheltenham
Glos
GL50 4AU

(Skin care and makeup)
RVB
Piana Cosmetici SPA
40024 Castel S. Pietro Terme
Bologna
Italy

(Makeup)
Linda Meredith Cosmetics
18 Rosedene Terrace
Leyton
London
E10 5LS

(Aromatherapy skin care
products)
House of Neroli
Oakelbrook Mill
Newent
Glos
GL18 1HD

Elizabeth of Schwarzenberg
The Coach House
Back Lane
Colsterworth
Grantham
Lincs
NG33 5HU

Pier Auge Cosmetics
Harbourne Marketing Associates
First Quarter
Blenheim Rd
Epsom
Surrey
KT19 9QN

(Skin care range)
Dr Cleor (UK) Ltd
59a Connaught St
London
W2 2BB

Remy Laure
520 Stockport Rd
Thelwall
Nr Warrington
Cheshire
WA4 2TJ

(Skin care range)
Rene Guinot
R. Robson Ltd
The Clock House
High Street
Ascot
Berkshire
SL5 7HU

(Skin care range)
Rose Laird
Sutton Fields
Hull
HU7 0XD

Clarins UK Ltd
150 High St
Stratford
London
E15 2NE

Equipment manufacturers and suppliers

Hairdressing and Beauty
Equipment Centre
262 Holloway Rd
London
N7 6NE

Carlton Professional
Carlton House
Commerce Way
Lancing
West Sussex
BN15 8TA

Salon System
1 Elystan Business Centre
Springfield Rd
Hayes
Middlesex
UB4 0UJ

Ionothermine Ltd
9–11 Alma Road
Windsor
Berks
SL4 3HU

Sorisa UK Ltd
212 Northenden Rd
Sale
Manchester
M33 2JP

Aston and Fincher
8 Holyhead Rd
Birmingham
B21 0LY

Trim-Tone
Clacton Rd
London
N17 6UG

Ellisons
Crondall Rd
Exhall
Coventry
CV7 9NH

Silhouette International Beauty
Equipment
York House
Vicarage Lane
Bowden
Altrincham
Cheshire
WA14 3BA

Depilex Ltd
Regent House
Dock Rd
Birkenhead
Merseyside
L41 1DG

George Solly Organisation Ltd
111 Watlington St
Reading
Berkshire

Salon work wear supplies
Florence Roby
Caddick Rd
Knowsley Industrial Park
Merseyside
L34 9HP

Gasper Career Apparel
217 Field End Rd
Eastcote
Pinner
Middlesex
HA5 1QZ

Ellisons Salon Wear
Crondal Road
Bayton Rd Industrial Estate
Coventry
CV7 9NH

D K Profashion (UK) Ltd
1 Bank St
Tonbridge
Kent
TN9 1BL

ABC Workwear
42 Lower Baggot Street
Dublin 2
Ireland

Conversion tables

Temperature Conversion

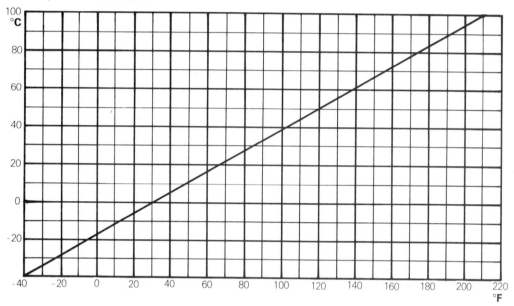

Height Conversion

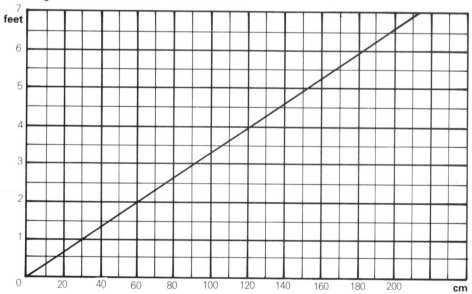

Measurements Conversion (inches/cm)

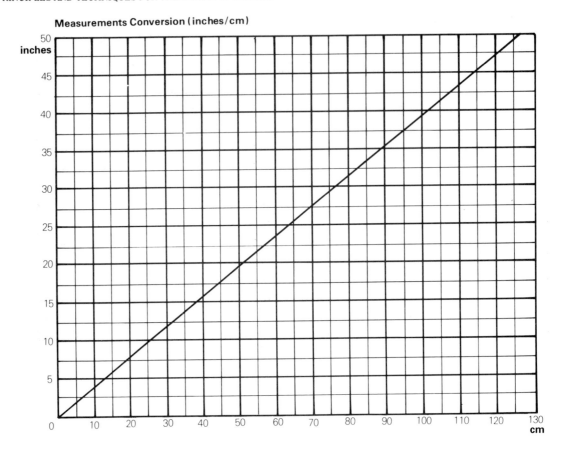

Volume Conversion

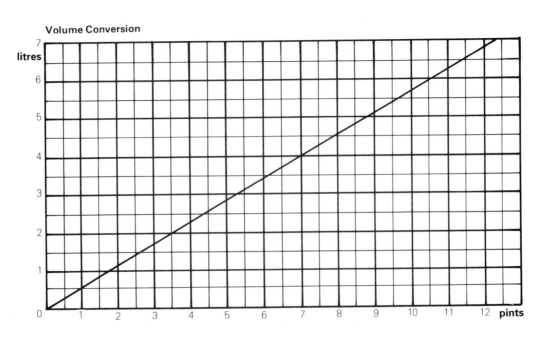

Weight Conversion

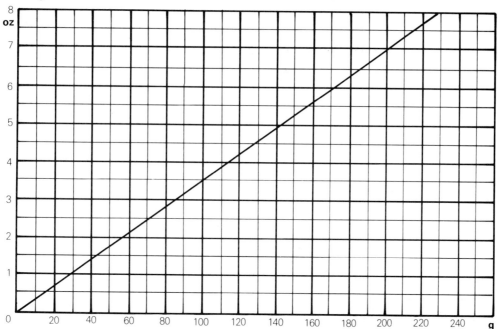

Index

Numbers in italic refer to illustrations
on that page.

abrasive peeling treatment 161–3, 215
abscess 89
acid mantle 26, 49, 50, 51, 208
acne 25, 26, 28, 102, 104, 164, 307;
   makeup 125, 126, 128, 148; post-
   acne treatment 158, 161, 173, 213,
   214, 215; rosacea 96, 154, 187;
   treatment 153, 154, 174, 182, 183,
   187, 188, 197–9, 216; vulgaris 68,
   95, 96, 178
adolescents 68, 69, 85, 96, 151, 174,
   215
African clients 88, 143, 144
Afro-Asian clients 143, 144, 146
age and ageing signs 24, 27–8, 31, 53,
   74, 135, 164, 168, 190, 191, 201,
   203, 206, 239, 241; mask therapy
   107, 108, 110
AHA (alpha-hydroxy acids) 31, 266, 273
AIDS 1, 286
air massage units 215
alcohol (ingredient) 32
allergic reactions 26, 53, 92–3, 125,
   151, 206, 208
ampoules 106, 125, 185, 186, 189,
   191–9 *passim*, 201, 203, 204, 205–6,
   207, 209, 210, 211, 212, 216
anidrosis 96
arms: massage 232, 233–7; waxing 281
aromatherapy 208, 216, 298
Asian clients 130, 143, 144, 145, 146
Asiatic clients 123
asthma 54, 151, 174, 183, 185, 188
astringents 32
audio-sonic vibrators 156–60

bacteria 29, 43, 50, 55, 89, 154, 287–8
birth marks 25, 126, 148
blackheads 193, 197, 213; *see also*
   comedones
blemished skin 26, 28–9, 32, 53, 68, 85,
   125, 126, 128, 145, 148, 154, 164,
   173, 176, 181, 185, 193, 194
blood pressure, high 151, 168, 174
blood spots 25, 167, 273, 279, 281
blood supply 51; head and neck 39–41
body odour 50, 96
body temperature 26, 39, 50–1

boils 89, 287, 290
bones: cranium 33–4, *34*; face 33,
   34–6, *34, 35*; feet 250–1, *250, 251*;
   forearm 218, *218*; hand and wrist
   217–18, *218*
bromidrosis 96
brush massage/cleansing 13, *21*, 160–1,
   187, 204, 205
bullae 87, 89
burrows 87, 91
business organisation: health authority
   legislation 20; salon hygiene
   291–5; standards/regulations 195,
   286–7; treatment charges and costs
   113, 123, 148, 244, 246, 267, 269,
   302, 303–4; treatments 302–7

capillaries 39, 42, *46*, 51; damaged 27,
   28, 191, 199, 202; dilated 25, 26,
   29, 94, 110, 129, 151, 164, 205, 208,
   210; split 70, 148; *see also*
   couperose skin
carcinogenic risks 156, 178, 195
cheeks 15, 64, 66, 128–9
chin 14, 26, 70, 79, 204, 267, 268,
   281–2, 284–5
chloasma 25, 94
cleansing 12–22; *see also* brush
   massage/cleansing; galvanic
   treatment; masks
cleansing milks 13, 21, 31, 106, 191,
   199
cleansing products 12–13, 14, 31–2
clients 1–11, 57, 302–4; hygiene of
   291; nervous (over-stressed/tense)
   13, 21, 53, 74, 108, 110, 117, 151,
   168, 173, 183, 185, 197, 206, 216;
   records and record cards 3, 4–7, 12;
   wearing glasses 117; *see also*
   adolescents; male clients; mature
   clients; young(er) clients
clinic 1–3, 4, 7–11, 190, 286; liability
   117
cold sores 90, 281, 284, 288, 290
combination skin 28, 32, 125, 307;
   masks 102, 104; treatment 68, 154,
   173, 176, 183, 185, 193–7, 213
comedones (blackheads) 26, 28, 88, 95,
   96, 197
consultation 1, 2, 3, 12

contact lens wearers 131
Continental facial massage 53, 73–84,
   201, 204
contra-indications 4, 12, 25–6, 89, 90,
   91, 216; makeup 116–18, 121; to
   electrical treatment 25, 151, 154,
   157, 164, 173–4, 187–8; to
   manicure 222; to mask therapy
   100, 108, 110; to massage 53–4,
   160; to ultraviolet 179
cosmetics 10, 26, 30–2; camouflage
   94, 126, 129, 148–9; sales 304–5
couperose skin (capillary damage) 25,
   103, 104, 191, 205, 208, 210–12,
   306–7
creams 13, 31, 69, 74, 124, 125, 162,
   191–7 *passim*, 200–12 *passim*, 216,
   266, 273
crepey skin 24, 74, 110, 126, 131, 164,
   200, 201, 205, 213
crust 88, *88*
cystic blockages 26, 197
cyst (wen) 87

dark skin 126, 143–8, 199, 282
delicate skin 13, 53, 56, 156, 157, 178
dental condition 151, 169, 172, 174,
   183, 185, 187, 188
depilatory treatments 265–85; *see also*
   waxing
dermatitis 92, 179, 188, 223
desincrustation, *see under* galvanic
   treatment
desquamation 28, 31, 47, 51, 53, 55,
   56, 101, 153, 158, 160, 173, 178,
   196, 199
diabetes 54, 151, 254, 268
diathermy (heat) coagulation treatment
   94, 95, 266
diet 24, 25, 26, 28, 191, 201, 208, 224,
   243, 290
dieting, effect on skin 24
drugs 179, 188, 216
dry/dehydrated skin 24, 27, 28, 31, 32,
   53, 88; contra-indications 162, 213,
   214; makeup 125, 128; masks for
   101, 102, 104, 105, 106; muscle
   toning 168; products for 306; treatment 109, 154, 157, 160, 164, 173,
   185, 187, 188, 200–3; waxing 241

Eastern clients 130, 131, 144
eczema 92, 117, 179, 188, 222
effleurage 14, 15, 54–5, 60–6 *passim*,
71, 73, 74–83 *passim*, 127, 207; arm
massage 233–7 *passim*; feet and
legs 257, 259, 261, 262
electrical equipment 108, 111, 153,
156, 160, 161, 162–3, 164, 166,
169–70, 174, 175, 179–80, 183–4;
home visiting 307; safety of 152–3
electrical treatment 3, 7, 12, 13, 20–2,
68, 123, 150–89; contra-indications
25, 151, 154, 157, 164, 173–4,
187–8; skin toning 30; *see also*
brush massage/cleansing; galvanic
treatment
electrolysis 266
enzyme peeler 196, 198
ephelides (freckles) 25
epilation 266
epilepsy 151, 173, 183, 185, 188
equipment 20, 115, 116, *121*, 304–7;
chairs/couches 10, *10*, 57, 305;
home visiting practice 307–8; and
hygiene 291–2; suppliers 317–20;
waxing methods 268–9, 270, 275,
284; *see also* electrical equipment
erythema 39, 56, 86, 89, 90, 109, 145,
157, 159, 160, 164, 168, 177–8, 194,
208
eyebrows 113–23, 131, 136; shaping
113–16; tinting 114, 115, 116–19,
120–1, 136; waxing 282–3
eyelashes: false 130, 132, 137–8, 139,
140, 141; individual 121–2, 132;
tinting 10, 119–20, 131, 132;
treatments 113–23
eyeline colour (permanent) 122–3
eyes 16, *16*, 17, 18, 65–6, 81, *81*;
makeup 129–32, 135, 137–41,
147–8

face: bones 33, 34–6, *34*, *35*; lymphatic
system 42–3; muscles 36–8, *36*, *38*;
muscles of facial expression 16, 24;
nerves 43–5
facial cubicle 297, 304–7
facial massage 53–84; basic 60–8;
Continental 73–84
facials 12, 192–3, 194, 201
facial vacuum/suction treatment 163–6
feet: bones 250–1, *250*, *251*; infections
of 89, 91; massage 257, 258–64;
muscles 252–3, *252*, *253*; pedicure
253–8
fibrous simplex and growths 26
forearm: bones 218, *218*; muscles
219–20
forehead 14, 16, *16*, 18, 65, 72, *72*, 80
freckles (ephelides) 93

friction gloves 266
fungal diseases 89–90, 288
furuncles 89

galvanic treatment 13, 20, 31, 32,
181–6, 189, 192, 193, 195, 197, 198;
desincrustation 13, 31, 32, 163,
164, 181, 182–5, 188, 189, 194,
196–7, 198, 199; galvanic and high-
frequency units combined 215;
iontophoresis (ionisation) 104, 106,
181, 185–6, 188, 189, 198, 199, 201,
203, 205
gels 69, 99, 195
germicidal effects 150, 172, 173, 175–6,
178, 180, 181
gland disorders 95–6

hair 26, 28, 50, 89
hair follicle *46*, 48–9; infections of 88,
89
hand mobility exercises 58–60
hands, bones 217–18, *218*; massage
232–3
head (cranium), blood circulation
39–41; bones 33–4, *34*; nerves
43–5, *43*, *44*
health, effects on skin 24, 26, 191, 201
health hydro 298
heart complaints 222, 223
heart pacemaker 151
hepatitis 288, 290
herpes simplex *see* cold sores
herpes zoster 90, 288
high-frequency treatment 20, 172–7,
188, 192, 196, 199, 209, 212
hives 93
HIV infection 288, 290
home care plans 12, 30, 32, 120, 149,
190–1, 192, 194, 197, 200, 202, 203,
204, 207, 209, 210, 211; depilatory
methods 265, 271; masks 99, 103,
104, 105; nail treatment 222, 226,
231–2, 242
home use of products 2, 3, 4, 7, 9, 13,
14, 17, 24, 31, 199, 201, 232, 303,
305
home visiting practice 297–8;
equipment 307–8
hormonal factors 22, 25, 28, 94
hormone therapy, effects of 118
hygiene 1, 8, 20, 74, 85, 267, 269,
286–95
hyperhidrosis 96
hypersensitive skin: contra-indicator
53, 100, 110, 151, 154, 164, 168,
183, 185, 187, 213, 268, 281, 284;
makeup 125
hypoallergenic products 125, 131

impetigo 89, 287, 290

Indian clients 123
infra-red 109–11
ingredients (of masks, products) 32,
99, 101, 102, 104, 105, 191, 194,
197, 199, 200, 202, 204, 206, 208,
210, 211
inverse square law 179, 180, *180*
iontophoresis (ionisation) *see under*
galvanic treatment

keloid 88, 145
keratin 46, 47
keratinisation 26, 28, 29, 47, 55, 197,
213
kneading 54, 76, *76*, 77, *77*, 79, *79*,
236, 260, *260*, 261, 262
knuckling 54, 63, *63*, 75, *75*, 83, *83*

lashes *see* eyelashes
legal position, tinting 117
legs: bones *250*, 252; massage 258–64;
muscles 252–3, *252*, *253*; waxing
methods 270–3, 276–8
leisure centres 301
lentigo 25, 94
lesions 86, 89
leuconychia 223
lice 91–2
lichenification 88
liposomes 31, 103, 104, 200, 201
lips: electrical treatment 172; hair
removal 26, 267, 268, 281–2;
284–5; lipstick 132–3, 142, 147;
massage (lip bracing) 80, *80*;
removing makeup 17–18, *18*
loose skin: contra-indications 54, 160,
164, 187; treatment 55, 56, 157,
205
lymphatic system: drainage 78, 166,
167, 195, 202, 205, 212, 215; effects
of treatment on 55, 156, 163, 198;
face and neck 42–3, 48; muscle
toning 168

macule 86, *86*, 90
makeup 10, 11, *11*, 29, 30, 124–49,
214, 143–8; removal and cleansing
13, 14, 15, 16, 17–19, *17*, 31;
television 298–9
male clients 69, 149, 226
manicure 222, 225–32, 237–9
masks 68, 84, 99–112; abrasive 160,
161, 199; biological 103, 104, 191,
192, 193, 196, 200, 201; clay 99,
100–2, 191, 192, 194, 195, 196, 198,
199, 209; contra-indications 100,
108, 110; for dark skin 145; geloid
103, 201, 207, 209, 212; ginseng
104, 202, 203; herbal 99, 104, 198;
liposome 103, 104, 200, 201;
natural products 105; paraffin wax

107–9; peel-off 105–6, *106*; phytotherapy 103–4, 194, 195, 196, 197,
198, 207, 212; products 216; royal
jelly/firming 104, 207; setting
100–1; skin preparation 100;
thermal/mineral 106–7, 207; warm
oil 109–11
massage 13, 202–3, 222, 271; contra-
indications 53–4; foot and leg 257,
258–64; manual movements 54–7;
technique 57–8; *see also* brush
massage/cleansing; effleurage;
petrissage; tapotement;
vacuum/suction treatment;
vibratory treatment
mature clients 13, 22, 27, 32, 53;
contra-indications 162, 213, 214;
makeup 118, 125, 126, 128; masks
104, 105, 106, 108, 109, 110;
massage treatment 53, 55, 74, 160;
muscle toning 168; nails 222;
products for 31, 32, 216, 306; skin
types 27–8; treatment for 154, 156,
157, 163, 164, 173, 185, 187, 188,
190, 200, 203–6, 215
medical agreement/advice (needed for
treatment) 4, 25, 68, 85, 89, 95, 96,
151, 168, 173, 174, 198, 222, 254
medical attention, refer client for 25,
85, 89, 90, 91, 92, 93, 157, 222, 223,
224, 225
medical history of client 3, 4, 179
medicated products 125, 128, 148, 282,
285
melanin 47, 51, 88, 145, 178
menopause 22, 28, 164, 203, 205, 206
migraine 151, 169, 174
miliaria (prickly heat) 96
milia (whiteheads) 88, 197
mineral water 30
mobile beauty specialists 153; home
visiting equipment 307–8
module 86, *86*
moles 25, 95, 97, 148, 268
muscles 15, 16, 54, 55, 56, 69; face and
neck 36–8, *36, 38*; forearm 219–20;
lower leg, ankle and foot 252–3,
252, 253
muscle toning 20, 167–72, 187, 193,
205

naevi 25, 95, 148, 205
nails: diseases and disorders 89, 93,
222–5; manicure 222, 225–32;
repairs and extensions 241–9;
structure and function 221–2
National Health Service 148
neck: blood circulation 39–41;
cleansing 15, *15*, 18; lymphatic
system 42–3; muscles 36–8, *36, 38*;
nerves 43–5

nerves, face and neck 43–5
nettle rash 93
normal skin 24, 25, 27, 28, 306; masks
102, 104; massage 53, 160; treatment 154, 157, 162, 164, 173, 176,
178, 182, 183, 185, 187, 188, 191–3,
213
nose 14, 15, *16*, 18, 70–1, 135, 204

oedema 86, 87, 96, 168, 174
oily skin 24, 25, 28, 307; makeup 125,
128; masks 101, 102, 104;
treatment of 13, 32, 68, 69, 153,
162, 163, 164, 173, 176, 182, 183,
184, 185, 187, 188, 193–7
ozone steaming (therapy) 153, 155–6,
164, 187, 194, 195, 196, 197, 198,
199

papilloma *see* moles
papules 86, *86*, 91, 92, 93, 96, 197; *see
also* warts
paraffin wax: hand and arm treatment
239–41; mask 107–9
parasitic skin problems 91–2
patch testing 117–18
pediculosis (lice) 91–2
pedicure 89, 253–8
petrissage 54, 55–6, 61, 63, 64, 65,
69–71, 72, 75–83 *passim*, 195
petrissage: arm massage 233, 236; legs
and feet 260, 262
pH balance 12, 22, 26, 29, 107, 108,
153, 154, 193, 198, 208
phytotherapy 32, 99, 192–3, 196, 302
pigmentary disorders 93–5
pigmentation 69, 86, 24–5, 127, 148,
178; senile 28, 222
pinching frictions 54
pinching movement 69, *69*
plaques 87, 93
pores 26, 197, 198; massage routine
68–73, 195, 196; treatment of 30,
53, 68, 69, 165, 167, 182, 183, 184
port wine stain 94
pregnancy 94, 118, 151; contra-
indicator 174, 188, 216; post-
pregnancy conditions 206, 279
prickly heat 96
products 3, 4, 30–2; suppliers 317–20;
see also ingredients
psoriasis 93, 117, 222, 223
pulsed air 166–7
pumice blocks 161
pustules 28, 68, 87, 96, 197, 198, 281,
284

qualifications 296, 297, 298, 303,
308–9

radiant heat irradiation 109–11
refining treatment 196–7

rejuvenation treatment 193, 206–7
rheumatism 222, 223
ringworm 89–90, 223, 224, 288
rollpatting 14, 15–16, *15, 16*, 54, 60,
64, 65, 67, 71, 80, *80*, 83

safety, in using equipment 111, 152–3,
156, 174–5, 176, 195, 241, 267,
268–9; *see also* hygiene
sales as a career 299–300
sales demonstrator 300–1
sallow skin 25, 28, 96, 125, 127, 145,
162, 176, 197, 213, 214
salon *see* business organisation; clinic
scabies 91
scales 87, *87*
scalp massage 158
scars and scar tissue 26, 29, 88, 90, 96,
157, 181; camouflage 126, 129, 148;
on darker skin 145; treatment of
68, 69, 162, 173, 175, 176, 193, 197,
198, 199, 213, 214, 215; *see also*
acne
sebaceous glands 14, 25, 26, 27, 28, 29,
46, 49, 50, 95, 173, 213
seborrhoea 25, 28–9, 95, 96, 197, 198,
199; masks 101, 104, 108; treatment of 153, 154, 162, 173, 178,
183
sebum 29, 49, 50, 52, 88, 95, 165, 182,
183, 197
sensitive skin 13, 20, 22, 25, 27, 30–1,
32, 55, 306–7; contra-indicator 162,
179, 214; makeup 125; masks 102,
103, 104, 105, 209, 212; treatment
53, 57, 157, 178, 187, 188, 208–10;
see also hypersensitive skin
sepsis 54, 85, 108, 151, 157, 183, 185,
268
shingles (herpes zoster) 90
shipboard therapists 301–2
shoulder, Continental massage 73–84
passim
sinus condition 54, 151, 154, 157, 169,
174, 183, 185, 187, 188
skin 12–32; anatomy 45–52; colour
24–5, 47; diseases and disorders 25,
85–98, 254, 268; functions of 50–2;
imperfections 5, 25–6; UV rays *177*
skin infection 54, 68, 100, 108, 151,
154, 157, 160, 162, 174, 183, 185,
214, 287
skin peeling treatment 213–15
skin tags 26, 88
snatching movement 263, *263*
spider naevus 94
sponges 20, 21, 30, 293
steaming 153–6, 163, 187, 192, 193,
195, 196, 198, 202, 207
sterilisation methods 160, 162, 237,
258, 288, 292–4

NSST

stock checking 4
strawberry mark 95
stress 53, 74, 208
stress therapy 208, 302
subcutaneous tissues 48, 51, 55, 69,
    110, 156
sudoriferous glands (eccrine, apocrine)
    49–50, 52
sun/sunburn 27, 28, 52, 88, 100, 154,
    160, 187, 201, 203, 210, 268;
    protection 124, 200, 201, 206, 207
suntanned skin, makeup for 125, 126,
    128
sweat glands (sweat) 26, 46, 49, 50, 51,
    52, 96, 110

tanning (UV) 178, 179, 180, 181
tapotement 54, 56, 61, 62, 66, 71, 73,
    82, 263
teaching 301
telangiectasia 25, 94
theatrical makeup 31, 126
thermal masks 106–7, 207
tinea (ringworm) 89–90, 223, 224, 288
tinting, of eyebrows and lashes 114,
    115, 116–21, 131, 132, 136

toning and toners 29–30, 31, 32, 68,
    192, 193
training 213, 298–9, 308–9;
    professional bodies and awards
    309–16
treatment plan, example of 6

ulcer 87, 88
ultraviolet 47, 51, 52, 94, 191, 200;
    used for sterilisation 292
ultraviolet treatment 153, 154, 156,
    177–81, 188, 199
urticaria 93

vacuum/suction treatment 20, 163–7,
    187, 192, 193, 195, 196, 198, 202,
    205, 209, 212
varicose veins 268
vascular skin 28, 53, 108, 110, 151,
    154, 157, 160, 168, 174, 183, 185,
    187, 188; vacuum treatment 164
vascular stimulation 54, 55, 56, 69,
    160, 163, 210
verrucas see warts
vesicles 87, 87, 89, 90, 91, 92

vibratory treatment 54, 56–7, 156–60,
    187, 209
Viennese massage 172, 174–5, 192,
    203, 209, 212
viral skin conditions 90–1
vitamins 204, 206; vitamin D 52, 178
vitiligo (loss of pigment) 24, 25, 94,
    144

warts (verrucae) 25, 26, 90–1, 175, 254,
    268, 290
waste disposal 106, 294–5
waxing 10, 265, 266, 267–85;
    abdominal 274, 278, 279–80; arm
    281; bikini 274–5, 278–9; of hand
    and arm 239–41; underarm 273–4,
    280–1
wen 87
whipping movement 54, 71, 263, 263
whiteheads see milia

young(er) clients 28, 110, 148, 155,
    213; cleansing 7, 12, 20, 31, 32;
    makeup 120, 128, 129, 131, 137,
    139, 140; massage treatment 53,
    55, 74; nails 247